Media Messages and Public Health

Media Messages and Public Health addresses the full range of methodological and conceptual issues involved in content analysis research, specifically focused on public health-related messages and behaviors. Uniquely tailored to the challenges faced by content researchers interested in the study of public health topics, coverage includes:

- conceptual and methodological foundations involved in the practice of content analysis research used to examine public health issues
- measurement challenges posed by the broad range of media
- use of content analysis across multiple media types
- the potential for individual differences in audience interpretation of message content
- case studies that examine public health issues in the media to illustrate the decisions that are made when developing content analysis studies.

The volume concludes with a set of guidelines for optimal content analysis research, and suggests ways in which the field can accommodate new technologies and new ways of using media. Developed for researchers in communication, media, and public health, this unique resource demonstrates how the variety of decisions researchers make along the way allows the exploration of traditions, assumptions, and implications for each varying alternative and ultimately advances the science of content analysis research.

Amy B. Jordan (Ph.D., University of Pennsylvania) is the director of the Media and the Developing Child research area of the Annenberg Public Policy Center of the University of Pennsylvania, where she studies children's media policy.

Dale Kunkel (Ph.D., Annenberg School, University of Southern California) is Professor of Communication at the University of Arizona, where he studies children and media issues from diverse perspectives.

Jennifer Manganello (M.P.H., Boston University; Ph.D., Johns Hopkins School of Public Health) is Assistant Professor of Health Policy, Management, and Behavior at the University at Albany. Her research interests include children's health and media effects on policy and health behavior.

Martin Fishbein (Ph.D., University of California Los Angeles) is the Harry C. Coles Jr. Distinguished Professor of Communication at the Annenberg School for Communication, and director of the Health Communications area of the Annenberg Public Policy Center, University of Pennsylvania. Developer of the theory of reasoned action and the integrative model, his research interests include communication and persuasion.

Communication Series
Jennings Bryant/Dolf Zillmann, General Editors
Selected titles in Applied Communication (Teresa L. Thompson, Advisory Editor) include:

Media Messages and Public Health

A Decisions Approach to
Content Analysis

**Edited by
Amy B. Jordan,
Dale Kunkel,
Jennifer Manganello,
Martin Fishbein**

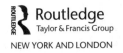

Routledge
Taylor & Francis Group
NEW YORK AND LONDON

First published 2009
by Routledge
270 Madison Ave, New York, NY 10016

Simultaneously published in the UK
by Routledge
2 Park Square, Milton Park, Abingdon, Oxon OX14 4RN

Routledge is an imprint of the Taylor & Francis Group, an informa business

© 2009 Taylor & Francis

Typeset in Galliard by
Bookcraft Ltd, Stroud, Gloucestershire
Printed and bound in the United States of America on acid-free paper by
Walsworth Publishing Company, Marceline, MO

Trademark Notice: Product or corporate names may be
trademarks or registered trademarks, and are used only for
identification and explanation without intent to infringe.

Library of Congress Cataloging-in-Publication Data
Media messages and public health: a decisions approach to
content analysis / by Amy B. Jordan ... [et al.].
  p. cm.
  1. Mass media in health education. 2. Content analysis
  (Communication) 3. Health behavior. 4. Communication in
  medicine. I. Jordan, Amy B. (Amy Beth)
  [DNLM: 1. Health Education. 2. Mass Media. 3. Attitude to
  Health. 4. Health Behavior. 5. Health Promotion. 6. Information Dissemination--methods. WA 590 M4879 2008]
RA440.5.M435 2008
362.1--dc22   2008013002

ISBN10: 0-805-86024-X (hbk)
ISBN10: 0-805-86025-8 (pbk)
ISBN10: 0-203-88734-4 (ebk)

ISBN13: 978-0-805-86024-5 (hbk)
ISBN13: 978-0-805-86025-2 (pbk)
ISBN13: 978-0-203-88734-9 (ebk)

Contents

PART 3
Case Studies 97

PART 4
The Big Picture 231

Illustrations

Tables

Contributors

Erica Weintraub Austin is Dean of the Edward R. Murrow College of Communication at Washington State University and a recipient of the Krieghbaum Under-40 Award from the Association for Education in Journalism and Mass Communication. Her research addresses individuals' uses of the media in decision-making.

Jay M. Bernhardt is the Director of the National Center for Health Marketing at the Centers for Disease Control and Prevention (USA). His research focuses on applying innovative information and communication technology to public health and social marketing efforts in the USA and around the world.

Elaine Chan is an Assistant Professor in the Broadcast and Electronic Communication Arts Department at San Francisco State University. Her research interests include social aspects of video game playing and interactive media.

Michael J. Cody is Professor of Communication at the University of Southern California. He is currently involved in a number of projects using entertainment as a means to educate viewers about breast cancer and infectious diseases. He is co-editor of *Entertainment-Education and Social Change: History, Research, and Practice* (2004).

Rebecca L. Collins is Senior Behavioral Scientist and Director of the Health Promotion and Disease Prevention Program at the RAND Corporation. She studies the social and cognitive factors that influence health risk behavior, including media effects on adolescent sexual health and underage drinking.

Ralph J. DiClemente is the Charles Howard Candler Professor of Public Health and Medicine, Department of Pediatrics (Division of Infectious Diseases, Epidemiology, and Immunology), Department of Medicine (Division of Infectious Diseases), and Department of Psychiatry and Behavioral Sciences (Child and Adolescent Psychiatry); and Associate Director at the Center for AIDS Research at the Rollins School of Public Health, Emory University.

Marc N. Elliott is a Senior Statistician at RAND. He has published more than 120 peer-reviewed journal articles including 'Use of a Web-based Convenience Sample to Supplement and Improve the Accuracy of a Probability Sample' (2007), 'Problem-Oriented Reporting of CAHPS Consumer Evaluations of Healthcare' (2007), and 'Are Finite Population Corrections Appropriate When Profiling Institutions?' (2006).

Martin Fishbein is the Harry C. Coles Jr. Distinguished Professor of Communication at the Annenberg School for Communication, and director of the Health Communications area of the Annenberg Public Policy Center, University of Pennsylvania. Developer of the theory of reasoned action and the integrative model, his research interests include communication and persuasion.

Pamela J. Fleischauer works in the Rollins School of Public Health, Emory University, as a research project manager for an adolescent sexual risk reduction program. She received her M.P.H. in Health Behavior and Health Education from the University of North Carolina-Chapel Hill in 2001.

Grace C. Huang is a Ph.D. student in Health Behavior Research at University of Southern California's Keck School of Medicine. She was formerly Research Specialist at Hollywood, Health & Society, a project of the USC Annenberg Norman Lear Center, and participated in over 20 studies on the impact of entertainment television.

Amy B. Jordan is the director of the Media and the Developing Child research area of the Annenberg Public Policy Center of the University of Pennsylvania. She is co-author of *Children, Adolescents, and the Media* (second edition, 2008) and co-editor of *Children in the Digital Age* (2002).

Dale Kunkel is Professor of Communication at the University of Arizona, where he studies children and media issues from diverse perspectives.

Jennifer Manganello is Assistant Professor of Health Policy, Management, and Behavior at the University at Albany School of Public Health. Her research interests include children's health, media effects on policy and health behavior, and health literacy.

Suzanne M. Martin has over 15 years' research experience, with a main focus on youth studies. She earned a Ph.D. in Educational Psychology, an M.S. in Marketing, and spent time as a post-doctoral fellow at Annenberg Public Policy Center. Before joining Just Kid Inc., she worked as a researcher at Harris Interactive.

Angela Miu received her M.S. in Biometry from the University of Southern California and is a senior research programmer analyst at RAND Corporation. She has extensive experience in database management and the statistical analysis of survey and claims data for interdisciplinary public policy research projects.

Sheila T. Murphy is an Associate Professor at the Annenberg School for Communication at the University of Southern California. Her research focuses on how people make decisions and the factors that influence them, including emotion, racial and gender stereotypes, cultural norms, and cognitive factors such as how information is framed.

Kimberly A. Neuendorf is Professor, School of Communication, at Cleveland State University. She researches the content and impacts of media with regard to marginalized populations, new technology adoption, and the use of humorous and other media content for mood management. Her methodology writings include *The Content Analysis Guidebook* (2002).

Katherine M. Pieper received her M.A. from the Annenberg School for Communication at the University of Southern California in 2006. Her research interests include the effects of entertainment media on children and using entertainment products for health and social change. She is currently serving with World Relief in Phnom Penh, Cambodia.

W. James Potter is a Professor in the Department of Communication at the University of California at Santa Barbara. He has published numerous scholarly articles and 15 books, including: *Arguing for a General Framework for Mass Media Research* (2008), *Theory of Media Literacy: A Cognitive Approach* (2004), *The 11 Myths of Media Violence* (2003), and *An Analysis of Thinking and Research about Qualitative Methods* (1996).

Srividya Ramasubramanian is Assistant Professor of Communication at Texas A&M University. Her research focuses on media psychology, with particular reference to race, gender, and sexuality in youth-oriented media. Her research appears in journals such as *Sex Roles, Media Psychology, Journalism and Mass Communication Quarterly*, and *Howard Journal of Communication*.

Laura F. Salazar is an Assistant Research Professor of Behavioral Sciences and Health Education in the Rollins School of Public Health, Emory University. She earned her Ph.D. from the Georgia State University Psychology Department in Community Psychology. Her areas of research interest are two intersecting epidemics: adolescent sexual health and violence against women.

Nancy Signorielli is Professor of Communication and Director of the M.A. program in Communication at the University of Delaware (USA). She has conducted research on images in the media and how these images are related to people's conceptions of social reality (cultivation analysis) for the past 35 years.

Stacy L. Smith is an Associate Professor at the Annenberg School for Communication at USC. Her research focuses on children's responses to media portrayals of violence, gender, and hypersexuality. Dr. Smith has written nearly 50 journal articles and book chapters on content patterns and effects of the media on youth. Her scholarly work has been published in *Communication Research, Journal of Communication, Journal of Broadcasting and Electronic Media,* and *Media Psychology.*

Lynn Sorsoli is a Research Associate at the Center for Research on Gender and Sexuality at San Francisco State University. She has published several articles and book chapters on adolescent sexuality and gender development, the disclosure of difficult or traumatic experiences, including the disclosure of sexual abuse, and research methodology.

Deborah L. Tolman is Professor of Urban Public Health at Hunter College and Professor of Psychology at the Graduate Center, CUNY. She has published many articles and book chapters on adolescent sexuality, gender development, and research methodology, as well as the award-winning *Dilemmas of Desire: Teenage Girls Talk about Sexuality* (2002/2005), and co-edited *From Subjects to Subjectivities: Interpretive and Participatory Action Methods in Psychology* (2000).

L. Monique Ward is an Associate Professor of Psychology at the University of Michigan. Her research examines parental and media contributions to gender and sexual socialization. Dr. Ward's work has been published in several academic journals, including *Developmental Review, Psychology of Women Quarterly,* and the *Journal of Research on Adolescence.*

Ellen Wartella is the Executive Vice Chancellor and Provost at the University of California, Riverside and a Distinguished Professor of Psychology at UCR. She is currently co-principal investigator on the National Research Foundation project "IRADS Collaborative Research: Influence of Digital Media on Very Young Children". She serves on the Board of Trustees of Sesame Workshop, the National Educational Advisory Board of the Children's Advertising Review Unit of the Council of Better Business Bureaus, and is a member of the National Academy of Sciences Board on Children, Youth, and Families.

D. Charles Whitney is Professor and Chair of the Department of Creative Writing and Professor of Media and Cultural Studies at the University of California, Riverside. His Ph.D. in Mass Communication is from the University of Minnesota, and his research specialties are in the sociology of mass media communicators and in political communication and public opinion. Currently associate editor of the four-volume *Encyclopedia of Journalism* (2009), he was editor of the research journal *Critical Studies in Mass Communication* from 1995 to 1998.

Holley A. Wilkin is an Assistant Professor in the Department of Communication and affiliate of the Partnership for Urban Health Research at Georgia State University. Her research focuses on increasing health literacy and reducing health disparities in diverse urban environments and on entertainment-education.

Preface

A few years ago, Martin Fishbein and Amy Jordan received one of the National Institute of Child Health and Human Development's (NICHD) multi-year grants to explore the relationship between young people's exposure to sexual content in entertainment media and their subsequent sexual beliefs and behaviors that might put them at risk for sexually transmitted infections, unwanted pregnancy, and HIV/AIDS. One of their first tasks was to devise and implement a plan to measure exposure to sexual media content. In order to do this, they first had to develop a method to assess the amount and type of sexual content that was present in the media to which young adolescents were exposed. Several similar projects also funded by NICHD were already well underway—including studies at Emory University, the University of North Carolina-Chapel Hill, the Rand Corporation, and San Francisco State University. Each of these projects incorporated substantial content analysis components to measure the sexual messages in television and other media.

Hoping to benefit from these previous investigations and to share the findings of their own formative research, Fishbein and Jordan decided to host a meeting of these NICHD-funded PIs at the University of Pennsylvania. This meeting was sponsored by NICHD and the Annenberg Public Policy Center (APPC). Like most working groups, this meeting raised more questions than it answered, but equally important, it suggested that the time was right to hold a larger conference focusing on the role of content analysis in media effects research that would bring together leading scholars with experience in several health-related areas of content analysis research.

Recognizing that this was a unique opportunity to convene a dynamic group of researchers facing common issues, Susan Newcomer of NICHD offered her agency's support for the conference, which was again co-sponsored by the Annenberg Public Policy Center. This conference, which was held in December 2003 and organized with the assistance of Dale Kunkel of the University of Arizona and Jennifer Manganello, then a post-doctoral fellow at APPC, generated intense discussion, debate, and novel ideas and approaches regarding the methodology of content analysis. In each session, the dialogue typically started with a practical question—such as what to measure, or how to measure —in the quest to identify sexual content. For example, one discussion focused on how best to compare portrayals across diverse media such as print, television, and the internet. But in the process of addressing those applied questions, the conversations consistently evolved into deeper analysis of the fundamental capabilities and limitations of content analysis research. The participants soon began to realize that most of their discussions had implications far beyond the realm of measuring sexual content. In fact, the issues faced by researchers interested in studying sexual content are not very different from the issues faced by researchers interested in examining media content for a wide variety of public health-related topics. While content analysis research originated in the field of communication, it is now practiced widely by researchers from a variety of disciplines. As we note in Chapter 1, many published content analysis studies—regardless of their field of origin or topic of interest—focus on a public health topic of some sort, addressing such issues as obesity, body image, suicide, violence, sexual behavior, unintentional injury, tobacco use, and substance abuse.

Like communication, public health is a multidisciplinary field made up of scholars from a wide range of areas, including medicine, sociology, economics, political science, anthropology, and psychology, among others. In addition, researchers from academic disciplines beyond both public health and communication now use content analysis regularly to examine health-related messages in the media. With that in mind, and with the growing recognition of the role of media as a factor that could potentially shape all aspects of health-related behavior, we decided to build the conversations that originated at the Annenberg conference into the book you see before you. Its goal is to offer a state-of-the-art discussion about the best practices and tactics for content analysis research as they apply to the examination of health-related behaviors, and to provide examples of how researchers have made decisions involved with planning and executing content analysis studies.

There are already excellent books available to instruct researchers about how to employ content analysis methodology. This volume, however, is uniquely tailored to the challenges faced by content researchers interested in the study of public health topics and presents actual case studies that outline decisions made throughout the research process. We begin by laying out the fundamental issues involved in the conceptualization and design of content analysis investigations for public health research. In Part 1, we lay the foundation for the careful and considered approach we believe content analysis can and should take in informing debates in many disciplines, including both communication and public health. In Chapter 1, Manganello and Fishbein argue for the role of theory in justifying the use of a content analytic approach, informing methodology, and interpreting results in content analysis studies. Kunkel's Chapter 2 addresses the reason why many (but not all) researchers undertake content analysis studies in the first place: they assume media content has an effect on the health beliefs and behaviors of audiences who are exposed to media messages.

Part 2 offers a conceptual perspective on the many decisions we make as we engage in content analysis research. In Chapter 3, Potter walks the reader through the process(es) of defining and measuring key content variables. Jordan and Manganello's Chapter 4 weighs the pros and cons of distinct sampling approaches, and argues for the need for empirical research to undergird sampling decision-making. In Chapter 5, Neuendorf offers thoughtful recommendations for tackling the often difficult task of assessing reliability for content measures. Finally in this section, in Chapter 6 Signorielli recognizes that although content analysis is rarely the concern of Institutional Review Boards (IRBs), it is almost always human beings who do the coding—human beings who must be considered and protected.

Part 3 offers fascinating case studies of content analyses in the public health domain. In the first chapter of this section, Ramasubramanian and Martin (Chapter 7) consider the many changes now underway in the media landscape—including the rapid technological revolution that has made media more portable and interactive and ultimately made media use more idiosyncratic—and the challenges this presents for researchers trying to measure messages and exposure. Part 3 also includes three chapters that address sexual content in media from very different perspectives. In Chapter 8, Salazar and colleagues describe the challenges and opportunities they have faced in content analyzing internet pornography with the goal of ultimately linking this exposure to internet porn messages to adolescent users' sexual beliefs and behaviors. In Chapter 9, Sorsoli, Ward, and Tolman describe the ways in which they examined how television provides adolescents with heterosexual relational scripts. In Chapter 10, Collins and her colleagues describe how they conducted a content analysis to assess sexual content in prime-time television, finding that exposure to sexual content is related to earlier onset of coital behavior among teens. This case study section also contains an ambitious study by Murphy and her USC colleagues (Chapter 11) in which they describe how they identified numerous health-related messages (such as those about cancer, healthy lifestyles, prevention of sexually transmitted diseases) and how these television portrayals have changed over time. Austin (Chapter 12) addresses the issue of examining how receivers' characteristics interact with the alcohol messages they are exposed to in magazines. In the final case study, Pieper, Chan, and Smith (Chapter 13) describe their experiences and make critically important observations as they describe their efforts to measure the violent content of video games.

Our book concludes with a consideration of several "big picture" issues that we believe are necessary as we ponder the audiences for, and the future of, content analysis research. Researchers invest many thousands of hours engaging in content analysis in order to describe the landscape of health messages that are "out there." The focus is typically on the potential deleterious effects of ubiquitous negative messages. Who, ultimately, benefits from what these studies reveal? Where does this information go? Whitney, Wartella, and Kunkel (Chapter 14) consider these questions in their chapter on the audiences for content analysis research. Finally, we—the editors of this volume—distill the many lessons our authors have contributed by proposing a set of guidelines for optimal content analysis research. In a concluding chapter that we hope will advance the science of content analysis (Chapter 15), we suggest ways for the field to accommodate new technologies and new ways of using media. We encourage content analysis researchers to be more deliberate in their use of theory and empirical research in developing their content analytic categories and to be more transparent in the hard decisions they must make about what media they look at, how they look at them, and why.

Content analysis appears on the surface to involve a straightforward categorizing and counting of content attributes in media messages. In other words, it seems simple. The collection of chapters in this volume suggests that studying public health messages through content analysis research is anything but simple. Our authors provide a rare opportunity to witness key decisions that need to be made in designing and conducting a content analysis study of mass media. This "decisions approach" to studying content analysis should be encouraged, particularly as we have seen the investigators' own recognition of the implications of their methodological choices. Laying out the variety of decisions researchers make along the way allows the exploration of traditions, assumptions, and implications for each varying alternative and ultimately advances the science of content analysis research.

The Editors

Part 1
Conceptual Issues

1 Using Theory to Inform Content Analysis

Jennifer Manganello and Martin Fishbein

Introduction

Content analysis is a research method used to analyze content in a variety of formats (e.g., books, newspapers, television, internet) to understand patterns of messages. Sometimes content analysis research is conducted to describe or compare messages without the immediate goal of implying media effects (Riffe, Lacy, & Fico, 1998). In many studies, though, it is assumed that messages being analyzed hold implications for audience effects. In some cases, the expectation of effects comes from existing empirical evidence that documents the audience response, while in others, the expectation is derived from theoretical perspectives. Of course, some studies are informed by both existing research and theory.

Although many content analyses are conducted because of the assumption that media content will influence the beliefs, attitudes, intentions, or behaviors of some audiences, it is interesting to note that most content analytic studies are not combined with other research efforts to also measure outcomes related to attitude, behavior, or policy change. Rather, they analyze what content is currently available in some medium, or they consider changes in content that occur over time. In either case, the assumption is that exposure to this content will affect one or more outcomes.

In the realm of health behaviors, this assumption has often been based on two theoretical perspectives—George Gerbner's cultivation theory and Albert Bandura's social learning and social cognitive theories. However, it is important to recognize that many different theories have been used in health-related content analysis studies, and that even more theories may be applied going forward.

Cultivation theory proposes that, through the process of socialization, people who are heavy television users are more likely to view the world in a way that is consistent with the messages seen on television (Gerbner, 1972; Gerbner, Gross, Morgan, Signorielli, & Shanahan, 2002). Originally introduced when there were only a small number of network television stations and programming was rather homogeneous, it followed that measuring the amount of television viewing could serve as an indicant of exposure to content that regularly appears on television, such as violence. The theory suggests that the more people are exposed to certain messages on television, the more likely they are to develop beliefs or perceptions about the real world that are consistent with those messages. Thus, content analysts assess the amount of a particular type of content present on television to understand the extent that viewers are exposed to that content. For example, if violence is the topic of interest, one could use content analysis to document the fact that there is a considerable amount of violence on television and/or that the amount of violence has increased over time. This would allow a researcher to better understand the potential influence of violent content on the perceptions of heavy television viewers.

While cultivation theory suggests that consistent patterns of messages portrayed on television affect perceptions of viewers, other theoretical perspectives are required to further explain how such content can influence behavior. For example, social cognitive theory (SCT) points to elements of the portrayals that must also be assessed. From this perspective, the likelihood that media portrayals of certain types of behavior will affect our behavior depends on a number of factors such as the characteristics of the actor and whether his or her performing the behavior results in reward or punishment (Bandura, 2002). SCT is a frequently used theory in studies of content analysis and media effects. According to this perspective, the media represent an environmental factor that can influence health attitudes and behaviors, especially when positive and negative consequences are observed with respect to the depicted behavior. Thus, many content analytic studies have counted the number of times a given behavior is reinforced or punished.

Another central element of SCT is the concept of modeling. Generally speaking it has been observed that people who view a role model engaging in a positively reinforced behavior may be more likely to engage in the behavior themselves (Bandura, 2002). However, the theory suggests that the similarity between the role model and the receiver significantly affects the extent to which a model's behavior influences a receiver's behavior; thus, various demographic and other characteristics of the model often serve as explicit content categories to help better inform the researchers about potential effects on various sub-groups within the audience.

This chapter discusses the application of theory to studies utilizing content analysis. We first provide information from reviews of content analytic studies to establish the prevalence of the use of theory. We then present some illustrations of how theory can inform content analytic studies. To conclude, we provide a specific example of how theory has been used to develop questions and content categories for a study exploring the effects of media on adolescent sexual behavior.

Theory used in Published Content Analysis Studies

In this section, we provide an overview of the presence of theoretical framing in published content analysis studies, and the types of theories that are most commonly incorporated. In 1994, Cooper and colleagues analyzed the methods used in research about mass communication (Cooper, Potter, & Dupagne, 1994). They sampled 1,236 articles that had been published in "major mass media" journals from 1965 through 1989 and found that 19.2% (n = 273) of studies used content analysis. Although they measured the use of theory, they did not specify theory used by data collection method. However, they found that less than 1% of all studies included a test of theory, and only 19.5% actually tested hypotheses.

Riffe and Freitag (1997) examined all content analysis articles in *Journalism & Mass Communication Quarterly* from 1971 to 1995. They included content analysis of all forms of media, and found a total of 486 articles using this methodology, approximately 25% of all articles published in the journal during that time. They found that 27.6% of articles mentioned theory, and that this percentage remained fairly stable during the period they examined. In the discussion, when talking about the growth in the number of studies using content analysis, they state "if growth reflects increased theoretical importance of content, it is all the more disconcerting that there is no clear parallel trend toward more theoretical rigor that would allow linkage of content to process and effects" (Riffe & Freitag, 1997, p. 879).

In a more recent study, Kamhawi and Weaver (2003) examined articles in 10 communication journals from 1980 through 1999. Only 39% of all studies mentioned a theory, and of these, 26.7% used content analysis methods. The authors did not provide a breakdown of which theories were used in the content analysis studies.

The above studies showed that theory is used in less than half of content analysis studies published in communication journals. However, content analysis studies focusing on health messages appear in journals from a wide range of disciplines including communication, medicine, and psychology. Manganello and Blake are currently conducting a review of content analysis studies focusing on health messages that appeared in journals from 1985 through 2005 (Manganello & Blake, 2008). For the purpose of the review, health issues include, among other topics: violence, sexual behavior, physical activity, nutrition, obesity, body image, injury, and substance use (tobacco, alcohol, and drugs). To date, over 300 articles have been identified.

In a preliminary examination of the use of theoretical concepts, the most common theories and models referred to either by name or cited in the reference list are social learning theory/social cognitive theory, cultivation theory, socialization, framing, and agenda setting. Some of the others mentioned include desensitization, feminist theory, schema theory, and script theory. At this time, it appears that theory is most often addressed in articles appearing in communication journals, and least often mentioned in studies published in journals from the medical field. In health or medical journals, study authors typically cite prior research findings which support media effects on attitudes or behavior as opposed to outlining the theoretical constructs explaining why the messages have the potential to influence behavior.

When comparing theory use across media, there appear to be some differences and similarities. Compared with other media types, a higher number of television and movie studies use theory, often citing cultivation theory and social learning theory/social cognitive theory. Newspaper studies most commonly reference agenda setting and framing. Studies looking at messages in magazines seem to refer to a larger mix of theories than other media, citing theories such as feminist theory, socialization, social comparison theory, and framing.

So far, a small number of the internet studies have incorporated theory, possibly because it is a newer medium that is more interactive, and thus harder to analyze, than other media types. In addition, interactive media users are not repeatedly exposed to a set of similar messages, making it harder to apply mass media theories such as cultivation theory to explain the potential effects of interactive media. Studies using content analysis for internet sites often focused more on assessing information available or ease of use than on measuring media effects. However, some studies have utilized behavior theories to assess the potential influence content could have on behavior. For example, Ribisl and colleagues (2003) examined websites (n = 30) with material related to smoking culture and lifestyle. The results suggested that websites often depicted smoking combined with alcohol use and sexual content, and that negative consequences were rarely presented. They also found that one third of the sites provided information about positive reasons to smoke. The authors suggest that such images and messages may encourage people to imitate the behavior.

In general, the above literature reviews have found that less than half of published content analysis studies mention theory in an explicit way. Although many articles do not specifically discuss theory, it is possible and likely that theory has been considered in some way during the conception and implementation of the study. Below, ways of using theory in content analysis studies are discussed.

Theory and Content Analysis

The use of theory for content analytic studies of public health messages is a crucial part of the "decisions approach" for several reasons.

1   Theory can be used for the justification of a content analysis study.

The use of theory is not necessary for content analysis, and is often not explicitly stated in papers, as described in the previous section. However, researchers often do rely on at least one theory or model when developing the rationale for a content analytic study that suggests a potential effect from the content being studied. For instance, someone interested in analyzing media messages because of the potential for children to imitate observed behaviors would, to some degree at least, justify their study with reference to SCT. Theories used in content analytic studies of public health topics have come from a wide range of disciplines, including communication, psychology, and public health. Even theories not commonly used in public health research could be applied to content analyses looking at health messages. Moreover, as Kunkel et al. (2007) argue, the clear specification of an effects theory can not only help to explain why a study should be conducted, but it can also inform the design of the study, thus guiding the decisions approach.

Bell and colleagues (2005) offer an example of a content analysis study specifically identifying a theory as a justification for conducting the research. According to the authors, cultivation theory suggests that people exposed to repeated messages about unhealthy eating and little or no exercise behavior are likely to believe that such behaviors are "normal." They thus conducted a content analysis of the 10 top grossing movies of each year from 1991 through 2000 in order to see the frequency with which these behaviors occurred. More specifically, they counted the incidents of healthy and unhealthy food or drink ingestion, as well as the number of times physical activity was shown.

2   Theory can be used to develop research questions and inform the methodological approach (i.e., sample, unit of analysis, content categories).

In some cases, it seems plausible that authors use theory to guide their study without clearly stating this in an article. For instance, Stockwell and Glantz (1997) conducted a content analysis of smoking in movies. They counted tobacco events, and for each smoking event, looked at location, positive or negative reaction to use, and presence of a minor. They also examined character variables, such as character type and role, gender, age and ethnicity, and analyzed the portrayal of the scene (e.g., stressful vs. relaxed). Although it could be argued that these types of content categories are derived from SCT or some other theory, no theory was mentioned.

Other authors clearly explain how theory informs their study design. For example, Roberts and colleagues (1999) examined substance use in movies and music. Explicitly referencing cultivation theory, they state that behaviors portrayed more frequently become more acceptable to the audience. To apply the theory, they counted the frequency of alcohol, tobacco, and illicit drug use as part of the content analysis. They also discuss how social cognitive theory emphasizes that behaviors portrayed with mostly positive outcomes as opposed to negative outcomes are more likely to be imitated. For this reason, they examined both short-term and long-term consequences of substance use as portrayed in media. In sum, they use the theories to link their assumption of effects with their observation of the portrayals of substance use presented in the media venues examined. Their theoretical foundation affords a strong expectation of effects even though their analysis is limited to content observations.

3   Theory can be used to test the effects of content exposure in different outcome domains.

Studies may employ theory to explain the link between content and outcomes, including policy or behavior outcomes. While some content analysis studies are mainly designed to assess, measure, and quantify media content from the premise that the messages can influence attitudes and behavior, others evaluate messages in order to directly link them to outcomes. In a study of media effects, one might use theory to inform both content categories and also survey questions for participants in order to make comparisons between the two sources of data. This comparison allows theory to guide the selection of other variables of interest that may have a moderating effect on the influence of media content on attitudinal or behavioral outcomes.

Media effects studies incorporate some sort of media use variables as predictors for an outcome, but do not always rely on content analysis to provide data about messages to which people are exposed. Typically, researchers will use time spent with media or with media genres as the predictor variables. For instance, Wingood and colleagues (2003) explored the relationship between viewing rap music videos and health risk behaviors among adolescent females. In the discussion, the authors suggest that SCT may help explain the mechanism behind the effect of videos on behavior, stating that music videos that "rarely show the potential long-term adverse effect of risky behavior, may influence adolescents by modeling these unhealthy practices" (Wingood et al., 2003, p. 438). Teens were asked how much time they spent watching music videos, what type of videos they watched, who they watched the videos with, and where they watched them, but the researchers did not examine the content of music videos.

There are some media effects studies that include content analysis as part of the research methods. They determine what media are used by the respondents, conduct a content analysis to examine messages, and then examine association of messages with behavioral outcomes. There is a wide variation of whether these studies mention specific models or theories to explain the role that media can play on behavior, and how theories shape such studies.

One example is a study by Dalton and colleagues (2003). The study examined the link between exposure to smoking in movies and initiation of smoking among adolescents. The researchers surveyed teens aged 10 to 14. Those teens who reported having never smoked were surveyed again one to two years later. A variety of risk factors were examined, one of which was movie viewing. For each survey, teens were provided with a list of 50 movies and asked which they had seen. The researchers then conducted a content analysis to count incidents of smoking in each movie. In the discussion, the authors mention that "more than 40 years of research shows that observers imitate specific behaviors they see modeled" (Dalton et al., 2003, p. 284). No specific theory is discussed to explain why movies might influence smoking behavior, but the mention of imitation suggests the ideas are coming from Bandura's theories. In the published paper that presented the content analysis findings, the authors reported examining character attributes, such as gender and race, as well as attributes of the tobacco use, such as frequency and reasons why tobacco was used (Dalton et al., 2002). However, it is unclear whether these additional character-level variables collected in the content analysis were incorporated into the media effects analysis conducted at a later time. The researchers mainly included information about the total number of smoking incidents per movie seen by the respondent for the media effects analysis (Dalton et al., 2003).

Some studies rely on theories to inform both the content analysis categories and questions for surveys administered to participants. Collins and colleagues studied the link between exposure to sexual content on television and sexual behavior (2004; see also Chapter 10 in this volume). The authors point to social cognitive theory as an explanation for why teens might be more likely to engage in sexual behavior if they see characters on television having sex without seeing negative consequences from the behavior. Teens were given a list of 23 television programs and asked how often they watched each program. A content analysis was conducted to assess sexual talk and behavior in a sample of episodes for each program. Messages about risk and safety were also analyzed. Results showed an association between greater exposure to sexual content and advances in sexual behavior during the following year. Links were found with risk messages and behavior only for African American youth, but the authors emphasize that risk messages were rare, possibly causing weaker effects.

Current Example

In a study currently underway at the Annenberg Public Policy Center of the University of Pennsylvania, researchers are examining the influence of five different types of media on risky sexual behavior among adolescents. Adolescents aged 14 to 16 at the time the study began completed surveys in years one, two, and three. The integrative model of behavior (IM) is being used to justify the need for the inclusion of content analysis in a mixed-method approach to answer the research questions. The IM also informs both survey questions and content analysis coding categories.

The IM, depicted in Figure 1.1, is an attempt to include the key concepts from many of the leading theories of behavioral prediction and behavior change within a single model (Fishbein, 2000). More specifically, it is based largely on the theories of reasoned action and planned behavior, SCT, and the health belief model. Generally speaking, the model assumes that intentions are the best predictors of any given behavior. It recognizes, however, that one may not always be able to act on one's intention, particularly if one doesn't have the necessary skills and abilities needed to perform the behavior or if one encounters barriers or other types of environmental constraints that can prevent behavioral performance. Thus skills and abilities, and environmental factors, may moderate the influence of intention on behavior.

A person's intention to perform a given behavior is viewed as a function of three variables: attitude toward performing the behavior, perceptions of the social pressure exerted upon them to perform the behavior, and perceptions

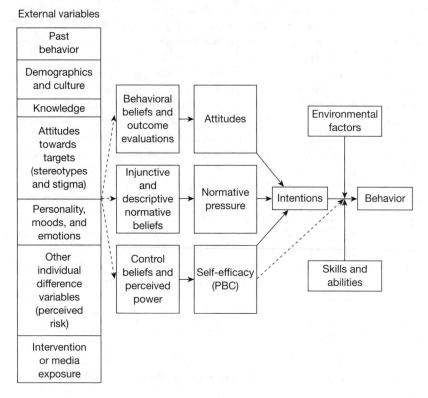

Figure 1.1 The integrative model of behavior change

of control or self-efficacy with respect to performing the behavior. The more positive one's attitude toward performing the behavior (i.e., the more favorably one feels about performing the behavior), the more one feels social pressure to perform the behavior (i.e., the more one believes that important others think one should or should not perform the behavior and/or that most of these important others are themselves performing the behavior). The stronger one's sense of self-efficacy or control over the behavior (i.e., the more one believes that they have the necessary skills and abilities to perform the behavior even under a number of difficult circumstances), the stronger should be one's intention to perform (and thus one's actual performance of) the behavior in question.

Attitudes, perceived social pressure, and perceived self-efficacy/control are themselves assumed to be based on underlying beliefs. More specifically, attitudes are assumed to be a function of beliefs that performing the behavior will lead to various outcomes. Referred to as *behavioral beliefs* in the theories of reasoned action and planned behavior, as *outcome expectancies* in SCT, and as *costs and benefits* in the health belief model, it is assumed that the more one believes that performing the behavior will lead to positive outcomes (and/or prevent negative ones), the more favorable will be the person's attitude. Perceived social pressure is viewed as a function of beliefs that specific individuals or groups think one should (or should not) perform the behavior as well as beliefs that these others are themselves performing (or not performing) the behavior. The more one believes that these referent others think one should perform the behavior and/or are themselves performing the behavior, the stronger will be the perceived social pressure to perform that behavior. Similarly, self-efficacy or perceived control is seen as a function of beliefs that, even in the face of specific barriers and impediments, one can perform the behavior. Thus, according to the IM, and as indicated previously, one's behavior is ultimately determined by one's beliefs concerning the behavior, and media messages may play an important role in shaping those beliefs.

Finally, as can also be seen in Figure 1.1, the theory recognizes that there are a large number of variables that may (or may not) influence these behavioral, normative, and control beliefs. Thus for example, rich and poor, old and young, high and low sensation seekers, those who are scared or not scared, anxious or relaxed, those who perceive they are or are not at risk for a serious illness, as well as those differing in ethnicity, age, and gender, may have similar beliefs with respect to some behaviors but very different beliefs with respect to others. Thus, in order to understand why some people do and some do not perform a given behavior, it is necessary to identify the beliefs that underlie that behavior.

The formative research that assisted with the design of the survey for the longitudinal study included focus groups with teens in the Philadelphia area. During the focus groups, we asked participants to complete several questionnaires. One had questions to assess various aspects of the IM model. For example, in order to identify salient beliefs underlying attitudes, teens were asked "If you were to have sex in the next year, what are some of the **good things** that might happen?" and "If you were to have sex in the next year, what are some of the **bad things** that might happen?" Questions were also asked about who would approve or disapprove if the teen had sex in the next year (normative beliefs) as well as about what things would make it easy or hard to have sex (control of efficacy beliefs) in the next year.

Responses from the open-ended questionnaires distributed during the focus groups were used to develop questions for the survey. For instance, responses about who would approve or disapprove included people like mothers, fathers, siblings, and friends. A section was added to the survey listing different types of people (parent, best friend). Teens were then asked to indicate, for each person listed, whether that person thought the teen should or should not have sex in the next year. Similarly, to assess behavioral beliefs, the teens were asked to indicate the likelihood that their having sex in the next year would lead to each of the salient outcomes identified in the elicitation study. And to assess control beliefs, they were asked to indicate how certain they were that they could have sex in the next year even if the salient barriers identified in the elicitation study were present. In addition, teens were asked to indicate their intentions to have sex in the next year, their attitudes toward having sex in the next year, the amount of social pressure they felt with respect to having sex in the next year, and their self-efficacy with respect to having sex in the next year.

Finally, questions were asked about specific media types used, frequency of use, and favorite media titles for each media type. Responses to these questions were used to develop a sample of media to be content analyzed. When developing the categories for the content analysis, the different aspects of the IM were taken into account. Categories similar to the belief questions that were developed for the survey were added into the content analysis codebook. More specifically, coders were trained to look for content that addressed salient behavioral, normative, and control beliefs related to sexual intercourse. For example, they would code whether referent others approve or disapprove of the characters' sexual behavior; whether the content provided information that performing the behavior would lead to the various positive and negative outcomes; and whether the content provided cues for over-coming barriers to engaging in sexual intercourse. While all sexual content was coded both in terms of talk and behavior, these more detailed contextual analyses were triggered if the media content portrayed or implied sexual intercourse.

By developing similar questions for both the survey and the content analysis based on the IM, it may be possible to assess, for example, whether teens exposed to content that has specific messages about a particular positive or negative outcome of engaging in sex are more likely to hold this belief than those who have not been so exposed. By considering the impact of the media on the full set of salient behavioral, normative, and control beliefs, we will also be able to begin to link media exposure to attitudes, perceived social pressure, self-efficacy, intentions, and behavior.

By using theory to inform both the survey design and the content analysis, we expect that our study will be able to connect media messages to attitudes and behaviors over time. Additional examples of the use of theory in content analysis research appear in several case studies presented in this volume. Gender schemas are addressed in Chapter 12, social learning theory is covered in Chapter 10, and desensitization appears in Chapter 8. Several theories are mentioned in Chapter 11, including cultivation theory, social learning theory, and the health belief model. In Chapter 9, the authors discuss script theory, socialization, and feminist theory.

Conclusion

The relevance and usefulness of a theoretical approach are not unique to content analysis studies. Public health research using any methodology often benefits from the guidance of theoretical perspectives. In addition, the practice of public health is heavily informed by behavioral theories. They provide a framework for understanding factors related to change in attitudes, knowledge, and behavior, offer a road map for designing interventions, and facilitate the design of scientifically sound evaluation strategies for intervention programs and policies (Glanz, Rimer, & Lewis, 2002; National Cancer Institute, 2005; Noar, 2006).

Much has been written to emphasize the need for theory in several areas of public health work. Fishbein and Yzer (2003) recommend the use of theory for informing the design of communication campaigns, and Fishbein (2000) discusses how theory is relevant to designing interventions to prevent the transmission of HIV. Baranowski and colleagues (2003) discuss the role of theory in obesity research, while Gielen and Sleet (2003) and Trifiletti and colleagues (2005) describe how theory can be utilized to inform injury prevention programs and research. Norman and colleagues (2007) reviewed studies specific to eHealth interventions for obesity-related issues, and found that a majority used theory to guide the design of the intervention. These are just some examples.

Although application of theory to content analysis research is not essential, and may not be necessary for some studies, it can provide a strong foundation for any content analysis study related to public health that has the ultimate goal of implying potential effects from the content being analyzed. Theory can provide the justification for research, offer a framework for linking content to effects, and serve as a guide for developing content categories. As Shoemaker and Reese (1990) suggest, studies of content and studies of media effects should be better integrated, and we believe that theory can play an important role in achieving this integration.

References

Bandura, A. (2002). Social Cognitive Theory of mass communication. In J. Bryant & D. Zillmann (Eds.), *Media effects: Advances in theory and research* (pp.121–153). Mahwah, NJ: Lawrence Erlbaum.

Baranowski, T., Cullen, K. W., Nicklas, T., Thompson, D., & Baranowski, J. (2003). Are current health behavioral change models helpful in guiding prevention of weight gain efforts? *Obesity Research, 11*(S), 23S–43S.

Bell, R. A., Berger, C. R., Cassidy, D., & Townsend, M. (2005). Portrayals of food practices and exercise behavior in popular American films. *Journal of Nutrition Education and Behavior, 37*(1), 27–32.

Collins, R., Elliott, M., Berry, S., Kanouse, D., Kunkel, D., Hunter, S. B., et al. (2004). Watching sex on television predicts adolescent initiation of sexual behavior. *Pediatrics, 114*, 280–289.

Cooper, R., Potter, W. J., & Dupagne, M. (1994). A status report on methods used in mass communication research. *Journalism Educator, 48*(4), 54–61.

Dalton, M., Sargent, J. D., Beach, M., Titus-Ernstoff, L., Gibson, J., Ahrens, M., Tickle, J. J., et al. (2003). Effect of viewing smoking in movies on adolescent smoking initiation: A cohort study. *Lancet, 362*, 281–285.

Dalton, M., Tickle, J., Sargent, J. D., Beach, M., Ahrens, M., & Heatherton, T. (2002). The incidence and context of tobacco use in popular movies from 1988–1997. *Preventive Medicine, 34*, 516–523.

Fishbein, M. (2000). The role of theory in HIV prevention. *AIDS Care, 12*(3), 273–278.

Fishbein, M., & Yzer, M. (2003). Using theory to design effective health behavior interventions. *Communication Theory, 31*(2), 164–183.

Gerbner, G. (1972). Violence in television drama: Trends and symbolic functions. In G. A. Comstock & E. A. Rubinstein (Eds.), *Television and social behavior* (Vol. 1). Washington, DC: US Government Printing Office.

Gerbner, G., Gross, L., Morgan, M., Signorielli, N., & Shanahan, J. (2002). Growing up with television: Cultivation processes. In J. Bryant & D. Zillmann (Eds.), *Media effects: Advances in theory and research* (pp.43–67). Mahwah, NJ: Lawrence Erlbaum.

Gielen, A. C., & Sleet, D. (2003). Application of behavior-change theories and methods to injury prevention. *Epidemiologic Reviews, 25*, 65–76.

Glanz, K., Rimer, B. K., and Lewis, F. M. (2002). *Health behavior and health education: Theory, research and practice* (3rd ed.). San Francisco, CA: John Wiley & Sons, Inc.

Kamhawi, R., & Weaver, D. (2003). Mass communication research trends from 1980 to 1999. *Journalism & Mass Communication Quarterly, 80*(1), 7–27.

Kunkel, D., Eyal, K., Donnerstein, E., Farrar, K., Biely, E., & Rideout, V. (2007). Sexual socialization messages on entertainment television: Comparing content trends 1997–2002. *Media Psychology, 9*(3), 595–622.

Manganello, J., & Blake, N. (2008). Two decades of studying health messages in the media: Where have we been and where should we be going? Unpublished manuscript.

National Cancer Institute. (2005). Theory at a glance: A guide for health promotion practice. Retrieved October 3, 2007, from http://www.cancer.gov/theory/pdf

Noar, S. (2006). A health educator's guide to theories of health behavior. *International Quarterly of Community Health Education, 24*(1), 75–92.

Norman, G. J., Zabinski, M. F., Adams, M. A., Rosenberg, D. E., Yaroch, A. L., & Atienza, A. A. (2007). A review of eHealth interventions for physical activity and dietary behavior change. *American Journal of Preventive Medicine, 33*(4), 336–345.

Ribisl, K., Lee, R., Henriksen, L., & Haladijan, H. (2003). A content analysis of web sites: Promoting smoking culture and lifestyle. *Health Education and Behavior, 30*(1), 64–78.

Riffe, D., Lacy, S., & Fico, F. G. (1998). *Analyzing media messages: Using quantitative content analysis in research*. Mahwah, NJ: Lawrence Erlbaum.

Riffe, D., & Freitag, A. (1997). A content analysis of content analyses: Twenty-five years of *Journalism Quarterly*. *Journalism & Mass Communication Quarterly, 74*(4), 873–882.

Roberts, D. F., Henriksen L., & Chistenson, P. G. (1999). *Substance use in popular movies and music*. Sponsored by Office of National Drug Control Policy and Department of Health and Human Services. Retrieved August 18, 2005, from http://www.mediascope.org/pubs/supmm.pdf

Shoemaker, P. J., & Reese, S. D. (1990). Exposure to what? Integrating media content and effects studies. *Journalism Quarterly, 67*(4), 649–652.

Stockwell, T., & Glantz, S. (1997). Tobacco use is increasing in popular films. *Tobacco Control, 6*, 282–284.

Trifiletti, L. B., Gielen, A. C., Sleet, D. A., & Hopkins, K. (2005). Behavioral and social science theories and models: Are they used in unintentional injury prevention research? *Health Education Research, 20*(3), 298–307.

Wingood, G., DiClemente, R., Bernhardt, J., Harrington, K., Davies, S., Robillard, A., et al. (2003). A prospective study of exposure to rap music videos and African American female adolescents' health. *American Journal of Public Health, 93*(3), 437–439.

2   Linking Content Analysis and Media Effects Research

Dale Kunkel

Content analysis research has a long history in the field of communication and related social sciences. More than 50 years ago, journalists were counting story topics and elements to track trends in newspaper coverage of various issues (Krippendorff, 2004). Following the advent of television, researchers began to explore entertainment program content, measuring character demographics as well as sensitive behaviors that might influence viewers (Cassata & Skill, 1983; Greenberg, 1980). Today, in an era of increasing media channels, content analysis research seems to be growing in popularity. It is applied across a broad range of new and old media forms, from newspapers and magazines to websites and chat rooms. Moreover, content analysis is frequently employed to examine all types of health-related behavior, from seat belts to substance use, body image, sexual risk taking, and a host of other important concerns (Kline, 2003, 2006).

Most content analysis studies are descriptive and often univariate. They report such findings as the number of violent acts in an hour of television (Gerbner, Gross, Morgan, & Signorielli, 1980), the frequency of sexual intercourse in soap operas (Greenberg & Buselle, 1996), and the percentage of characters featured in motion pictures who smoke cigarettes (Dalton et al., 2002). The relevance of such research is underscored by substantial evidence documenting the contributions of entertainment media to people's social knowledge, beliefs, attitudes, and behaviors. But when a researcher's data are limited to identifying patterns in message content, the critical challenge is to effectively link the content-based evidence to other existing studies that illuminate the implications for communication processes and effects. This chapter considers how content analysis researchers can most effectively meet that challenge.

The Growth of Health-related Content Studies

Content analysis studies are traditionally associated with the field of communication, an academic discipline that emerged in the 1950s (Glander, 2000; Schramm, 1997). Research reviews that tally methodological tactics in the field generally estimate that content analysis evidence is found in at least

20–30% of all published articles in leading mass communication journals (Cooper, Potter, & Dupagne, 1994; Kamhawi & Weaver, 2003; Riffe & Freitag, 1997; Wimmer & Haynes, 1978). The field of communication has long used content analysis to investigate a broad range of issues, including the prominence of different types of news coverage and the nature and extent of political campaign advertising (Neuendorf, 2002).

Reflecting a growing awareness of the role of mass communication as a potential factor shaping people's health-related beliefs, attitudes, and behaviors, researchers in the fields of both communication and public health began to actively pursue content analysis studies of health-related topics in the media in the 1980s. Such studies were a major thread in the growing fabric of "health communication" research, which encompassed issues ranging from patient-provider interaction to "entertainment-education" health information campaigns. The synergy in this domain led to the establishment of specialized divisions in professional associations (e.g., International Communication Association, National Communication Association, American Public Health Association) and the creation of multi-disciplinary support groups (e.g., Coalition for Health Communication). Complementary journals were also launched, such as *Health Communication* in 1989 and *Journal of Health Communication* in 1996 (Thompson, Dorsey, Miller, & Parrott, 2003). Both regularly publish content analysis research conducted by scholars from a wide range of disciplines, most notably public health and medicine. It seems clear that content analysis research of health-related media messages is pursued widely today by scholars both within and outside of the field of communication, and published in a diverse range of journals.

Differing Approaches to Content Analysis Research

Regardless of the disciplinary background of the investigator, there are two primary ways in which content analysis data can be situated in a research study. First, content patterns can be conceptualized as an implicit dependent variable, with the investigation seeking to examine the likely influence of causal factors that might account for an increase or decrease in certain types of messages. This tactic can be employed in a wide range of different scenarios. For example, media sociologist Muriel Cantor spent decades exploring how media industry organizational structures and processes helped to shape the nature of prime-time television programming on the broadcast networks (Cantor, 1971, 1982; Cantor & Cantor, 1992). Her work helped to explain how and why shifts occurred over time from one genre of popular television show to another.

Similarly, other researchers have used content analysis data in an effort to identify the influence of government policy or regulation on television content. Rowland (1983) observed that the frequency of televised violence dropped significantly in years immediately following major Congressional hearings on the topic, while Kerkman, Kunkel, Huston, Wright, and Pinon (1986) documented a significant decline in children's educational programs shortly after the Federal Communications Commission deregulated its requirement for such material on broadcast channels. However, content analysis studies that posit message patterns as dependent variables are relatively sparse, as compared to the alternative perspective (Shoemaker & Reese, 1996).

The more common tactic adopted by content analysis researchers is to conceptualize message patterns as a putative independent variable, or potential cause of media effects (Shoemaker & Reese, 1996). For example, studies might examine the amount of violence on television, and if the data indicate a high frequency of violent behavior, then the conclusion is drawn that the evidence gives cause for concern. Such a conclusion is typically derived by implicitly linking the evidence about content patterns to previous studies that demonstrate adverse effects of exposure to media violence. In other words, the content analysis data derive their primary meaning from their implications for audience effects.

The Problem of Weak Linkage

Depending upon the design of the study, this latter approach to content analysis research may leave "weak links" in the chain connecting the content patterns observed with their relevant implications for effects. For example, many studies seem to assume that all instances of a media character smoking, or drinking, or having sexual intercourse are essentially equivalent in terms of their implications for audience influence. Yet media effects theory and research make clear that this is not always the case.

There is no question that the growing number of content studies that examine media portrayals pertaining to health issues such as tobacco use, alcohol consumption, or safe sex have generated a great deal of knowledge about the frequency with which such messages appear. This chapter raises the question of whether the utility of such studies has been needlessly constrained. To the extent that a content analysis study seeks to draw implications for audience influence, it is essential that the design of the message analysis be sensitive to existing knowledge regarding media effects. The goal of this chapter is to encourage content analysis researchers to establish greater linkage between the nature of the content patterns observed and the relevant theory and evidence regarding audience effects. When this strategy is successful, the content analysis researcher stands on more solid ground in drawing implications for likely influence based upon audience exposure to the message patterns identified.

Some content researchers might object to this prescription, arguing that their investigations are purely descriptive, such that they could be applied equally well in either of the modes described above; that is, as either an independent or dependent variable in a broader approach to understanding media processes and effects. This position, however, ignores the framing that is used to present and indeed legitimize the value of content analysis research published in academic journals that are largely committed to "explaining and predicting" as opposed to simply "describing" the variables under examination. For example, if a study investigates how physical exercise is portrayed on prime-time television, the implication is likely to be that more frequent portrayals are better and that fewer portrayals are worse in terms of increasing the visibility and attractiveness of physical activity. But are all portrayals the same in terms of such implications for effects? What if a featured character who starts an exercise regimen constantly complains of sore muscles and experiences frustration from the lack of any weight loss after several weeks of activity? Such a portrayal clearly holds different implications for audience effects, as compared to one in which the featured character encounters more positive outcomes from engaging in exercise.

For content analysis studies that hope to draw implications for audience effects, there is generally more to be done than a simple counting of the frequency of targeted behaviors. The content measures employed in the research should incorporate detailed aspects of the ongoing narrative that help to establish the interpretation and meaning that viewers will likely ascribe to each relevant portrayal. To accomplish this typically requires the careful consideration of the *context* in which targeted behaviors occur. The following sections demonstrate how content analysis research can employ measurement of contextual features that should enhance a study's ability to draw implications for audience effects, and explain why such measurement is important. To make this case, we will consider several health-related behaviors, starting first with the depiction of televised violence.

The Importance of Context: Lessons from Televised Violence

If content analysis has long been one of the favored methods employed in mass communication research, the topic of television violence has long been one of the most popular targets of content analysts (Comstock & Scharrer, 1999). Violence is considered a public health issue because of its implications for medical treatment and morbidity, and it is no coincidence that early research in this realm was shepherded by the U.S. Surgeon General (Surgeon General's Scientific Advisory Committee, 1972). Since then, the topic of media violence has attracted significant attention from such professional groups as the American Academy of Pediatrics, American Medical Association, and American Psychological Association (Joint Statement, 2000).

What are the implications for effects on viewers, especially children, who observe a mediated depiction of violence? It is well established that heavy exposure to televised violence poses a risk of harmful effects, including exaggerated fear, desensitization, and subsequent aggressive behavior (Anderson et al., 2003; Comstock & Scharrer, 2007; Wilson et al., 1997). A broad base of evidence including cross-sectional surveys, longitudinal panel studies, and experiments all contribute to conclusions in this realm. But a critical question for the content analyst is: Are all acts of violence the same in terms of their implications for effects?

In most cases the answer is no, but the response is always contingent upon the dependent variable of interest. A substantial collection of experimental studies, most of which were conducted in the 1970s and 1980s, identified a number of key contextual features that help to shape most effects of exposure to televised violence (Wilson et al., 1997). Violence may occur on-screen and be shown graphically or it may occur off-screen but be clearly implied. Violent acts may be shown close-up or at a distance. There are differences in the types of characters who commit violence and their reasons for doing so. And there are differences in the outcomes of violence. Some depictions focus on the pain and suffering of victims, whereas others avoid showing the negative consequences of physical aggression. Simply put, not all portrayals of violence are the same; their context can vary on many important dimensions. These differences matter because there is substantial experimental evidence that such differences in the message characteristics hold important implications for the impact of particular violent scenes on viewers (Kunkel et al., 1995; Smith et al., 1998; Wilson et al., 1997).

In the mid-1990s, a large-scale project called the National Television Violence Study (NTVS) reviewed all existing effects research that had previously examined the influence of various contextual features, and devised a content analysis framework that measured attributes known from previous studies to either increase or diminish the likelihood of one of the three basic types of harmful influence: exaggerated fear, desensitization, or increased aggression (Wilson et al., 1997). For example, Berkowitz and his colleagues (Berkowitz & Geen, 1967; Berkowitz & Powers, 1979; Berkowitz & Rawlings, 1963) established through numerous lab studies that violence perceived as justified from a societal perspective causes more subsequent aggression in viewers than violence perceived as unjustified. Similarly, violence that is rewarded or shown without punishment was found to increase the likelihood of subsequent viewer aggression based upon numerous empirical studies by Bandura and his colleagues (Bandura, Ross, & Ross, 1961, 1963a, 1963b), whereas violence that is punished diminished the risk of such effects.

Yet another important contextual factor is the perceived realism of violent portrayals. Numerous experimental studies have presented the same media content and framed it as either something that really happened (i.e., news, documentary) or as fictional entertainment. Following exposure, viewers were significantly more aggressive when the content was perceived as realistic, rather than fiction or fantasy (Berkowitz & Alioto, 1973; Feshbach, 1972; Geen, 1975). This outcome has been linked in part to increased physiological arousal associated with violent scenes perceived as more realistic (Geen, 1975; Geen & Rakosky, 1973).

Employing an analytical framework based upon a comprehensive review of the relevant effects literature, the NTVS researchers were able to measure a broad range of contextual features such as the justification for violence, the rewards or punishments for violence, and the degree of realism. By incorporating these and other important context factors known to shape the effects of exposure, the NTVS content-based data could effectively identify depictions of violence with the greatest risk of harm, and differentiate them from portrayals that were less likely to lead to adverse effects. For example, violent portrayals that were glamorized (i.e., committed by attractive role models who are often rewarded and rarely punished for their violent acts) and sanitized (i.e., depicting unrealistically mild harm to victims, little pain and suffering) were judged to pose the greatest risk of harmful influence on child viewers.

A Contrasting Perspective: Emphasizing Prevalence

In the 1970s and 1980s, George Gerbner's cultural indicators project dominated the study of violence on television (Gerbner, Gross, Morgan, & Signorielli, 1986; Signorielli, Gerbner, & Morgan, 1995). In reporting his content-based findings, Gerbner consistently emphasized evidence assessing the overall prevalence of violence on television. Across most of their studies, Gerbner and his colleagues reported findings of approximately five to six violent acts per hour of television (Signorielli, 1990). Other scholars who employed broader definitions of violence, including actions that cause psychological or emotional harm rather than purely physical damage, reported higher averages ranging from 18 to 38 violent acts per hour (Greenberg, 1980; Potter et al., 1995; Williams, Zabrak, & Joy, 1982). Still other researchers counted violence differently, measuring the number of scenes with violent behavior, rather than the number of violent acts. For example, Lichter and Amundson (1994) reported that an average of 10.7 scenes per hour of prime-time programming contained violence. Note that a scene could contain 1, 5, 10, or any number of violent actions and it would still be coded identically as simply "contains violence" under this approach.

The noteworthy point across all of these studies is that they tend to employ a highly reductionistic approach in framing their central findings, which means that their summary statistics count all acts of violence as equivalent to one another in generating the totals. This common tactic poses a significant validity problem if one is trying to draw implications for some types of effects, as opposed to others.

The cultivation theory developed by Gerbner and his colleagues emphasized the influence of media exposure on viewers' beliefs and perceptions, rather than on any attitudinal or behavioral outcomes. Given that Gerbner was interested in explaining media influence on beliefs and perceptions about social reality, it makes sense that his content data about violent depictions were aggregated collectively for his key analyses. The focus was on studying people's perceptions of the frequency or likelihood of actually encountering violent activity.

While it may have been prudent to employ this perspective given Gerbner's particular interest in beliefs and perceptions, many readers of this research at the time—including the press and public policy-makers—sought to apply it more broadly to draw implications for other types of effects, such as an increase in aggressive behavior following exposure to media violence (Kunkel, 2003). Yet shifting the application of the content data from one possible dependent variable to another in this case is highly problematic.

There is a fundamental disconnect between content analysis evidence that treats all depictions of violence the same in terms of their implications *for behavioral effects*, when in fact there is substantial knowledge from experimental lab research establishing that certain contextual features significantly enhance the risk of exposure to such media content for subsequent aggressive behavior. Simply put, not all violence is the same in terms of its risk of influencing aggressive attitudes and behaviors, as established in the previous section.

This example clarifies that the content analysis researcher can hardly afford to be agnostic in terms of drawing implications for effects. Rather, if a content researcher conceptualizes message patterns as an implicit independent variable, then the nature of the content categories measured in the study must be sensitive to what is known about predicting the dependent variables of interest. In the case of televised violence, counting all acts of violence in the same way may be sensible for inferring influence on a variable such as beliefs, while using the same measurement tactic would hardly be optimal for inferring effects on attitudinal or behavioral outcomes, as the experimental lab studies explicated earlier demonstrate.

The Importance of Context: Examples from Sexual Content Studies

Regardless of the specific topic area, content analysis of health-related behavior can benefit from more careful consideration of contextual factors. Important lessons can also be drawn from the study of sexual content in the media, another issue that fits squarely in the public health domain (Office of the U.S. Surgeon General, 2001).

Numerous content analysis studies over the years have examined various types of sexual portrayals in television programming. Early studies demonstrated that sexual behavior is common in prime-time shows (Franzblau, Sprafkin, & Rubinstein, 1977; Lowry & Shidler, 1993; Sapolsky & Taberlet, 1991), as well as in soap operas (Greenberg & Buselle, 1996; Greenberg et al., 1993; Lowry & Towles, 1989). Just as with the topic of violent portrayals, early research exploring the effects of viewing sex on television found that heavier viewers had increased perceptions of the frequency with which sexual behaviors occur in the real world (Buerkel-Rothfuss & Mayes, 1981; Buerkel-Rothfuss & Strouse, 1993).

Like the study of media violence, early content analysis research of sexual behavior devoted little attention to contextual features that might be instrumental in shaping the audience's interpretation of the portrayals. While it was common for analyses to differentiate the type of sexual behavior depicted—such as kissing, fondling, or intercourse—it was rare to consider contextual features such as one partner's knowledge of the other's sexual history. The emphasis was initially placed on analyzing the overall frequency of sexual portrayals, and the question of whether the volume was increasing or decreasing over time (Greenberg & Buselle, 1996; Sapolsky & Taberlet, 1991).

Consistent with the trend described above in the study of televised violence, the examination of sexual media content has now evolved to reflect greater emphasis on contextual features or cues that can in some way help to establish linkages with potential effects. For example, a series of content-based studies entitled "Sex on TV" supported by the Kaiser Family Foundation (Kunkel et al., 1999, 2001, 2003, 2005) included measures that help to establish the positive or negative consequences associated with sexual activity. This element is derived from social cognitive theory (Bandura, 1986; 2002), and has also been linked empirically as a moderator of sexual media effects (Eyal & Kunkel, 2008).

Another contextual feature that has received increasing attention involves the examination of "safe sex" messages incorporated into televised scenes with sex. Several recent experimental studies document significant effects on attitudes and behavioral intentions when such messages are included in television comedies or dramas (Collins, Elliott, Berry, Kanouse, & Hunter, 2003; Farrar, 2006). Early content studies that examined this issue, however, measured such messages at only a rudimentary level (Kunkel et al., 1999; Lowry & Shidler, 1993), identifying the mere presence of any sexual risk and responsibility topic (e.g., sexual patience, sexual precautions such as condoms and birth control) simply to gauge their visibility among viewers. In terms of implications for effects, content-based evidence at this rudimentary level could only be tied to a cultivation perspective that might posit influence on people's awareness of or concern about sexual risk issues.

In order to draw implications for attitudinal or behavioral effects on the audience, it would be essential to know more about the context of such portrayals. Thus, more recent content studies have also measured such factors as the positive or negative valence associated with each risk or responsibility depiction (Kunkel et al., 2003, 2005). Without the valence measure, a portrayal in which a teenager refuses to use a condom because it "takes the fun out of sex" would be counted the same as one in which a woman tells a man with whom she is about to engage in intercourse for the first time that "I never have sex without a condom." By adding more contextual richness to the content measures, the implications for audience effects are clearly enhanced. Other recent content research in this realm (Eyal, Kunkel, Biely, & Finnerty, 2007; Fisher, Hill, Grube, & Gruber, 2004) also reflects a similar sensitivity to contextual features that are expected to be important in shaping the meaning of "safe sex" messages for viewers.

Beyond Implications: Directly Linking Content Analysis Measures with Exposure Effects

The discussion so far has been directed to the most common form of published content analysis research, and that is a stand-alone study that strictly identifies patterns in message characteristics. This prototype encompasses studies that document the nature and extent of portrayals of smoking, or eating, or driving after drinking alcohol, or performing any health-related behavior—but where the empirical data gathered for the investigation are limited solely to content-based observations. Such content analysis studies leave it to others to measure possible outcomes from exposure to these messages, such as increased smoking rates, levels of obesity, or drunk driving incidents.

Given that a primary motivation for pursuing most content analysis research is the implicit assumption that media message patterns hold important implications for audience effects, it should be apparent that the optimal research design in this realm would be one in which content analysis data are linked directly with measures of viewers' exposure to such messages, as well as with the hypothesized outcome variables (e.g., viewers' beliefs, attitudes, behaviors). Of course, such a design is hardly a novel suggestion. For example, most of Gerbner's content analysis data examining televised violence was presented in tandem with survey evidence that established linkages between people's time spent viewing television and their beliefs about the frequency of crime and violence in the real world. When Gerbner discovered significant correlations between people's television viewing and their estimates of the frequency of crime and violence, his content analysis data documenting the heavy presence of violence on television provided a plausible mechanism to account for this relationship.

Unfortunately, employing this same tactic today is problematic because of the profound change that has occurred in the media environment since the 1970s and 1980s, when most of Gerbner's cultivation research was conducted. At that time, the media environment was characterized by a limited number of channels and the programming content was quite homogeneous. In contrast, the contemporary media landscape offers a plethora of television channels exceeding the capacity of Gerbner's era by numbers in the hundreds, not to mention the existence of many other sources of electronic mass media available via the internet.

The bottom line is that the media environment today has grown so large and diverse that a researcher can no longer be safe in assuming that one heavy user of a medium will be exposed to a similar type of content as compared to another heavy user, whether the medium of interest is film, television, or the internet, among other sources. On television, the proliferation of niche-oriented specialty channels means that audience members can readily indulge their unique preferences and predilections (see Chapter 7 in this volume). In other media, the diversity of content may well be even greater than that found on television. Consequently, a researcher interested in establishing an effect from media exposure today must measure more carefully the specific nature of the media content to which each individual is exposed, rather than simply relying upon estimates of people's overall time spent with a given medium.

Collins et al. (Chapter 10 in this volume) report a successful example of this tactic. In their study of adolescents, Collins and her colleagues initially gathered content analysis evidence assessing the sexual portrayals presented on a broad range of the most popular programs available on television, and then married that data with information about each individual subject's viewing patterns. This yielded an index of exposure to sexual content on television for each subject that is much more valid and precise than any estimate of total time spent with television could ever be, given the diversity of program options available.

Statistical analyses of these viewing indices yielded significant findings about the effects of watching sex on television, with causal conclusions made possible because of the longitudinal design of the study. Adolescents who viewed heavier amounts of sexual content at Time 1 were significantly more likely to engage in intercourse a year later at Time 2, as compared to those who saw light amounts of sexual material. Consistent with the point raised above about the increasing diversity of media content, the same data from the Collins study revealed no significant relationship between total television viewing and sexual behavior (Collins et al., 2004). In other words, the effects of exposure to sexual content on television could only be identified by carefully scrutinizing the amount of sexual content included in each individual's diet of programs, but not by considering their total amount of time spent watching television.

Interestingly, while the Collins study benefited from its precise assessment of the amount of sexual content included in each subject's media exposure, it failed to employ any sophisticated examination of contextual features in that same content. Had that study incorporated more elaborate contextual information such as the consequences of the sexual liaisons viewed or their degree of realism, its findings might well have been more robust. In fact, however, Collins and her colleagues did identify one significant finding linked to a key contextual feature of the content viewed by different individuals. In their examination of the effects of viewing sexual risk or responsibility messages, Collins et al. (2004) found that increased exposure to such content reduced the risk of teenage intercourse, but only for African Americans. Because research examining the impact of "safe sex" messages is still in its infancy, this finding offers more questions than answers. Yet this outcome leads us to another important consideration for the content analysis researcher: the prospect that important differences exist in the way that different audiences "see," or interpret, media content.

The Issue of Varying Audience Interpretations

In order to posit the effects of media messages on an audience, it is critical to take into account the meaning of the message as understood by the receiver. Krippendorff (1980, 2004) has long been at the forefront in emphasizing the point that meanings do not reside inherently in messages. Rather, the meaning of each message is generated by the receiver based upon his or her comprehension of the words or pictures that form the message content, which may vary according to differences in background or experiences. Indeed, Krippendorff's

(2004) observation that "meanings invoked by texts need not be shared" by all who perceive them poses a challenge for content researchers (p. 23).

The utility of content analysis evidence is generally grounded in the assumption that there is largely shared meaning associated with the message patterns identified by the research. Without such an assumption, one set of content analysis data would hold little value. Instead there might be a need for multiple datasets for differing audiences with different interpretive predilections.

Fortunately for the content researcher, it seems likely that there is a lot of shared meaning in how people make sense of a wide range of behaviors portrayed in the media, at least at a rudimentary level. When a police officer shoots a mentally ill suspect who is wielding a knife and threatening others, almost any observer would interpret this as a violent act. This is manifest content. Where the issue becomes more complicated is in the realm of latent content, which requires more interpretation on the part of the receiver. The question of whether or not the officer was justified may be more subtle and nuanced, and might be judged differently by a diversity of viewers.

The case studies in this volume present a number of strategies that are relevant in considering the issue of varying audience interpretations. For example, Austin (Chapter 12 in this volume) employs receiver-oriented message analysis, in which content analysis data are generated by members of the particular target audience of interest for the research. Thus, Austin relies upon young adults to classify content judgments about alcohol advertisements targeted at young adults. She finds this strategy particularly useful for measuring latent variables such as identifying an advertisement's intended target demographic.

Another perspective is offered by Pieper, Chan, and Smith (Chapter 13 in this volume), who tackle the task of performing content analysis on interactive video games. Perhaps the biggest challenge in this media environment relates to the fact that there is no linear content, with the actions of the "player" determining the flow of messages encountered. Pieper and colleagues observe that many aspects of the content of video games will vary according to individual differences between players, such as their degree of game experience. In some of their studies, they specify the degree of experience of their coders, but they also discuss the prospect of conducting multiple investigations with coders of varying levels of experience and comparing the findings accordingly.

Another strategy that a content analyst may employ involves the use of distinct content measures that are uniquely tailored to reflect particular audiences' interpretive capabilities or predilections. An example from the NTVS illustrates this tactic. Given the importance of consequences associated with depictions of violence in predicting effects, the NTVS project measured the extent to which violence was rewarded or punished within each program. However, because young children were an audience of particular concern for this study, and because this age group has only limited capacity to draw cause-and-effect conclusions across disparate scenes (Collins, 1979, 1983), the study employed a content measure uniquely relevant for child viewers: the extent to which violence was rewarded or punished in the same scene, or an immediately adjacent scene. While adults can understand that punishments at the end of a show are linked to acts that occurred right at the beginning, young children cannot. But that "problem" for the content analyst who is focused on implications for effects is ameliorated simply by adding supplementary content measures that better reflect the child's information processing capabilities. Such child-sensitive content measures can then be applied to analyze the patterns of violence across all programming as they would likely be interpreted by the child audience; or conversely, applied to programming primarily directed at children to better assess its sensitivity to the comprehension capabilities of the target audience.

Whether the strategy is to apply different measures that are uniquely applicable to different audiences, or to employ different demographic groups to conduct the message analysis, content analysis researchers are increasingly tailoring their studies to take into account the prospect of varying audience interpretations of media messages. Such tactics are another mechanism that can be employed to enhance the sophistication and rigor of content analysis investigations.

Conclusion

This chapter focuses primarily on content analysis research that seeks to draw implications for audience effects. Given this emphasis, it is critical to underscore the importance of audience exposure patterns in one's initial approach to a content-based study. We live in an age when the mass media deliver an unprecedented number of messages. Some of these media vehicles attract large audiences, but many do not. Content analysis researchers cannot simply assume an audience is present for the message environment that they choose as their target for investigation. Meticulously coded, highly reliable data that are based upon television programming aired on Channel 172 at 3:00 a.m. may have a critical problem. What if the program failed to attract any viewers? Try drawing effects implications from those message patterns!

In previous decades, content studies of television programming typically sampled network prime-time shows on the presumption that they were the most heavily viewed. But those assumptions are barely tenable today, and completely irrelevant to the world of video games and websites, among other new media. The increasing number and diversity of media channels and venues place a heavier burden than ever before on content researchers to ascertain that the content they choose to study is indeed the media environment that is frequented by their audience of interest. Without attention to this critical detail, the connection between message patterns observed and any likely audience influence can be left hanging by a thread, when it deserves to be an important link in the chain between content and effects.

This chapter's key conclusion is that content-based research benefits from the use of measures that offer greater contextual richness. That richness may provide greater clarity about the likely interpretations derived by audience members with differing backgrounds, or in optimal circumstances, may strengthen the linkage between the content patterns observed and their implications for effects. The latter outcome occurs when the design of the message analysis framework has been carefully crafted in advance to match the findings from existing theory or empirical evidence, such as has been done in the area of televised violence. It seems that many of the same types of lessons already learned in the realm of violent portrayals could be applied in the examination of a broader range of health-related behaviors in the media.

The perceived realism of media characters' actions as well as the consequences of their behavior both help to shape the meaning of the message for the audience, and are two examples of important contextual features that are typically worthy of attention in content-based studies because of their widespread utility in media effects research. While there are certainly many others, it is impossible to craft a comprehensive list because of the situational specifics associated with differing health behaviors. Indeed, there seems to be ample opportunity for enterprising health communication researchers to further probe in the laboratory to discover the influence of important contextual features on the outcomes of exposure to portrayals of sexual behavior, drinking alcohol, and smoking cigarettes, among others. Such laboratory effects evidence could strengthen the hand of subsequent content investigations in identifying more precisely the particular types of portrayals most likely to lead to adverse influence on viewers' health-related beliefs, attitudes, and behaviors.

This chapter's prescription to emphasize context in the pursuit of content analysis research is important but not necessarily novel. There are strong examples to point to where content investigators have already employed such emphasis quite successfully. In her examination of television programs popular with youth, Monique Ward (1995) designed her content measures to assess "talk about sex" according to meaningful scripts commonly employed by adolescents, as identified by previous literature in the area of sexual socialization. This tactic reflects sensitivity not only to message context, but to the interpretive predilections of the audience of interest, another important theme in this chapter. Similarly, in their study of tobacco use in movies, Dalton and colleagues (2002) measured such contextual factors as character smokers' motives for use, affective experience, and consequences encountered. Studies such as these maximize their utility by gathering content evidence in such depth that one can have very high confidence regarding the implications for effects of the message patterns identified.

When the measures employed in a content analysis design are linked effectively with a solid, consistent body of media effects research, a content-based study can serve as a perfect complement to extend the value of that effects evidence in practical, real-world terms. The effects studies establish the risk of particular types of influence from exposure to certain types of portrayals; then the content analysis tracks media industry performance to determine whether the type of portrayals deemed to be problematic are common or infrequent, increasing or decreasing, widely viewed or unpopular, and so on.

Such contributions from content analysis researchers can provide invaluable insight into the role that media play in shaping health-related behaviors.

As long as the public continues to devote extraordinary amounts of time attending to entertainment media, there will be a critical need for two important types of scientific evidence: studies of media effects on health behavior, and studies of media content that identify message patterns likely to trigger those effects. Striving to link these two types of research together clearly offers great advantages to the content analysis investigator.

References

Anderson, C., Berkowitz, L., Donnerstein, E., Huesmann, L. R., Johnson, J., Linz, D., et al. (2003). The influence of media violence on youth. *Psychological Science in the Public Interest, 4*, 1–41.

Bandura, A. (1986). *Social foundations of thought and action: A social cognitive theory.* Englewood Cliffs, NJ: Prentice-Hall.

Bandura, A. (2002). Social cognitive theory of mass communication. In J. Bryant & D. Zillmann (Eds.), *Media effects: Advances in theory and research* (pp. 121–154). Mahwah, NJ: Lawrence Erlbaum Associates.

Bandura, A., Ross, D., & Ross, S. (1961). Transmission of aggression through imitation of aggressive models. *Journal of Abnormal and Social Psychology, 63*, 575–582.

Bandura, A., Ross, D., & Ross, S. (1963a). Imitation of film-mediated aggressive models. *Journal of Abnormal and Social Psychology, 66*, 3–11.

Bandura, A., Ross, D., & Ross, S. (1963b). Vicarious reinforcement and imitative learning. *Journal of Abnormal and Social Psychology, 73*, 601–607.

Berkowitz, L., & Alioto, J. (1973). The meaning of an observed event as a determinant of its aggressive consequences. *Journal of Personality and Social Psychology, 28*, 206–217.

Berkowitz, L., & Geen, R. (1967). Stimulus qualities of the target of aggression: A further study. *Journal of Personality and Social Psychology, 5*, 364–368.

Berkowitz, L., & Powers, P. (1979). Effects of timing and justification of witnessed aggression on the observers' punitiveness. *Journal of Research in Personality, 13*, 71–80.

Berkowitz, L., & Rawlings, E. (1963). Effects of film media on inhibitions against subsequent aggression. *Journal of Abnormal and Social Psychology, 66*, 405–412.

Buerkel-Rothfuss, N., & Mayes, S. (1981). Soap opera viewing: The cultivation effect. *Journal of Communication, 31*(3), 108–115.

Buerkel-Rothfuss, N., & Strouse, J. (1993). Media exposure and perceptions of sexual behaviors: The cultivation hypothesis moves to the bedroom. In B. Greenberg, J. Brown, & N. Buerkel-Rothfuss (Eds.), *Media, sex, and the adolescent* (pp. 225–247). Cresskill, NJ: Hampton Press.

Cantor, M. G. (1971). *The Hollywood TV producer. His work and his audience.* New York: Basic Books.

Cantor, M. G. (1982). The organization and production of prime-time television. In D. Pearl, L. Bouthilet, & J. Lazar (Eds.), *Television and behavior: Ten years of scientific progress and implications for the eighties* (pp. 349–362). Rockville, MD: National Institute of Mental Health.

Cantor, M. G., & Cantor, J. M. (1992). *Prime-time television: Content and control.* Newbury Park, CA: Sage Publications.

Cassata, M., & Skill, T. (1983). *Life on daytime television: Tuning in American serial drama.* Norwood, NJ: Ablex.

Collins, R., Elliott, M., Berry, S., Kanouse, D., & Hunter, S. (2003). Entertainment television as a healthy sex educator: The impact of condom efficacy information in an episode of "Friends." *Pediatrics, 112,* 1115–1121.

Collins, R., Elliott, M., Berry, S., Kanouse, D., Kunkel, D., Hunter, S., & Miu, A. (2004). Watching sex on TV affects adolescent initiation of sexual intercourse. *Pediatrics, 114*(3), e280–e289.

Collins, W. A. (1979). Children's comprehension of television content. In E. Wartella (Ed.), *Children communicating: Media and development of thought, speech, understanding.* Beverly Hills, CA: Sage Publications.

Collins, W. A. (1983). Interpretation and inference in children's television viewing. In J. Bryant & D. Anderson (Eds.), *Children's understanding of television: Research on attention and comprehension* (pp. 125–150). New York: Academic Press.

Comstock, G., & Scharrer, E. (1999). *Television: What's on, who's watching, and what it means.* New York: Academic Press.

Comstock, G., & Scharrer, E. (2007). *Media and the American child.* New York: Academic Press.

Cooper, R., Potter, J., & Dupagne, M. (1994). A status report on methods used in mass communication research. *Journalism Educator, 48,* 54–61.

Dalton, M., Tickle, J., Sargent, J., Beach, M., Ahrens, B., & Heatherton, T. (2002). The incidence and context of tobacco use in popular movies from 1988 to 1997. *Preventive Medicine, 34,* 516–523.

Eyal, K., & Kunkel, D. (2008). The effects of sex in television drama shows on emerging adults' sexual attitudes and moral judgments. *Journal of Broadcasting & Electronic Media, 52,* 161–181

Eyal, K., Kunkel, D., Biely, E., & Finnerty, K. (2007). Sexual socialization messages on television programs most popular among teens. *Journal of Broadcasting & Electronic Media, 51,* 316–336.

Farrar, K. (2006). Sexual intercourse on television: Do safe sex messages matter? *Journal of Broadcasting & Electronic Media, 50,* 635–650.

Feshbach, S. (1972). Reality and fantasy in filmed violence. In J. Murray, E. Rubinstein, & G. Comstock (Eds.), *Television and social behavior* (Vol. 2, pp. 318–345). Washington, DC: U.S. Government Printing Office.

Fisher, D., Hill, D., Grube, J., & Gruber, E. (2004). Sex on American television: An analysis across program genres and network types. *Journal of Broadcasting & Electronic Media, 48,* 529–553.

Franzblau, S., Sprafkin, J., & Rubinstein, E. (1977). Sex on TV: A content analysis. *Journal of Communication, 27,* 164–170.

Geen, R. (1975). The meaning of observed violence: Real vs. fictional violence and consequent effects on aggression and emotional arousal. *Journal of Research in Personality, 9,* 270–281.

Geen, R., & Rakowsky, J. (1973). Interpretations of observed violence and their effects on GSR. *Journal of Experimental Research in Personality, 6,* 289–292.

Gerbner, G., Gross, L., Morgan, M., & Signorielli, N. (1980). The "mainstreaming" of America: Violence profile No. 11. *Journal of Communication, 30*(3), 10–29.

Gerbner, G., Gross, L., Morgan, M., & Signorielli, N. (1986). Living with television: The dynamics of the cultivation process. In J. Bryant & D. Zillmann (Eds.), *Perspectives on media effects* (pp. 17–40). Hillsdale, NJ: Erlbaum.

Glander, T. (2000). *Origins of mass communications research during the American cold war*. Mahwah, NJ: Lawrence Erlbaum Associates.

Greenberg, B. (1980). *Life on television: Content analyses of U.S. TV drama*. Norwood, NJ: Ablex.

Greenberg, B., & Buselle, R. (1996). Soap operas and sexual activity: A decade later. *Journal of Communication, 46*(4), 153–160.

Greenberg, B., Stanley, C., Siemicki, M., Heeter, C., Soderman, A., & Linsangan, R. (1993). Sex content on soaps and the prime-time television series most viewed by adolescents. In B. Greenberg, J. Brown, & N. Burkel-Rothfuss (Eds.), *Media, sex, and the adolescent* (pp. 29–44). Cresskill, NJ: Hampton Press.

Joint Statement on the Impact of Entertainment Violence on Children. (2000, July 26). Congressional Public Health Summit, Washington, DC. Retrieved January 31, 2005, from http://www.aap.org/advocacy/releases/jstmtevc.htm

Kamhawi, R., & Weaver, D. (2003). Mass communication research trends from 1980 to 1999. *Journalism & Mass Communication Quarterly, 80*, 7–27.

Kerkman, D., Kunkel, D., Huston, A., Wright, J., & Pinon, M. (1990). Children's television programming and the "Free Market Solution." *Journalism Quarterly, 67*, 147–156.

Kline, K. (2003). Popular media and health: Images, effects, and institutions. In T. Thompson, A. Dorsey, K. Miller, & R. Parrott (Eds.), *Handbook of health communication* (pp. 557–581). Mahwah, NJ: Lawrence Erlbaum Associates.

Kline, K. (2006). A decade of research on health content in the media: The focus on health challenges and sociocultural context and attendant informational and ideological problems. *Journal of Health Communication, 11*(1), 43–59.

Krippendorff, K. (1980). *Content analysis: An introduction to its methodology*. Newbury Park, CA: Sage Publications.

Krippendorff, K. (2004). *Content analysis: An introduction to its methodology* (2nd ed.). Thousand Oaks, CA: Sage Publications.

Kunkel, D. (2003) The road to the V-chip: Media violence and public policy. In D. Walsh & D. Gentile (Eds.), *Media violence and children* (pp. 227–246). Westport, CT: Praeger.

Kunkel, D., Biely, E., Eyal, K., Farrar, K., Donnerstein, E., & Fandrich, R. (2003). *Sex on TV 3*. Menlo Park, CA: Henry J. Kaiser Family Foundation.

Kunkel, D., Cope, K., Biely, E., Farinola, W., & Donnerstein, E. (2001). *Sex on TV 2: A biennial report to the Kaiser Family Foundation*. Menlo Park, CA: Henry J. Kaiser Family Foundation.

Kunkel, D., Cope, K., Farinola, W., Biely, E., Rollin, E., & Donnerstein, E. (1999). *Sex on TV: Content and context*. Menlo Park, CA: Henry J. Kaiser Family Foundation.

Kunkel, D., Eyal, K., Finnerty, K., Biely, E., & Donnerstein, E. (2005). *Sex on TV 4*. Menlo Park, CA: Henry J. Kaiser Family Foundation.

Kunkel, D., Wilson, B., Donnerstein, E., Linz, D., Smith, S., Gray, T., Blumenthal, E., & Potter, W. (1995). Measuring television violence: The importance of context. *Journal of Broadcasting & Electronic Media, 39*, 284–291.

Lichter, S. R., & Amundson, D. (1994). *A day of TV violence*. Washington, DC: Center for Media and Public Affairs.

Lowry, D. T., & Shidler, J. A. (1993). Prime-time TV portrayals of sex, "safe sex," and AIDS: A longitudinal analysis. *Journalism Quarterly, 70*, 628–637.

Lowry, D. T., & Towles, D. E. (1989). Prime-time TV portrayals of sex, contraception, and venereal diseases. *Journalism Quarterly, 66*, 347–352.

Neuendorf, K. (2002). *The content analysis guidebook.* Thousand Oaks, CA: Sage Publications.

Office of the U.S. Surgeon General. (2001). *The Surgeon General's call to action to promote sexual health and responsible sexual behavior.* Rockville, MD: U.S. Department of Health and Human Services.

Potter, W. J., Vaughan, M. W., Warren, R., Howley, K., Land, A., & Hagemeyer, J. C. (1995). How real is the portrayal of aggression in television entertainment programming? *Journal of Broadcasting & Electronic Media, 39*, 496–516.

Riffe, D., & Freitag, A. (1997). A content analysis of content analyses: Twenty five years of *Journalism Quarterly. Journalism & Mass Communication Quarterly, 74*, 873–882.

Rowland, W. (1983). *The politics of TV violence: Policy uses of communication research.* Beverly Hills, CA: Sage Publications.

Sapolsky, B., & Taberlet, J. (1991). Sex in prime-time television: 1979 vs. 1989. *Journal of Broadcasting & Electronic Media, 35*, 505–516.

Schramm, W. (1997). *The beginnings of communication study in America: A personal memoir.* Thousand Oaks, CA: Sage Publications. [Edited by S. H. Chaffee & E. M. Rogers, published posthumously.]

Shoemaker, P., & Reese, S. (1996). *Mediating the message: Theories of influence on mass media content* (2nd ed.). White Plains, NY: Longman.

Signorielli, N. (1990). Television's mean and dangerous world: A continuation of the Cultural Indicators perspective. In N. Signorielli & M. Morgan (Eds.), *Cultivation analysis: New directions in media effects research* (pp. 85–106). Newbury Park, CA: Sage Publications.

Signorielli, N., Gerbner, G., & Morgan, M. (1995). Violence on television: The Cultural Indicators project. *Journal of Broadcasting & Electronic Media, 39*, 278–283.

Smith, S., Wilson, B., Kunkel, D., Linz, D., Potter, W. J., Colvin, C., & Donnerstein, E. (1998). Violence in television programming overall: University of California, Santa Barbara study. *National television violence study* (Vol. 3). Thousand Oaks, CA: Sage Publications.

Surgeon General's Scientific Advisory Committee on Television and Social Behavior. (1972). *Television and growing up: The impact of televised violence.* Washington, DC: U.S. Government Printing Office.

Thompson, T., Dorsey, A., Miller, K., & Parrott, R. (Eds.). (2003). *Handbook of health communication.* Mahwah, NJ: Lawrence Erlbaum Associates.

Ward, L. M. (1995). Talking about sex: Common themes about sexuality in prime-time television programs children and adolescents view most. *Journal of Youth & Adolescence, 24*, 595–615.

Williams, T., Zabrak, M., & Joy, L. (1982). The portrayal of aggression on North American television. *Journal of Applied Social Psychology, 12*, 360–380.

Wilson, B., Kunkel, D., Linz, D., Potter, W. J., Donnerstein, E., Smith, S., Blumenthal, E., & Gray, T. (1997). Violence in television programming overall: University of California Santa Barbara study. *National television violence study* (Vol. 1). Thousand Oaks, CA: Sage Publications.

Wimmer, R., & Haynes, R. (1978). Statistical analyses in the *Journal of Broadcasting,* 1970–1976. *Journal of Broadcasting, 22*, 241–248.

Part 2
Research Design Issues

3 Defining and Measuring Key Content Variables

W. James Potter

When designing content analyses, social scientists construct coding rules to define the measurement categories that will be used in their investigation of media message patterns. The goal of coding rules is to fully specify the task of determining which messages fit into which content categories. When the coding task is fully specified, coders are able to make decisions that are consistent throughout the sample and over time. This results in high reliability of a dataset that can then be considered to be systematically generated and hence scientific. However, when the coding rules do not work well, the degree of consistency in classifying messages across coders, across types of content, and over time is low; thus reliability and hence validity are low, and the resulting data must be regarded as having little scientific worth. Constructing good coding rules that fully specify the coding task is fundamental to a scientific content analysis.

This chapter focuses on what it means to construct coding rules and how those constructions contribute (or fail to contribute) to fully specifying the research design. Content analysts are often limited by the belief that they need to construct a complete set of prescriptive rules in order to reach the goal of fully specifying the coding task. There is the strong temptation to continue to construct additional coding rules when coder reliability is low. That is, content analysts believe that the only way to increase inter-rater consistency is to continue adding rules in order to gradually reduce and eventually eliminate the chance for individual coders to deviate in their interpretations from other coders. However, adding more coding rules does not always serve to provide useful guidance to coders such that all coders are able to converge in their decisions and thereby exhibit a high degree of consistency. Furthermore, the increase in the number of rules beyond a certain point is likely to reduce the ecological validity of the data, confuse coders, and even reduce the reliability.

This chapter argues that when reliability is low, there are alternatives to the writing of more and more coding rules. This argument begins with an analysis of the debate over what types of content are optimal or even appropriate for examination by content analysis. The chapter then examines the purpose of coding rules, the nature of coding decisions, and the types of rules. This builds to the final section, which explicates how to make good design decisions by matching the type of rule to the type of coding task.

Manifest Versus Latent Content Coding

There is a long-standing debate about whether content analysts should limit themselves to coding manifest content or whether they should also consider latent content. This debate is interesting because it implicates more than the mere categorization of different forms of content; rather, the debate is really about the purpose of content analysis, its limits, and the roles of both the scholars who design content analysis studies and the coders who generate data as part of such research. The issues raised in this debate are fundamental to the kinds of rules we construct to guide our coders.

A good starting place for this analysis is Holsti (1969), who observed that a "major source of disagreement among those defining content analysis is whether it must be limited to manifest content (the surface meaning of the text) or whether it may be used to analyze the deeper layers of meaning embedded in the document" (p. 12). Manifest content is typically regarded as content elements that are relatively discrete symbols that lie on the surface of the content and are easy for coders to recognize. In contrast, latent content is something—like a pattern or a theme—that must be inferred from the discrete symbols. For example, let's say we want to look at risky behaviors of teens as portrayed on television shows, and we are most concerned with the element of humor in those portrayals. We could treat humor as manifest content and direct our coders to focus on whether there is a laugh track on a television program. When coders hear a laugh track behind a risky portrayal, they code it as humorous; when there is no laugh track, the portrayal is coded as serious. This is a relatively easy task of recognition and recording of manifest content.

Continuing with this example, let's say a content analysis project is interested in the type of humor, reasoning that there is a difference between *laughing at* a risky behavior and *laughing with* a character who is about to perform a risky behavior. If the humor in the show makes us *laugh at* the foolishness of a character, the humor is being used in a prosocial way, that is, to denigrate the risky behavior. In contrast, if the humor in the show makes us *laugh with* a character as she leaps into a risky behavior, the humor is being used in an antisocial manner, that is, to trivialize the risk and make the character's risky behavior seem like fun. Distinguishing the underlying intention of someone's behavior is a much more challenging task than coding whether or not there is a laugh track present. The audience's interpretation of humor lies in the way the humor is portrayed, and it requires a significant degree of interpretation on the part of coders to make decisions about classifying the type of humor being presented. As designers of such a content analysis, we may ask our coders to pay attention to laugh tracks and whether characters laugh, or whether characters say something is funny, but none of these symbols is necessarily the indicator of a particular type of humor. Coders need more guidance to help them "read" all the relevant symbols specified in their coding rules, then construct a judgment of type of humor from this information. The goal is to do this in a way that is consistent with the message interpretations likely to be derived by the audience of interest for the study.

In addressing the debate about the use of content analysis to measure latent content, Holsti (1969) argued that the distinction between manifest and latent content takes place at two levels. One level involves the coding task in which coders record whether certain symbols are present in the text. If they are, those symbols are classified as being present in a certain category. This is manifest content. But coders can also be asked to "read between the lines" (p. 12) and code latent content. Regardless of whether content analysis focuses on manifest or latent content, Holsti identified another issue that has to do with extending the quantitative analysis beyond simply describing the results and interpreting those results. But there seems to be a confounding of two dimensions in his argument. One of these dimensions focuses on the type of content being analyzed (manifest or latent) while the other dimension focuses on the purpose of the analysis and tone of the reporting (descriptive or inferential). Figure 3.1 separates these two concerns and illustrates the key differences between them.

In the upper left quadrant of Figure 3.1, coders are regarded as clerks, and analysts are regarded as scribes. This is the simplest form of content analysis, and that content must be manifest. Coders receive simple training on easy-to-recognize symbols; their task is to count the occurrence of these symbols. The only significant threat to reliability is fatigue. Analysts (scholars who design the study, analyze the results, and report the findings) write simple coding rules, run simple quantitative tests (counts and percentages) on the data, and describe the summary statistics. Very little interpretation is required from either the coders or the analysts. This is the way in which a variety of scholars

Coders: clerical recording Analyst: faithful reporting of counts and summaries	Coders: clerical recording Analyst: positioning findings in a larger context
Coders: inducing patterns Analyst: faithful reporting of counts and summaries	Coders: inducing patterns Analyst: positioning findings in a larger context

Figure 3.1 Alternative roles for coders and analysts

(Berelson, 1952; Kaplan, 1943; Kerlinger, 1973; Janis, 1949) conceptualize content analysis research. For example, Berelson (1952) defines content analysis as "a research technique for the objective, systematic and quantitative description of the manifest content of communication" (p. 18). Notice that he limits the technique to examining manifest messages. Kerlinger (1973) defines content analysis as "a method of studying and analyzing communications in a systematic, objective, and quantitative manner to measure variables" and added that most content analysis has been used "to determine the relative emphasis or frequency of various communication phenomenon" (p. 525) and not to make inferences from the data patterns.

The argument that Holsti makes is that content analysts need to move to the right side of Figure 3.1. The role of the coders does not change. But the role of the analyst is expanded in the reporting of findings, that is, the analyst is seen as having an obligation to contextualize the results either in terms of relating the found content patterns to the senders of the message (i.e., their motives, conventions, formulas) or to the audience (i.e., connecting content patterns to possible effects on people exposed to those patterns). For example, Osgood (1959) reflects this upper right position when he defines content analysis "as a procedure whereby one makes inferences about sources and receivers from evidence in the messages they exchange" (p. 13). Also, Stempel (1981) has defined content analysis as "a formal system for doing something that we all do informally rather frequently, drawing conclusions from observations of content" (p. 119). Budd, Thorp, and Donohew (1967) say that because the ultimate goal of communication scholars is to predict behavior, they must relate the findings of content analyses to effects on the communicators. Riffe, Lacy, and Fico (1998) say the purpose of content analysis is "to describe the communication, draw inferences about its meaning, or infer from the communication to its context, both of production and consumption" (p. 20). All of these scholars argue for the importance of drawing inferences, but they assign that task to the analyst who designs the study, not to the coders. Their point is that unless content analysts can move beyond the simple reporting of frequencies of manifest messages, the results of their studies will not be very interesting. Analysts have the responsibility, in their view, to move beyond data counts by drawing inferences about content patterns and relating those inferences to values of the producers and/or effects on the audiences.

Holsti's own view is also positioned in the upper right. He defines content analysis as "any technique for making inferences by objectively and systematically identifying specified characteristics of messages" (p. 14), which puts the focus on the coding of manifest content and positions him in the upper half of Figure 3.1. In addition, Holsti also argues that once the coding is finished and quantitatively analyzed, the researcher makes inferences about the results—either inferences about the causes of the communications analyzed or inferences about the effects of those messages. For example, a content analysis study that reports high frequencies of violence on television programs could be linked to the idea that violent entertainment is profitable or that exposure to violence is heavy and widespread for most TV viewers.

At the time Holsti made his argument to push the focus of content analysis from the upper left to the upper right quadrant of Figure 3.1, there was already reason to believe that a shift was underway. For example, Danielson (1963) wrote about a trend away from purely descriptive content analysis towards the testing of hypotheses. However, several decades later, Shoemaker and Reese (1990) observed that most content analyses are not linked "in any systematic way to either the process that created the content or to its effects" (p. 649). In 1996, Riffe and Freitag examined 25 years of published content analyses in *Journalism & Mass Communication Quarterly*. They identified 486 content analyses over that period, which indicates that it is a popular method, but they also observed that 72% of those content analyses lacked a theoretical framework linking their findings to either the antecedents or the effects of the content. Instead most content analyses are fairly descriptive in nature and are limited to manifest content or at least content that is treated as if it were manifest, which puts most content analyses squarely in the upper right quadrant of Figure 3.1.

Moving from the upper level to the lower level in Figure 3.1 shifts the focus from manifest content to latent content; it also shifts the focus from the analyst to the coder. When we shift from manifest to latent content, the role of the coder changes from that of a clerk who records occurrences of symbols in the content and instead requires the coder to be more of an interpretive instrument. To highlight this difference in coder roles, consider the use of two different terms to define the coder's orientation. With manifest content, coders are "decision-makers"; with latent content, coders are "judgment-makers." Decision-making involves selecting among a finite set of options in a relatively automatic, standard manner. Coders rely on simple prescriptive rules that are based largely on denotative meanings. For example, coders read newspaper articles and make a mark on a coding sheet every time a source is quoted in a story. Also, coders may be asked to select a code from a list of sources by type (e.g., 1 = government official; 2 = spokesperson for a commercial business; 3 = spokesperson for a non-profit organization; 4 = private citizen, etc.) and record the type of source on the coding sheet. Another example is coders watch an hour of television and make a mark on a coding sheet every time there is a commercial ad. Also, coders may be asked to select a code from a list of types of commercial products and record the judgment on the coding sheet. With manifest content, the symbols are fairly salient and discrete. The coder must only recognize certain symbols and record their presence. The skill used by coders is simple deduction, where the coding rule is the major premise, the symbols in the content are the minor premises, and the coder deduces a simple conclusion of whether the symbol fits the rule.

In contrast to coding decisions, there also are coding judgments. Judgments occur as the result of an inductive process of surveying symbols in the flow of content and inferring patterns, which are perceived connections among the individual symbols. Coders are provided with rules to guide them in searching for certain symbols while ignoring other symbols. Coders are also provided with examples that illustrate how particular configurations of symbols should be judged as a pattern, but these examples can never be exhaustive. Thus, coders will be continually confronted with novel configurations of symbols in the content they must code, and those coders must judge whether the configurations are alike enough to the example in order to be assigned the particular code suggested by the example. Clearly, the coding of latent content requires much more mental effort from coders as they make their judgments. The judgment-making process is susceptible not just to fatigue but is also sensitive to the relative degrees of skill across coders (i.e., ability to perceive symbols and ability to construct patterns systematically) in mastering the classification system, not to mention the individual differences in coders' idiosyncratic knowledge about the content being coded. The threats to reliability and validity are much more severe when coding latent content compared to manifest content.

Despite the challenges inherent in coding latent content, there are big payoffs if it is done well. For example, it is more valuable to know how much dangerous driving behavior there is in the movies than to know how many times characters fastened their seat belts. It is more valuable to know how much sexual activity there is in movies than to know how many times one character kissed another.

Some scholars argue strongly for the coding of latent content. For example, Krippendorff (1980, 2004) has consistently argued for a wider range of forms of content. Also, Merton (1991) said, "Content analysis is a method for inquiring into social reality that consists of inferring features of a nonmanifest context from features of a manifest text" (cited in Krippendorff, 2004, p. 25). In fact, Krippendorff has taken such a strong position on this matter that it appears that he believes there is no such thing as manifest content. To illustrate this, he has laid out a strong constructivist epistemology that is based on principles such as: "Texts have no objective—that is, no reader-independent qualities," "Texts have meanings relative to particular contexts, discourses, or purposes," and "The nature of text demands that content analysts draw specific inferences from a body of texts to their chosen context" (pp. 22–24). I agree with Krippendorf that content analysts must be more sensitive to the way coders construct meaning and that these constructions can differ significantly across coders. However, there are many types of content where coders do not significantly differ in their meaning construction, that is, the symbols in the texts are salient and those symbols trigger the same meaning construction across coders. Examples of such manifest content coding on television include whether a character is animated or live action, the gender of a character, whether there are words on the screen or not, whether the picture is color or black and white, to name a few.

All four quadrants of Figure 3.1 represent important areas for scholarship. Not all content is the same; there are differences in the degree to which symbols are salient and discrete. There are differences in the meaning of texts depending on how deeply they are analyzed and who does the analysis. A deeper analysis is not necessarily more valuable than a recording of symbols on the surface. It depends on the purpose of the analyst.

The central concern of this chapter is how designers of content analyses can make better decisions in creating coding rules, such that coders can consistently make good judgments. It seems that this is the least developed area in all of the writings about the content analysis method. It is perhaps ironic that it is so underdeveloped, because this is the font of reliability and validity. The lack of a good set of coding rules is a sign that the designers may lack a clear understanding of the purpose of their study. This ambiguity is passed along to the coders who amplify it in the form of inconsistent coding.

Constructing Coding Rules

Scholars writing about the content analysis method provide little guidance regarding the construction of sets of coding rules. Those who do write about it focus their efforts on defining different types of rules—but not what makes a good rule or set of rules. Moreover, most methodological scholarship regarding content analysis focuses only on the coding of manifest content. For example, Holsti (1969) suggests that manifest content can be studied with a quantitative method, but that latent content requires a qualitative method. He reminds designers of content analyses that the data generated must be valid, reliable, and reflect the investigator's research question—which is generic advice to a scholar designing any scientific study regardless of method.

Riffe, Lacy, and Fico (1998) observe that the "heart of content analysis is the content analysis protocol or codebook that explains how the variables in the study are to be measured and recorded" (p. 50). The key to the coding lies with what they call "context units" that they define as "the elements that cue researchers to the context that should be examined in assigning content to categories" (p. 61). In describing how a coder might infer socio-economic status (SES) when classifying characters appearing on television, they say that context units such as a character's dress, language skills, friends, and surroundings may be important elements. They argue that study designers need to provide coders with a list of these context units for each variable, but their example stops short of providing the calculus about how these context units are assembled in making an overall judgment of SES.

It is unrealistic to expect any study to provide detailed guidance to help analysts construct rules for every kind of latent content. The quality of the set of rules comes from the details, and they change from study to study. However, there needs to be more guidance than "do a qualitative analysis" or "let the coders make judgments." The remaining sections of this chapter seek to provide more clarity and advice about how researchers should construct coding rules such that a scientific content analysis can be designed and executed in all four quadrants of Figure 3.1. This effort begins by first considering the purpose for the coding rules.

Purpose of Coding Rules

The fundamental purpose of crafting coding rules is to achieve full specificity of the coding task. If the content analysis is to generate scientific data, the research study must be designed so that all coders are given sufficient direction such that coding decisions are made consistently across coders, across content, and across time. Consistency is the key to reliability, and reliability is one of the major components in achieving validity in the data. The key to achieving consistency lies in fully specifying the coding tasks.

A fully specified task is one where all the information that is needed to solve a problem is available to the person. For example, consider the following problem:

$$6 + 18 = \underline{\hspace{1cm}}$$

This task is fully specified, because a person has enough information to solve the problem.

Now consider this problem:

$$Y + Z = 24$$

This problem has two unknowns—Y and Z—so there is not enough information to arrive at one solution with confidence. One person could answer 6 and 18, while another might answer 10 and 14, and both would be right. There are also many other correct answers to this problem, because it is only partially specified. To most of us, each of these "answers" intuitively seems faulty. Because many answers are possible, can any one of them be regarded as "the solution?" Key information is missing from the problem that once included would help us all arrive at the one and only correct solution with confidence.

When we approach content analysis from a social science perspective, we do not want each coder to arrive at his/her own unique interpretation of the content, even if each coder's judgment is a reasonable and defensible one. Instead we want convergence; we need to provide enough rules so that all coders make the same decisions and all arrive at the same "solution" when encountering equivalent content. When a study's pilot test finds that the consistency in judgments across coders is low, a natural response is to assume the task is not yet fully specified and there is a need to construct more rules. However after constructing more rules and re-training the coders, the consistency might not increase; indeed, sometimes it decreases. There are several possible reasons why reliability may decrease when adding more depth and detail to coding rules. One is that the additional complexity puts too much of a burden on coders, so fatigue increases. Another is that a large rule set might serve to *over*-specify the task. That is, the greater number of rules raises an even greater number of sub-questions that are left unanswered. Yet a third reason is that coders may struggle with the dialectic between the rule set and their own intuitive understanding of the phenomenon they are asked to code.

It is possible for social scientists to approach full specification on most content analysis projects. However, the strategy to close the specification gap rests less with the number of rules and more with the type of rules that are constructed.

Types of Rules

A narrow conception of rules is most often employed in the design of content analysis studies, thinking of rules only as prescriptions. Prescriptive rules tightly channel coders into one system of decision-making that is largely external to their own natural ways of making decisions about meaning. By crafting prescriptive rules, the content analysts are moving the locus of meaning away from the individual coders and more into a system of rules. This is done in an effort to eliminate individual interpretations as much as possible. The belief is that individual interpretations involve error because they are variations from the "true judgment," which is the one accurate application of the rule. The more variation in judgments across coders, the more error and the lower the reliability coefficients. Under the prescriptive conception of rules, social scientists must tighten their rules so as to eliminate fluctuations across coders as much as possible. The goal is to train people to be interchangeable recording devices.

Two other conceptions of rules can be offered: rules as guides and rules as cues. Rules as guides are suggestions rather than prescriptions. They are based on the assumption that content analysis requires human interpretation and trusts that there is a relatively large degree of systematicity to human interpretation, that is, it is not purely idiosyncratic. If you give five people the same interpretation task, there will be considerable overlap in their interpretations; all five will not have radically different, mutually exclusive interpretations. Under this conception of a rule, there is some tolerance for individual differences in interpretations as long as there is fundamental agreement. Also, under this conception of rules, the designer of coding rules needs to be careful not to "over-rule" the task. There is a value to writing enough rules to provide clarity in guidance but not too many rules that may confuse coders. Designers must ask if the addition of a guidance rule has marginal utility, that is, if the addition of another rule and its subsequent addition in complexity will be paid back in terms of increases in coding agreement. If the answer is yes, the guidance rule has marginal utility and should be included. If the answer is no, then the increase in complexity would result in less, not greater coder agreement, and hence should not be added. There are projects that are so driven in their sincere quest to provide coders with enough guidance so they can be consistent in their coding that they end up being "over-ruled." By this I mean that beyond a certain point, the addition of coding rules drives the costs of the study beyond its benefits.

A third conception for a rule is as a cue. When constructing a cue rule, a designer must think about what coders already know, that is, what interpretive schemas they are already likely to possess. Designers must recognize which of those schemas are substantially shared, then write their rules as cues to activate those existing schemas. For example, recall the example above of $6 + 18 = \_\_$. This example fully specifies the problem by leaving only one unknown. However, one should not ignore what the solvers of the problem must bring to the task. Solvers of this problem must bring to it their mathematical schema in order to understand that "6" and "18" represent numbers with particular values and that the symbol "+" means addition. Even though the problem was constructed with only one unknown, the problem is not fully specified unless people come to it with a good mathematical schema. If people do not have this schema, the designers of the problem need to provide additional rules in order to fully specify the task; that is, they must train people in addition.

With content analysis projects, the designer of the study must ask: What schemas do people bring to the coding task? If this is not considered, it may at minimum make the design task much more difficult than it need be and at maximum result in writing large rule sets to try to overcome people's naturally occurring schema, thereby diminishing claims for the ecological validity of the results. When social scientists design a content analysis of latent content, they need to consider carefully what coders bring to the task.

Coding Decisions

Designers of content analysis need to carefully consider the characteristics of the content they are analyzing and their purpose when deciding what kinds of rules to construct. Some coding tasks lend themselves to prescriptive rules, while others do not. The question now is: How can one tell if a coding task lends itself to prescriptive rules? The answer lies in the characteristics of the content units, the content phenomenon, and the definition of the content elements.

Content Units

The units of analysis can be either natural or constructed. Naturally occurring units present symbols for boundaries within the content itself. For example, a newspaper story is a naturally occurring unit; it begins with a headline of larger font, then proceeds paragraph by paragraph, sometimes jumped to a subsequent page and ending with the last paragraph as indicated by a change in content (e.g., another headline, picture, end of page with no indication of a jump). Television programs, theatrical films, and songs on the radio are also examples of naturally occurring content units.

Some unitizing is done with grids—such as space or time—that are natural. For example, newspaper stories might be unitized by the column inch with each story divided into inches and each inch coded for the presence or absence of some content. Television shows and radio programs can be divided into 60-second units. Magazines can be divided by page.

There are times when a naturally occurring unit is not useful for a particular coding purpose, and the designer of the study must provide rules for coders to construct smaller units of content in their coding procedure. An example of this is typically found in studies that code for violence in television programs. In these studies, the television program is regarded as being too large a unit to be the focus of the entire analysis, so the researchers will construct smaller units, typically the scene. In this construction, researchers must provide clear rules to identify the beginning and ending of a relevant unit.

There are also times when a unit of analysis may at first appear as a naturally occurring unit but in the design of the content analysis, the researchers begin constructing rules to "clarify" the unitizing and end up with a highly constructed unit. An example of this is characters in films. At first consideration, character appears to be an easily recognized symbol and in some content analyses, it may simply be treated as a naturally occurring unit. But what if the researchers want to avoid including every single character appearing in a film? What if there is a restaurant scene; do the waiters get counted? The busboys? The receptionist? All the customers? What do you do if a character in a movie has three distinct personalities; is this one or three characters? What about inanimate objects as characters, such as HAL in *2001*? Once researchers start asking these kinds of questions, they journey down a very long and winding path that requires them to begin constructing a rather large set of complicated rules for what the unit is. In their everyday lives people can recognize characters in narratives, and they do not ask a long series of questions, because they are not usually interested in making fine discriminations. If designers of content analyses are interested in making such fine discriminations, they need to have a clear reason that resides in the purpose of their study. If they have a compelling reason, then they must ask the series of questions, make fine discriminations, and then construct a set of rules for coders. These rules are likely to be prescriptive in order to move coders away from their natural schema that identifies media characters for them in their everyday exposures.

Coding Variables

Once the content has been unitized, coders turn to the task of coding variables in the content. For example, if a study is interested in the sources used in news stories, it would have a variable called "news source."

Each coding variable has values. In the simplest case, a variable has only two values – presence or absence – of evidence of the variable's concept. In the example of the use of sources in news stories, these could be two values: 0 = no source mentioned in story; 1 = source acknowledged. A more ambitious approach would incorporate a variable called "type of news source" and this would require a longer list of values such as: 0 = no source mentioned in story; 1 = government official, 2 = spokesperson for a commercial business; 3 = spokesperson for a non-profit organization; 4 = private citizen.

The key to writing a good set of coding categories on a variable is that they be exhaustive, mutually exclusive, independent from one another, and be derived from a single classification principle (Budd, Thorp, & Donohew, 1967; Holsti, 1969). Methodologists are good at presenting guidance on how to achieve these characteristics of coding categories, but they are less forthcoming in addressing how to help coders make decisions about selecting among the categories when they must assign a code to a specific piece of content. Budd, Thorp, and Donohew (1967) say that designers of content analyses need to provide what they call "indicators" which are descriptions of the values on a coding variable. These indicators are like operational definitions of the values (Cartwright, 1953). Berelson (1952) calls these standards, because they are the criteria that coders use to make their decisions; that is, if a piece of content exhibits the characteristics to meet the standard as specified by a coding variable's value, the coder assigns that value to that piece of content.

Definition of Content Elements

An essential task in designing coding rules is to construct a clear definition of content elements. Consider definitions in a three-dimensional manner. One dimension is the "primitive to constructed" continuum. Primitive definitions are those with a high degree of common agreement. These are used constantly in everyday language and there is no need to define them. Once learned, people automatically use these primitive terms with confidence that others will understand their intended meaning. At the other end of this continuum is the constructed definition. These are the technical terms in theories, or the use of a common-looking term applied in a special manner. For example, most people recognize the term "reliability" and use it in everyday language to mean something like dependability. Content analysis researchers, however, have a special, technical meaning for this seemingly common term.

A second dimension about definitions is the simple to the complex. Complex definitions are of course much more difficult to communicate. Definitions vary in complexity not just in terms of the number of elements in the definition but also in the way the elements work together in defining the concept. For example, the following is a simple coding rule: Code X when Y appears in the content. A more complex rule is: Code X when Y or A or B appears in the content. A more complex rule is: Code X when Y or A or B but not C appears in the content. An even more complex rule is: Code X either if: (1) A and B appear together, (2) if A appears with Y—but not if A and B appear together without Z. This last rule is complex not only because of many elements and many conditions, but it also has some holes that require the coder to fill with his/her own judgment; that is, what should you do if A and B do appear together but not Y? Or more concretely, a rule for coding violence in movies might say: Code the scene as violent when one character physically harms another character. But this rule does not account for intentionality, so we could revise the rule to state: Code the scene as violent when one character intends to harm another character physically and carries out actions to do so, even if the target character is not actually physically harmed; also, code acts of God and accidents where a character is physically harmed even if there is no clear intention to harm that particular character. These progressions of making rules more elaborate are illustrations of how making a rule more complete to cover more conditions makes the rule more complex, but not necessarily more complete in terms of guidance to coders. And it certainly makes the coding more complex for coders.

The third dimension is the form of the definition. The best form can be labeled the "clear boundaries" definition. This is where the definition focuses on classification rules so clearly that a user of the definition knows when any specific example should be ruled in or ruled out as meeting the definition. A less useful, but often used form of defining content, is the process or component definition. The process definition focuses on steps in a process. Its weakness is that the definition does not also include classification rules for what constitutes inclusion in each step in the process. Thus if something exhibits all the steps in the process, it should be regarded as an example of that which is being defined in the process definition. However, what if content X exhibits four of the five steps (or components) presented in the definition? Clearly X mostly fits the definition but how much of the definition (if any) can one ignore and still conclude that X qualifies as meeting the coding rule? To illustrate, let's say a content analyst has defined "healthy behavior" as consisting of avoidance of illegal drugs, not smoking tobacco, exercising, and eating healthy meals. What if a character on a television series is never shown using illegal drugs and tobacco, regularly shown exercising, but never shown eating anything at all? Are these three characteristics enough for this character to get coded as exhibiting healthy behavior?

The least useful type of definition, used all too often, is the ostensive definition. This is when researchers construct their definitions through examples. With ostensive definitions, researchers expect coders to compare and contrast across those examples and infer the classification rules, instead of the researchers providing clear rules themselves. When coders see a pattern that all examples have in common, they infer an inclusion rule; when coders see a pattern that separates examples from non-examples, they infer an exclusion rule. This form of definition provides a concrete approach to acquainting coders to the essence of the content. This is how children learn the meanings of words. For example, parents point out examples of dogs and non-dogs and through this procedure of using examples, children learn to recognize dogs with great accuracy. This is a very successful way of teaching everyday language, but it lacks the precision necessary for scientific coding of content, and is generally a strategy to be avoided.

Achieving Scientific Credibility

In reading the conceptualizations and advice provided by content analysis methodologists over the years, one clear trend emerges. A strong premium is placed on achieving scientific credibility. When a study has scientific credibility it has greater believability and therefore typically enjoys increased prospects for enhancing public knowledge as well as informing policy. The findings are not merely one person's opinion.

Achieving scientific credibility requires demonstrating strong reliability and validity—characteristics that are directly traceable to the quality of coding rules. The greatest threat to these qualities is coder idiosyncrasies that lead one coder to categorize cases differently from another, typically because of differing interpretations of the message content under examination. In essence, designers of content analysis try to write rules that enable their coders to be micro-decision-makers rather than macro-judgment-makers. An interesting example of methodologists doing this comes from a study by Budd, Thorp, and Donohew (1967), who measured the "direction" of news stories. By direction, they mean whether the stories have a positive bias, negative bias, or are neutral or balanced in their coverage. Rather than have coders actually make this overall judgment about a story, they break the story down into content units and have the coders evaluate each content unit as negative or positive. Then they employ a quantitative formula to compute a coefficient of balance. They present this procedure as a highly scientific one that frees coders from making judgments about latent content – in this case news balance. But all they have really done is to remove the need for coder judgment at the aggregate level; coders still had to make judgments of negative–positive for each content unit. This is a typical example about how content analysts try to systematize coding by developing rules and quantitative formulas to help coders, but rather than eliminate the need for judgments, they drive the judgment-making process to a more detailed level. Coders still must make judgments; the need for coder judgment is not eliminated. The fundamental issues here are whether it is easier for coders to make judgments at the macro or micro level and at which level coders are able to exhibit a higher degree of agreement in their coding patterns.

The following section offers some guidance to help content analysts construct coding rules that can help increase the reliability and validity of the data by shifting coders away from broad-based judgment-making and toward more narrow, focused decision-making. Reducing the scope of the judgment offers many benefits, which should include an increased probability of inter-coder agreement.

Matching Type of Rules to Tasks

The potential for fully specifying the coding task with prescriptive rules is highest when coding units are naturally occurring, when the content phenomenon is manifest, and when the definition of coding categories is primitive and simple. The more the task elements deviate from these characteristics, the less potential there is for prescriptive rules to be successful in fully specifying the task. Gaps will remain, no matter how many rules are written and no matter how formally our procedures are explicated. Examples of content that would lend itself to prescriptive rules are things such as type of news (local, regional, national, international), genre of entertainment program, format of radio playlist, type of products advertised in internet pop-ups, body type of characters in films, and type of selling appeal in ads.

There are many content analysis projects that do not lend themselves well to the use of prescriptive rules. It can be argued that most content analysis of popular media fits in this category. For example, the analysis of violence in the media does not lend itself well to prescriptive rules. There are several major reasons for this. First, there are no natural units for violence. Second, violence as perceived by the public and people in the media industries is not a simple manifest act; instead its essence lies in narrative structures, which are a challenging form of latent content. Third, it is not possible to write a simple set of boundary conditions for a definition of violence; instead, people understand what violence is largely through examples. Their collective experience has resulted in a schema for violence. When we take people with such a schema and try to train them to code violence with a set of complex coding rules that ignore—and often contradict—their learned schema, it poses a very difficult training challenge that often results in failure to get all coders to follow the complex set of rules consistently. Hence reliability coefficients are likely to be suppressed.

Violence is only one example; there are many others, such as sex, character attractiveness, and affluence, among others. But the problem of the low utility of prescriptive rules does not automatically prevent us from developing fully specified designs for the coding of such content. Instead of trying to write more and better prescriptive rules, researchers should consider changing focus to a different kind of rule. As an example to illustrate this, consider the idea of a sexy kiss. If we were committed to using prescriptive type of rules we would have to write all kinds of rules about who is the kisser and who is the kissee; the relationship between the two people; what part of the body is kissed; and why? Does length of kiss matter? Is it more sexy if the lips are open? If so, open how much? In considering questions such as these, it seems that we are trying to capture an overwhelming and probably unnecessary level of micro-detail. However, it is likely that people have a well developed and shared schema for what constitutes a sexy kiss. While no one may be able to define it using elaborate written rules, most would be likely to achieve high reliability in identifying it as a coding task. As a designer of a content analysis of sexy kissing, would it not be far easier to write a simple rule to cue the schema? Such a rule would make the coding task far easier for coders and likely result in high reliability. Moreover, the subsequent reporting of the findings would have high ecological validity for readers.

Avoiding a Critical Trap

In content analysis, as with any scientific study, high value is placed on the characteristics of reliability and validity. Reliability refers to the degree to which coders consistently agree in their coding decisions. Validity refers to the degree that coders are capturing the meaning in the content accurately in their coding decisions. Both are important, and the goal of designers of scientific content analysis is to maximize both reliability and validity.

There is, however, a trap along the path to maximizing both reliability and validity. This trap lies much more in the coding of latent content than in the coding of manifest content. To illustrate, designers who are faced with low reliability in a pilot test are inclined to regard the low reliability as being due to the more difficult coding decisions where coders facing the same content are coding it differently. The normal response to this is for the study designers to write more coding rules to help their coders all converge to the same decisions. Sometimes this works, and the reliability increases. But there are times when this does not work, especially when coders must make a judgment about a pattern for which there is no simple set of rules to fully specify the coding problem. In this case, the creation of more coding rules makes the coding decision more complex without making it more consistent across coders. The additional rules may confuse or fatigue some coders who try to work around the rules. Other coders who really get into the additional rules want more precision and they experience the perimeter problem. The additional rules are creating divergence rather than convergence. This divergence also impacts the validity because as reliability is reduced, so necessarily is validity. But even more profoundly, validity can go down with the addition of more coding rules, because the additional rules further remove the coding decision from the way people perceive the content in their everyday lives. This is the issue with ecological validity. If the content analysis is a purely technical one where the audience for the research is only highly trained researchers, then the issue of ecological validity is not very important. However, if the content analysts see as their audience policy-makers or the public, then it is important that their findings be grounded in definitions of forms of content that resonate with people's everyday definitions of those content forms. When designers of content analyses add more rules and conditions as guidance for the coding, they are removing the decision-making procedure from everyday experience and this directly impacts the ecological validity.

Conclusion

If one is committed to designing projects using only prescriptive rule sets, then it is best to select projects where the units are naturally occurring, where the content phenomenon is manifest, and where the definition is primitive, simple, and clearly specifies classification rules. However, most of the interesting content analysis projects do not fit this profile. So what to do? Should researchers try to translate complex profile projects into a more simple design? I would argue no, because that would violate the content we are trying to capture in the more complex profiles. Then we are left with the challenge of dealing with partially specified problems, and this seems to be a challenging path to travel.

Are researchers doomed to constructing large, complex sets of prescriptive rules in order to fully specify most coding tasks? Again, my answer is no, if one is willing to consider other types of rules, such as guidance rules and cue rules. However, these latter two types of rules present their own considerable risks. Before constructing content analysis using these other types of rules, one needs to think carefully about what experiences and perspectives coders bring to the task, and how content characteristics shape the challenges faced by coders.

It is likely that people have a considerable number of shared schemas that can be tapped by designers of content analysis. Think about how formulaic most of the media content is and how much familiarity people in our culture have accumulated as they age. The key argument of this chapter is that researchers should trust that these shared schemas exist, and rely upon them when devising coding designs. By doing so, designers of content analysis projects will be able to create simpler coding schemes, achieve high reliability among coders, and generate data with strong ecological validity.

References

Berelson, B. (1952). *Content analysis in communication research.* New York: Free Press.

Budd, R. W., Thorp, R. K., & Donohew, L. (1967). *Content analysis of communications.* New York: Macmillan.

Cartwright, D. P. (1953). Analysis of qualitative material. In L. Festinger & D. Katz (Eds.), *Research methods in the behavioral sciences.* New York: Holt, Rinehart and Winston.

Danielson, W. (1963). Content analysis in communication research. In R. O. Nafzinger & D. M. White (Eds.), *Introduction to mass communications research.* Baton Rouge, LA: Louisiana State University Press.

Holsti, O. R. (1969). *Content analysis for the social sciences and humanities.* Reading, MA: Addison-Wesley.

Janis, I. L. (1949). The problem of validating content analysis. In H. D. Lasswell, N. Leites, R. Fadner, J. M. Goldsen, A. Gray, I. L. Janis, A. Kaplan, D. Kaplan, A. Mintz, I de S. Pool, & S. Yakobson (Eds.), *The language of politics: Studies in quantitative semantics* (pp. 55–82). New York: George Stewart.

Kaplan, A. (1943). Content analysis and the theory of signs. *Philosophy of Science, 10,* 230–247.

Kerlinger, F. N. (1973). *Foundations of behavioral research* (2nd ed.). New York: Holt, Rinehart and Winston.

Krippendorff, K. (1980). *Content analysis: An introduction to its methodology.* Beverly Hills, CA: Sage Publications.

Krippendorff, K. (2004). *Content analysis: An introduction to its methodology* (2nd ed.). Thousand Oaks, CA: Sage.

Merton, K. (1991). *Inhaltsanalyse: Eine Einführung in Theorie, Methode und Praxis.* Opladen, Germany: Westdeutscher Verlag.

Osgood, C. E. (1959). The representational model and relevant research methods. In I. De S. Pool (Ed.), *Trends in content analysis* (pp. 33–88). Urbana: University of Illinois Press.

Riffe, D., & Freitag, A. (1996, August). Twenty-five years of content analyses in *Journalism & Mass Communication Quarterly.* Paper presented to the annual convention of the Association for Education in Journalism and Mass Communication, Anaheim, CA.

Riffe, D., Lacy, S., & Fico, F. G. (1998). *Analyzing media messages: Using quantitative content analysis in research.* Mahwah, NJ: Erlbaum.

Shoemaker, P. J., & Reese, S. D. (1990). Exposure to what? Integrating media content and effects studies. *Journalism Quarterly, 67,* 649–652.

Stempel, G. H. III. (1981). Content analysis. In G. H. Stempel III & B. H. Westley (Eds.), *Research methods in mass communication* (pp. 119–131). Englewood Cliffs, NJ: Prentice-Hall.

4   Sampling and Content Analysis

An Overview of the Issues

Amy B. Jordan and Jennifer Manganello

One of the first decisions facing content analysis researchers is to determine the most appropriate strategy for sampling media messages. This can be a daunting task, as the cultural environment offers an almost boundless universe of media titles and infinite ways of parsing the content. In this chapter, we consider two distinct ways in which samples can be constructed. Specifically, decision-making about sampling is of critical importance, and often reflects the compromise that the content analyst makes between what is *available* within the media landscape and what is *consumed* by the audience(s) of interest. A health communication researcher interested in magazine articles that focus on diet and exercise as part of a healthy lifestyle will find, in the universe of magazines, hundreds of titles from which to sample (from *Ebony* to *Men's Health*, to *CosmoGirl!*, to *The Economist*). Depending on the objectives of the research and the theoretical underpinnings of the presumed effects, the researcher may want a sub-sample of titles—for example, those magazines that are most likely to be consumed by a segment of magazine readers (for example, adolescent girls or adults at risk for cancer)—in order to narrow his frame.

Capturing messages that are relevant to public health may be particularly challenging for those who wish to sample across the landscape of messages that are "out there" and to which audiences may be "exposed." Public health messages are embedded in entertainment narratives (for example, Russell Crowe's portrayal of a tobacco company whistleblower in *The Insider*). They appear in government-sponsored public service campaigns (such as the White House Office of National Drug Control Policy's *Parents: The Anti-Drug*). They may be subtle cues in a character's behavior (for example, *Sex and the City*'s Carrie Bradshaw, portrayed as a writer who smokes and then struggles to quit). Or they may be explicit information in news media about risks of excessive sun exposure and skin cancer (e.g., Stryker, Wray, Hornik, & Yanovitsky, 2005). For each public health concern the content analyst wishes to address, decisions must be made about which medium (or media) to examine, which genre (or genres) to include, how large the sample can reasonably be, and what temporal period should be sampled. With either approach—sampling what is available vs. sampling what is consumed— researchers are challenged to create samples that are generalizable to the population of interest even as they struggle to ensure that their sample is a valid reflection of the audiences' experiences with media content in their day-to-day lives.

Consider, for example, the researcher who is interested in "junk food" marketing to children. She determines that her sampling frame is "children's television shows" and sets about recording the programs airing in her market on commercial broadcast and cable television during the fall semester of her academic year. It takes some time to identify all of the programs, and by the time she has prepared a sampling frame, it is nearly the end of October. She proceeds with recording a random sample based on this frame over the next two months. After analyzing all the ads on the programs, she determines that toy ads outnumber junk food ads by a ratio of two to one.

Though this researcher was careful to construct a comprehensive list of children's programs and to randomly sample from that list, the mere fact that she recorded them during prime holiday toy-hawking season calls into question the extent to which her sample is reflective of what children see over the course of a year. Using the non-program advertising breaks will necessarily preclude her ability to assess junk food products that may be shown during the show. Even the decision to sample only shows specifically designed for children limits what she can say about the "junk food" ads children see in the larger television landscape, as children watch general audience programs like *American Idol* as much as if not more than they watch children's shows.

This hypothetical example illustrates the challenges of stepping into a steadily flowing stream of media messages, where potential threats to validity and generalizability lurk around every corner. We make this point not to discourage the use of content analysis methodology, but rather to encourage researchers to consider the implications of their sampling decisions for the data patterns they ultimately observe. In this chapter we explore the variety of approaches researchers have taken to sampling, particularly as it relates to public health, and explore the strengths and weaknesses of these approaches. We contrast approaches to sampling "what's available" with sampling "what's consumed," and we provide examples from content analyses of public health as illustrations. Ultimately, we do not argue for a "gold standard" that might dictate how researchers should select their sample. Rather, we encourage the research community to devote more resources to formative and basic research to inform sampling decisions and to offer greater explication of the sampling decision-making process.

Sampling

Sampling is the process of selecting a sub-set of units for study from a larger population (Neuendorf, 2001). By definition, therefore, one must make decisions about this process of selection. Generally this involves determining how best to winnow to a manageable proportion a sample of the population in a way that it remains valid and representative of what is *available* in the media landscape and/or what is *consumed* by audiences of interest. The size of a media sample is often determined by resources available to the research project (e.g., budget, time, number of coders). In addition, our sampling decisions reflect the theoretical framework of the study, the conceptualization of audience exposure to message, and the extent to which one wishes to generalize findings. (Later in the chapter we argue that researchers should also be making evidence-based decisions about samples. For example, researchers have recently looked at sample size with an interest in being able to report standard error and confidence interval [Stryker et al., 2006].)

For most media-based content analyses, it is neither feasible nor efficacious to attempt to code an entire population (i.e., a census). The enormous amount of media available to audiences today means that it is frequently impossible to analyze every item, regardless of the medium.

Social science convention dictates that probability (random) sampling, wherein each unit has an equal chance of selection, offers the firmest ground on which the content analyst can say that his or her data are generalizable to a broader population (Stryker et al., 2006). Random sampling may include *simple* or *systematic* sampling, or may involve attempts to gain an accurate *representation* of the different types of media content available. Alternatively, researchers may want to use a stratified sampling procedure to cull a media sample that reflects the *proportion* with which a particular type of genre appears in the greater population. For instance, if a researcher knew that 25% of all movies for one year were comedies, he/she would ensure that 25% of the sample consisted of this genre. Though probability samples allow for greater statistical inferences, content analyses will most often rest on non-probability sampling procedures. Purposive or convenience samples include media titles that are specifically selected on the basis of a particular attribute. Riffe and Freitag (1997) examined all content analysis articles appearing in *Journalism & Mass Communication Quarterly* from 1971 through 1995 and found that more than two thirds used purposive sampling (a sub-set of the population as defined by the researcher; for instance, the top grossing movies), while about 10% used convenience sampling (a set of easy to access materials) and 22% used "census" sampling (all possible units are included in the analysis). From this research, one can deduce that the sampling of what is consumed is more common than using a census or randomly selecting items based on what is available.

Researchers sometimes find it necessary to create a sub-sample or a set of sub-samples of media titles. A study might use a sample of magazines from the population of all magazines published using a purposive sampling procedure to select only the most popular ones. However, once this sampling frame is created, it is neither feasible nor always relevant to examine every issue of the magazines in the sample. A sub-sample is drawn (using random sampling or some other sampling method) to create a body of articles for inclusion in the analysis (see, for example, Andsager & Powers, 1999). Indeed, multistage sampling in content analysis research is a common procedure (Riffe, Lacy, & Fico, 1998).

Generating a Sample Frame

Ideally, one will sample from the universe of media by creating lists of all available media (or media titles that have the content of interest) during a particular time frame. This has been possible with video games (e.g., Beasley & Standley, 2002; Thompson & Haninger, 2001), movies (e.g., Goldstein, Sobel, & Newman, 1999; Pearson, Curtis, Haney, & Zhang, 2003), broadcaster websites (e.g., Chan-Olmsted & Park, 2000; Potter, 2002), and TV advertisements (Media Information Services, 2007). In the latter example, researchers obtained a list of all TV ads appearing during a specified time period from Advertising Information Services (now known as Media Information Services).

Typically, however, the vast number of media products available precludes researchers' ability to create a census list. Indeed, in some cases, a sampling frame is not necessarily the equivalent of a clearly articulated population. As Riffe et al. (1998) point out, a sampling frame may not even be known ahead of time. Moreover, Stryker and colleagues (2006) write that one of the limitations of using a database such as LexisNexis to identify articles containing cancer-related information is the fact that print publications have been forced to choose between removing electronic traces of articles by freelancers, or to pay royalties to those freelancers. According to Stryker, many have chosen to remove those freelance articles (p. 424). In order to prospectively randomly sample television episodes from a season, moreover, the total number of episodes for the season would need to be known in advance (Manganello, Franzini, & Jordan, 2008). This information typically is not available until the season has concluded.

Options for Sampling Media Content

Sampling Based on What's Available

As the number of media platforms and media titles proliferate, so too have the challenges facing researchers who seek to describe the public health-related messages that are available to audiences. Indeed, the vehicles through which mediated messages are delivered have changed so dramatically that it is often difficult to draw even the contours of the media landscape. One might argue a distinction between "scheduled" media and "interactive" media. For example, television offers audiences a schedule of programming from which to choose, and this schedule can be used to define the sampling frame from which to draw programs. Alternatively, films are released in theatres and also made available through DVD rental services and through cable systems that hold vast libraries of movie titles. Though researchers continue to make these distinctions, revolutions in the way television is offered may force us to reconsider media-determined vs. audience-determined media titles. Network television shows, once only available on certain channels during certain times, can now be purchased, rented, or viewed online.

Sampling Based on Composite Time Periods

Despite this revolution, one often-used approach to sampling scheduled programming is the creation of a "composite" sample. Several major studies of television content have used a *composite week* to comprise a sample (Kunkel et al., 2003; National Television Violence Study [NTVS], 1998; Wallack, Grube, Madden, & Breed, 1990). This typically involves creating a temporal grid and filling in the time periods of interest (e.g., the prime-time hours for all major television networks) with programs that air during those times. The programs are sampled over the course of several weeks or months until all time blocks are filled in for all of the days of the week and the channels of the sample. In addition to television programming, composite week samples have also been used for newspaper content analysis (Riffe, Aust, & Lacy, 1993) and television advertising research (Larson, 2001; Wallack & Dorfman, 1992).

The use of a "composite week" that addresses temporal variations may improve the generalizability of a given study (Kunkel et al., 2003). For example, sampling an entire issue of the *Philadelphia Inquirer* on a day in which an inordinate number of articles are focused on the Philadelphia Phillies making the playoffs for the World Series in baseball might be misleading, since this is a highly unusual event for the city. In addition, by not sampling "intact" units one can create a more valid picture of the unit that is the focus of the study (i.e., the television program, or the newspaper story). However, even studies using composite week sampling may leave out key viewing hours (if, for example, they are limited to prime time) or programs (if, for example, the TV market under study has different syndicated programming schedules).

Sampling Based on Search Engines

Researchers sometimes examine relevant units in media by searching with specific key words. This has been done with text-based media, including: magazines (e.g., Hust & Andsager, 2003), websites (Hong & Cody, 2002; or Ribisl, Lee, Henriksen, & Haladjian, 2003), and newspapers (Stryker et al., 2006). It might also be done with analyses of audio-visual media, particularly if the researchers can use plot summaries to direct the search, as Comstock and Scharrer (2007) did in their analysis of the of popular movies and television shows.

Stryker et al. (2006) looked at newspaper coverage of cancer information by using a LexisNexis search for the year 2003. By developing a creative and rigorous process for testing the reliability and validity of the search terms they used, they were able to highlight the opportunities and limitations of using search engines for sampling. Their review of content analysis articles published in communication journals from 2000–5 found that almost half (43%) sampled from databases yet only one third of these studies even revealed search term(s) used (and almost none articulated how they had arrived at their term(s)).

Sampling Based on What's Consumed

As Kunkel writes in Chapter 2 in this volume, content analyses are carried out on the assumption that exposure to media messages affects audiences. With this assumption in mind, researchers may seek out media content that is more likely to reach a broad audience (and hypothetically reflect or shape the larger culture or broader swaths of an audience) or is more likely to reach an audience of particular interest (which may be uniquely vulnerable to the messages under analysis).

Sampling Based on Popularity

Content analysts may decide to use publicly available audience research data, such as that provided by Nielsen or Billboard, to construct a sample from what ratings companies indicate are most frequently watched, read, played or used by audiences—in other words, that which is most popular with the audience of interest (see, for example, Ward, 1995; Collins and colleagues, Chapter 10 in this volume). Purposive samples drawn from ratings data might include media titles used by the entire US population, or can focus on specific sub-groups of audiences (such as African Americans or teens). This approach has been used to select samples for studies involving television (e.g., Franzini, 2003; Greenberg & Smith, 2002; Ward, 1995), movies (e.g., Bufkin & Eschholz, 2000; Hedley, 2002; Pardun, 2002; Stockwell & Glantz, 1997), magazines (e.g., Signorielli, 1997; Tulsyan, Brill, & Rosenfeld, 2002), music (e.g., Gentile, 1999; Roberts, Henrikson, & Christenson, 1999), and video games (e.g., Dietz, 1998; Smith, Lachlan, & Tamborini, 2003).

While examining the most popular media is a common sampling method, it can be difficult to obtain information regarding certain media or certain audiences. This is especially true if one is interested in media and audiences for whom ratings data are not generally available. In the case of movies, for example, lists of the top grossing films or most often rented DVDs are easy to access, but data reflecting favorites among specific age and/or racial groups may need to be purchased from marketing firms at a cost that is prohibitive to academic researchers. Similarly, data on website traffic are not easily accessed, particularly since internet users are so idiosyncratic.

Sampling Based on Survey Data

Analysis of content may be driven by researchers' interest in how the media (and the messages contained therein) are used by a *specific* audience, often because the researcher is interested in how the media influences an identified behavioral outcome. For this purpose, a content analysis would not be conducted on an entire population of media, or even on media titles based on national ratings data, but rather on that sub-sample of content used by individuals with a particular demographic profile. Such studies may approach the construction of a sampling frame by asking participants to report what media they most commonly use, and then developing samples from the participants' reports (see Sorsoli, Ward, & Tolman, Chapter 9 in this volume).

One challenge in this approach is the ability of respondents to recall and report their media use accurately. Both memory and social desirability may impact the reporting by study participants, and adequate pretesting, such as test-retest reliability checks, are important (see, for example, Sargent et al., 2005). Another challenge lies in the respondents' shared definition of media and media use. For instance, one might ask teens about their favorite "television" shows, but, as Ramasubramanian and Martin (Chapter 7 in this volume) point out, a television series may be viewed on an iPod, a computer, a DVD player, or even a cell phone.

Creating Sub-samples from Samples

Numerous studies have employed some combination of probability and nonprobability sampling techniques to look at particular content, audiences, or historical time periods. In a study examining women and smoking, for example, researchers selected 10 top movie actresses and randomly selected five movies in which each actress had played a main role (Escamilla, Cradock, & Kawachi, 2000). In another, the amount and context of television violence was examined based on a sample of prime-time dramas airing in a one-week period but across different years (Signorielli, 2003; Signorielli & Bacue, 1999). The content analysis described by Murphy, Wilkin, & Cody in Chapter 11 (this volume) is concerned with the inclusion of health content on TV. In this study, the researchers sampled the top five shows for the general population, African Americans, and Hispanics. In addition, they selected shows that they believed were likely to have health content.

A Critical Decision: Depth vs. Breadth

Regardless of the approach one takes to constructing a sampling frame, content analysis researchers must always be concerned about whether the sample is representative of the population and a valid portrait of what media are available and what audiences consume. Consider a hypothetical study in which a researcher is interested in newspaper coverage of the "obesity epidemic" in the U.S. The researcher uses a search engine to examine *New York Times* articles over a two-year period that mention "obesity." The search engine comes up with 100 articles and the researcher randomly selects 50% of them to content analyze. He draws conclusions about newspapers' framing of the problem based on the 50 articles that make up his sample. While the sample may be representative of how the *New York Times* covers the issue, it says very little about how "newspapers" cover obesity. To be able to make this argument, the researcher would need to create a sampling frame in which national and regional newspapers are included. That is not to say the study is useless—it is important in terms of coverage of the topic by an "opinion leader" and it spotlights potential effects of the coverage on policy-makers or *New York Times* readers. However, the content analyst must be careful not to overgeneralize or to extend his conclusions beyond the findings of the analysis.

A similar issue lies in whether it is more useful (or valid) to obtain a fuller picture of a smaller number of media that are presumably more influential due to their broad audience reach. Studies that focus on a single medium—for example, television—allow resources to be concentrated on developing measures that offer a deeper assessment of the object of study. By focusing on all episodes in a season of a limited number of teen-oriented television dramas, Franzini (2003) offered a portrait of the development of characters' romantic relationships over the course of a season in order to contextualize sexual content portrayals. Sampling from all TV shows or randomly selecting a limited number of episodes from the series would have precluded this analysis.

The decision to focus on depth over breadth, however, means that the content analysis cannot account for the multiple messages audiences receive from different media on the same subject. In the hypothetical *New York Times* study of obesity coverage, the researcher might have decided to include more local newspapers in his sample, or to add television news coverage of the topic to broaden his sampling frame. But if the researcher achieves greater breadth—for example, by including multiple media—it is not clear that all media messages would have equal weight for the audiences that ultimately receive them. Determining this would be predicated on the theoretical foundation of the study and the researcher's hypothesized mechanisms for how content might have an effect. As Manganello and Fishbein point out in Chapter 1 of this volume, even within a medium, some theoretical frames suggest that audiences have greater affinity to one kind of program— for example, a popular program with teen characters with whom the audience identifies—suggesting that messages from these programs should receive greater weight.

Accounting for the Nature of the Medium

The form of a medium plays a critical role in many sampling decisions. Traditional media, such as magazines or movies, may make it easier to generate a sampling frame because all users receive the same static content. Static content may be simply captured and easily shared among coders. In contrast, newer media, including video games and websites, offer interactive or fluid content. With fluid content, media messages are determined by the individual user (for example, depending on the skill of the gamer or the click-throughs of the web-surfer). Of all of the media types, it is perhaps the internet that poses some of the most significant challenges. Even though researchers have been conducting content analyses of websites for over a decade, "there is currently no standardized method of sampling content featured on the World Wide Web" (Ribisl et al., 2003, p. 66). Mitra and Cohen (1999) also discuss the challenges in examining text on the internet, suggesting that there is no specific "beginning" and "end." The interactive nature makes it difficult to capture with confidence the messages that a typical user (if such a person exists) would encounter (Livingstone, 2003).

Determining an adequate sampling frame can be extremely difficult, especially as the number of websites is continuously increasing and the landscape is ever-changing (Riffe et al., 1998; Stempel & Stewart, 2000). Even using search terms to identify relevant sites is problematic, as each search engine uses different procedures for identifying websites (Martin-Facklam et al., 2002). Although a researcher may decide to examine only websites that are commonly used by study participants, the fact that website content is constantly updated may affect what people see when they visit websites, which of course impacts what researchers can capture. In addition, there is often unintentional exposure to various websites, either through spam or links. A web user may be exposed to certain material, even though he or she did not visit a particular website—something which traditional content analysis cannot capture. A web user may not even be able to report the URL (web address) that s/he visits, particularly since many users get to sites through search engines such as Google.

Beyond the challenges researchers face building samples from the web, the changing platforms of media make it difficult to know how users may be accessing media content. In the case of music, researchers must decide whether to sample from a radio station, a CD, a music video, or some combination of music platforms. Their choices have implications for their data too. Music on the radio may be "cleaner" than music on CDs, since the Federal Communications Commission fines broadcasters for the use of profanity or indecent language (www.fcc.gov). Music videos may add a layer of visual codes that appear to add to the sexual content of the same lyrics presented in audio-only formats. In addition, audience members who watch a movie on DVD will have more than the movie itself available to view, since DVDs provide additional content such as out-takes and "previously unseen" footage. Finally, even within a medium, a television series may be presented with different levels of graphic content depending on the type of television channel on which it airs. A researcher interested in the analyzing the program *Sex and the City* may include the sexier version originally shown on HBO or the tamer version aired in reruns on a different network.

Accounting for Fluctuations in Media

Media content can change quickly, making it imperative to pay attention to potential temporal fluctuations. The top music videos change on a weekly basis and top songs change fairly quickly as well. Although the list of the most popular magazines may be more stable over time, the content of individual issues of magazines may fluctuate by month or season. Larry and Grabe (2005), Johnston and Swanson (2003), and Walsh-Childers, Gotthoffer, and Lepre (2002) selected the most popular magazines and then sampled across seasons. Other researchers have sampled popular magazines in specific years or groups of years to look at trends over time (Garner, Sterk, & Adams, 1998; Walsh-Childers et al., 2002). Even the collection of a sample of television programs can prove problematic. Networks may use more provocative content to draw greater ratings during premiere weeks (Manganello et al., 2008). And blockbuster movies, which may have distinct content aimed at demographically defined audiences, tend to be released to coincide with summer and holiday vacations.

The Necessity of Formative Research in Content Analysis

Very few studies make decisions about sampling through formative research. No serious researcher would present results for a content analytic variable without reliability testing, yet few people have tested the superiority of one sampling approach over another before embarking on the creation of a sample for a particular study. In developing a sampling strategy for an analysis of sexual content in teen media, we set out to test various sampling strategies. In particular, we were interested in assessing the validity of the standard practice of using three randomly selected episodes to assess a season's worth of content (see, for example, Jordan, 1996). Using the program *Friends, season 9* as a test case, we trained coders to assess the amount and types of sexual behaviors in each episode of the series. The content categories used were based on Kunkel's widely used categories (Kunkel et al., 2003), which included indicators ranging from flirting and passionate kissing to intercourse. Each of the 23 episodes was coded for amount and type of sexual behavior, producing an assessment of the series as a whole and assessment of each individual episode. We also looked at data collected on the same program (*Friends, season 9*) and other programs by another researcher (Franzini, 2003) who focused on characters' sexual activity across the season (see Franzini, 2003). We looked at different sampling strategies separately for each dataset by drawing 50 random samples for each of the following methods: random sample (episodes 1, 3, 5 and 7) and specific episodes (premiere, finale, sweeps, and fifth episode). Analyses revealed that in the realm of sexual behavior, three randomly selected episodes are reliable indicators of the overall series' content of sexual behavior (five for variables with greater variation). However, to reliably assess a character's level of sexual activity, seven random episodes are needed (Manganello et al., 2008).

Formative research is also necessary to determine the number of media items needed to accurately assess sampling error and achieve a 95% confidence interval in probability sampling. Stryker et al. (2006) present a methodological study of approaches to validating search terms when sampling electronic databases. A critical first step, they argue, is to determine the extent to which search terms lead to a satisfactory level of recall ("recall" meaning the precision with which the search terms pull up the right stories for the analysis). They argued the yield of relevant stories generated should be about 93%. Predicting the yield will determine the number of articles that should be randomly selected from a computer database (they used LexisNexis) in order to set a confidence interval at 95% (plus or minus 5%). Their formative research found that one out of every 3.4 stories was relevant to cancer information. Having set their recall at .93, and their confidence interval at 95%, they knew they needed 225 relevant stories in their sample. This meant they needed to retrieve 765 (3.4 × 225) stories for the validation process.

Formative research such as that described here is time-consuming and expensive, but it is necessary for the advancement of the science of content analysis. Budgets must include time and dollars to develop and test sampling approaches, much as budgets accommodate pre-testing and piloting of instruments for human subjects research.

Conclusion

Our review highlights the numerous strategies that have been used to create samples for content analysis. The structure of this chapter is based on a heuristic approach that suggests that the content analyst may decide to sample the media content that is *available to* audiences or sample the media content that is *consumed by* audiences (one might consider this to be the distinction between "what's on" and "what's watched"). Clearly, media samples should aim to be both reliable and valid indicators of the media content that exists in the culture and to which audiences are exposed and we should base some element of sampling decisions on these considerations. More often than not, however, we neglect to clearly articulate the theoretical and conceptual under-pinnings of our sampling decisions. In addition, it is critical to consider how the sampling frame or the sample itself may contribute to the patterns of observed data.

Our review of sampling approaches highlights the need for the development of a base of empirical data that can inform the methodology. Additional studies content analyzing a large (all movies released in one year) or set number of units (all episodes of a television season), and then testing different sampling strategies, will provide valuable information for future research. Such studies must also be undertaken for various topics in public health. What may work for sexual behavior on television may be very different from the best strategy for analyzing substance use or physical activity.

Although we may develop recommendations for sampling procedures that increase validity and generalizability and decrease bias, we must not forget that sampling decisions must always be tied to the goals of the research as informed by theory (see Manganello & Fishbein, Chapter 1 in this volume). Sampling for content should also reflect a conviction that media content is the precursor to media effect (see Kunkel, Chapter 2 in this volume). For example, if a researcher seeks to gain information about female characters in video games, she might use a simple random sample of a census of video games available on the market. However, if the goal of a study is to look at teenage girls' exposure to images of females in video games—and hypothesize links between exposure and attitudinal or behavioral outcomes—it makes more sense to design a purposive sample of the video games that teenage girls play most often.

In conclusion, we would like to emphasize that there are no "right" or "wrong" sampling strategies. Instead researchers should consider their sample from various angles, and be sure they are using the "best" sample for their study. Additional formative research and dissemination of such findings will provide researchers with information to help guide such decisions.

References

Andsager, J. L., & Powers, A. (1999). Social or economic concerns: How news and women's magazines framed breast cancer in the 1990s. *Journalism & Mass Communication Quarterly, 76*(3), 531–550.

Beasley, B., & Standley, T. C. (2002). Shirts vs. skins: Clothing as an indicator of gender role stereotyping in video games. *Mass Communication & Society, 5*(3), 279–293.

Bufkin, J., & Eschholz, S. (2000). Images of sex and rape: A content analysis of popular film. *Violence Against Women, 6*(12), 1317–1344.

Chan-Olmsted, S. M., & Park, J. S. (2000). From on-air to online world: Examining the content and structure of broadcast TV stations' web sites. *Journalism & Mass Communication Quarterly, 77*(2), 321–339.

Comstock, G. & Scharrer, E. (2007). *Media and the American Child.* San Diego, CA: Academic Press.

Dietz, T. L. 1998. An examination of violence and gender role portrayals in video games: Implications for gender socialization and aggressive behavior. *Sex Roles, 38*(5/6), 425–442.

Escamilla, G., Cradock, A. L., & Kawachi, I. (2000). Women and smoking in Hollywood movies: A content analysis. *American Journal of Public Health, 90*(3), 412–414.

Franzini, A. (2003). Sex on television programming popular among teens: Correlates and consequences. Unpublished dissertation, Temple University, Philadelphia, PA.

Garner, A., Sterk, H. M., & Adams, S. (1998). Narrative analysis of sexual etiquette in teenage magazines. *Journal of Communication, 48*(4), 59–78.

Gentile, D. (1999, July 15). *Teen-oriented radio and CD sexual content analysis.* National Institute on Media and the Family. Retrieved October 9, 2003, from http://www.mediafamily.org/research/report_radiocontentanalysis.pdf

Goldstein, A. O., Sobel, R. A., & Newman, G. R. (1999). Tobacco and alcohol use in G-rated children's animated films. *JAMA, 281*(12), 1131–1136.

Greenberg, B. S., & Smith, S. W. (2002). Daytime talk shows: Up close and in your face. In J. D. Brown, J. R. Steele, & K. Walsh-Childers (Eds.), *Sexual teens, sexual media* (pp. 79–93). Mahwah, NJ: Lawrence Erlbaum Associates.

Hedley, M. (2002). The geometry of gendered conflict in popular film: 1986-2000. *Sex Roles, 47*(5-6), 201–217.

Hong, T., & Cody, M. J. (2002). Presence of pro-tobacco messages on the web. *Journal of Health Communication, 7,* 273–307.

Hust, S. J., & Andsager, J. L. (2003). Medicalization vs. adaptive models? Sense-making in magazine framing of menopause. *Women & Health, 38*(1), 101–122.

Johnston, D. D., & Swanson, D. H. (2003). Invisible mothers: A content analysis of motherhood ideologies and myths in magazines. *Sex Roles, 49*(1/2), 21–33.

Jordan, A. (1996). *The state of children's television: An examination of quantity, quality and industry beliefs* (Report no. 2). Philadelphia: The Annenberg Public Policy Center of the University of Pennsylvania.

Kunkel, D., Biely, E., Eyal, K., Cope-Farrar, K., Donnerstein, E., & Fandrich, R. (2003, February). *Sex on TV 3*. Report to the Kaiser Family Foundation. Available at: http://www.kff.org/content/2003/20030204a/Sex_on_TV_3_Full.pdf

Larry, A., & Grabe, M. (2005). Media coverage of sexually transmitted infections: A comparison of popular men and women's magazines. *Journal of Magazine & New Media Research, 7*(2), 1–23.

Larson, M. S. (2001). Interactions, activities and gender in children's television commercials: A content analysis. *Journal of Broadcasting & Electronic Media, 45*(1), 41.

Livingstone, S. (2003). Children's use of the internet: Reflections on the emerging research agenda. *New Media & Society, 5*(2), 147–166.

Manganello, J., Franzini, A., & Jordan, A. (2008). Sampling television programs for content analysis of sex on TV: How many episodes are enough? *Journal of Sex Research, 45*(1), 9–16.

Martin-Facklam, M., Kostrzewa, M., Schubert, F., Gasse, C., & Haefeli, W. (2002). Quality markers of drug information on the internet: An evaluation of sites about St. John's wort. *American Journal of Medicine, 113*, 740–745.

Media Information Services. (2007). *A brief history*. Retrieved September 19, 2007, from http://web.misnyc.com/default.asp?flash=True&wm=True&width=1024

Mitra, A., & Cohen, E. (1999). Analyzing the web: Directions and challenges. In S. Jones (Ed.), *Doing internet research: Critical issues and methods for examining the net* (pp. 179–202). Thousand Oaks, CA: Sage Publications.

National Television Violence Study (NTVS). (1998, April). *National television violence study* (Vol. 3). Available at: http://www.ccsp.ucsb.edu/execsum.pdf

Neuendorf, K. A. (2001). *The content analysis guidebook*. Thousand Oaks, CA: Sage Publications.

Pardun, C. (2002). Romancing the script: Identifying the romantic agenda in top-grossing movies. In J. D. Brown, J. R. Steele, & K. Walsh-Childers (Eds.), *Sexual teens, sexual media* (pp. 211–225). Mahwah, NJ: Lawrence Erlbaum Associates.

Pearson, D. W., Curtis, R. L., Haney, C. A., & Zhang, J. J. (2003). Sport films: Social dimensions over time, 1930–1995. *Journal of Sport & Social Issues, 27*(2), 145–161.

Potter, R. F. (2002). Give the people what they want: A content analysis of FM radio station home pages. *Journal of Broadcasting & Electronic Media, 46*(3), 369–384.

Ribisl, K. M., Lee, R. E., Henriksen, L., & Haladjian, H. H. (2003). A content analysis of web sites: Promoting smoking culture and lifestyle. *Health Education and Behavior, 30*(1), 64–78.

Riffe, D., Aust, C. F., & Lacy, S. R. (1993). The effectiveness of random, consecutive day and constructed week sampling in newspaper content analysis. *Journalism & Mass Communication Quarterly, 70*(1), 133–139.

Riffe, D., & Freitag, A. (1997). A content analysis of content analyses: Twenty-five years of *Journalism Quarterly*. *Journalism & Mass Communication Quarterly, 74*(4), 873–882.

Riffe, D., Lacy, S., & Fico, F. G. (1998). *Analyzing media messages: Using quantitative content analysis in research*. Mahwah, NJ: Lawrence Erlbaum Associates.

Roberts, D. F., Henriksen, L., & Christenson, P. G. (1999, April). *Substance use in popular movies and music*. Report for Mediascope. Available at: http://www.mediascope.org/pubs/supmm.pdf

Sargent, J. D., Beach, M. L., Adachi-Mejia A. M., Gibson, J. J., Titus-Ernstoff, L. T., Carusi, C. P., Swain, S. D., Heatherton, T. F., Dalton, M. A. (2005). Exposure to movie smoking: Its relation to smoking initiation among US adolescents. *Pediatrics, 116*(5), 1183–1191.

Signorielli, N. (1997). *A content analysis: Reflections of girls in the media.* Report for the Kaiser Family Foundation. Available at: http://www.kff.org/content/archive/1260/gendr.html

Signorielli, N. (2003). Prime-time violence 1993–2001: Has the picture really changed? *Journal of Broadcasting & Electronic Media, 47*(1), 36–57.

Signorielli, N., & Bacue, A. (1999). Recognition and respect: A content analysis of prime-time television characters across three decades. *Sex Roles, 70*(7–8), 527–544.

Smith, S. L., Lachlan, K., & Tamborini, R. (2003). Popular video games: Quantifying the presentation of violence and its context. *Journal of Broadcasting & Electronic Media, 47*(1), 58–76.

Stempel, G., & Stewart, R. (2000). The internet provides both opportunities and challenges for mass communication researchers. *Journalism & Mass Communication Quarterly, 77*(3), 541–548.

Stockwell, T. F., & Glantz, S. A. (1997). Tobacco use is increasing in popular films. *Tobacco Control, 6*, 282–284.

Stryker, J. E., Wray, R., Hornik, R., & Yanovitzky, I. (2006). Database search terms for content analysis: The case of cancer news coverage. *Journalism & Mass Communication Quarterly, 8*(2), 413–430,

Thompson, K., & Haninger, K. (2001). Violence in E-rated video games. *JAMA, 286*(5), 591–598.

Tulsyan, V., Brill, S., & Rosenfeld, W. D. (2002). A content analysis: Dieting, exercise, and weight loss messages in teen magazines. Abstract appearing in *Journal of Adolescent Health, 30*(2), 123.

Wallack, L., & Dorfman, L. (1992). Health messages on television commercials. *American Journal of Health Promotion, 6*(3), 190–196.

Wallack, L., Grube, J. W., Madden, P. A., & Breed, W. (1990). Portrayals of alcohol on prime-time television. *Journal of Studies on Alcohol, 51*(5), 428–437.

Walsh-Childers, K., Gotthoffer, A., & Lepre, C. R. (2002). From "just the facts" to "downright salacious": Teens' and women's magazine coverage of sex and sexual health. In J. D. Brown, J. R. Steele, & K. Walsh-Childers (Eds.), *Sexual teens, sexual media* (pp. 153–171). Mahwah, NJ: Lawrence Erlbaum Associates.

Ward, L. M. (1995). Talking about sex: Common themes about sexuality in the prime-time television programs children and adolescents view most. *Journal of Youth and Adolescence, 24*(5), 595–615.

5   Reliability for Content Analysis

Kimberly A. Neuendorf

One of the critical standards in quantitative, scientific research is the reliability of measures. Most basically, reliability is the extent to which measurement error is absent from the data (Nunnally, 1978). A widely accepted definition of reliability is that of Carmines and Zeller (1979): the extent to which a measurement procedure yields the same results on repeated trials. This chapter considers a type of reliability known as inter-coder reliability, which is a central concern in most content analysis research utilizing human coders. Inter-coder reliability assesses the consistency among human raters involved in a content analysis of messages. For such human coding, reliability is paramount (Neuendorf, 2002). If a content analytic measure is dependent upon the skills of a particular individual, the investigation has not met the standards of scientific inquiry.

Many decisions are made with respect to reliability in content analysis. This chapter covers the most critical among them, including: the selection of sub-samples for reliability coding, the training of coders, the task of unitizing media content for coding purposes, and the selection of reliability coefficients. Each of these issues is assessed in terms of the decisions approach, in particular decisions that weigh rigor against expediency. Finally, because researchers' approaches to assessing and reporting reliability are often inconsistent, this chapter concludes with recommendations for standards that researchers should use as they grapple with best practices for reliability in content analysis studies.

Rigor Versus Expediency: Overall Thematics for a Decisions Approach

It is hard to argue against rigor in a scientific investigation. However, at every turn there are decisions to make that seem to invite a trade-off between rigor and expediency. For example, a person's age measured in days is more precise than when measured in years. Yet, few researchers avail themselves of this precision, easily tapped by asking a subject's date of birth. It is more practical to ask age in years. It is an expected measure, unlikely to cause surprise or other heightened response. And, it requires no calculation by the researcher.

Measuring age in years is easier, though less precise and hence rigorous, but still gets the job done in a reasonable fashion. It is more expedient.

A well-rounded decisions approach to the assessment of inter-coder reliability in content analysis studies will involve a similarly pragmatic weighing of rigor and expediency. For example, while the most rigorous test would be to analyze 100% of the study sample for inter-coder reliability, this is rarely done, because of issues of practicality, including cost and time constraints. Similarly, using multiple, diverse coders rather than the minimal two may be a more rigorous tactic, guaranteeing that the coding scheme is not limited in its utility to certain individuals or certain types of coders (e.g., doctoral-level students, or individuals from a particular culture). However, the practical reality is that most content analysis projects are unfunded or have only limited means, and/ or are on a schedule that imposes some limitations on the project's workload. Coders are typically obtained where we can find them—often in the classroom or the office next door.

Throughout the sections that follow, both rigor and expediency will be considered when recommendations are offered for various decisions to be made by the content analyst with regard to inter-coder reliability.

Practical Decision-making About Reliability Assessment

The achievement of acceptable levels of reliability for a content analysis is intimately related to the coder training process. A thorough training and reliability assessment typically involves the following processes (Neuendorf, 2002):

1   development of the coding scheme—including discussion with coders and revisions of the scheme as necessary
2   practice coding (both group and independent coding)—followed by revisions of the coding scheme as necessary
3   initial or pilot reliability test—followed by revisions of the coding scheme as necessary
4   final training and actual coding of data
5   reliability testing with a sub-sample of units—executed throughout the actual coding process.

Note that there are at least three stages at which coding scheme changes should be considered: (1) the development stage; (2) after-practice coding; and (3) after an initial/pilot reliability test. Unfortunately, the third opportunity is rarely used. One example that did so successfully is a study of health representations in the Dutch press by Commers, Visser, and De Leeuw (2000), who condensed their coding categories to "minimize potential ambiguity" after pilot reliabilities proved to be unacceptably low.

The goal of completeness in describing message patterns may be tempered by the practicality of having to design and conduct a content analysis project on a given schedule. Content analysis can be a particularly time-consuming research method, often taking months or even years to execute. However, reliability should ideally be assessed both before coding begins as well as at regular intervals while ongoing coding of data is occurring.

Selecting the Reliability Sub-sample

The process recommended above includes two reliability sub-samples, one for an initial or pilot reliability test and one for a final reliability test. Two schools of thought prevail as to how to select reliability sub-samples. The more popular perspective focuses on the random, and therefore representative, selection of a reliability sub-set. Another is more concerned with testing the content analysis instrument on the widest possible variety of cases, and so involves the selection of a set of cases that typify the full range on the variables under investigation. Potter et al. (1998) call this the selection of a "good coding challenge" (p. 85). A good compromise would be to use a "rich range" sub-sample for the practice coding, and random sub-samples for both the pilot and the final reliability tests. Hubbell and Dearing's (2003) study of news coverage of health improvement projects employs this latter approach.

How large must each reliability sub-sample be? Rules of thumb range from 10% to about 20% of the full sample (Neuendorf, 2002). Lacy and Riffe (1996) proposed a method for determining sub-sample size based on a desired level of sampling error, but their consideration of the topic was limited to a single dichotomous variable and two coders. Their work seems to indicate that the reliability sub-sample should never fall below 50 cases, nor should it need to exceed about 300 cases. A large sub-sample (at the high end of this range) would be indicated by (a) a large full sample for the study, and (b) a low assumed level of reliability in the full sample.

Another issue to consider is whether the reliability sub-sample is used as part of the final dataset. Usually it is, although some intrepid researchers have used another, separate random sample of messages from the population under investigation to conduct reliability analysis. Chory-Assad and Tamborini (2001) employed this tactic in their study of portrayals of doctors on TV. However, this approach does not seem to add substantial rigor, and indeed some scholars would find it inappropriate (Fan & Chen, 2000), notwithstanding that it adds a burdensome task to the research protocol.

Coder Selection

The role of the coder should be seen as a part of the coding instrument or scheme. Coders should be relatively interchangable. That is, the written coding scheme consisting of a codebook and coding form, along with a standard coder training for that scheme, should be so carefully planned and well documented that: (a) the research is fully replicable by others; (b) nearly any individual might serve as a coder; and (c) the data generated by the analysis do not vary regardless of which coder is assigned to analyze any given piece of content.

Conversely, if the coding is dependent on the participation of particular individuals as coders, then the investigation ought not be considered a content analysis, but, rather, an expert analysis.

Number of Coders

At least two coders must be employed in any human-coded content analysis in order for inter-rater reliability to be assessed. Just as all variables in a study should be subjected to reliability assessment, all coders whose data are used in the study should be part of the reliability assessment. It is not generally acceptable to use only a sub-set of coders in reliability assessment, although this tactic may occasionally be found in the health media content analysis literature (e.g., Fouts & Burggraf, 2000; Myhre, Saphir, Flora, Howard, & Gonzalez, 2002).

The use of multiple coders is an attractive option for several reasons. It allows splitting of the often tedious task of coding, reducing the volume of material that must be reviewed by each individual. It also has the added advantage of assuring the researcher that the successful application of their coding scheme is not limited to just two individuals, enhancing confidence in the replicability of the data. Content analysts should not fall into the trap of believing that using a limited number of coders will make their measures more reliable. Indeed, a review of health media content analyses conducted for this chapter found two studies in which the authors used only one coder "to avoid reliability problems" (Mercado-Martinez, Robles-Silva, Moreno-Leal, & Franco-Almazan, 2001, p. 239) or to overcome "the problem of inconsistency between coders" (Batchelor, Kitzinger, & Burtney, 2004, p. 671). This shows a gross misunderstanding of the nature and purpose of inter-coder reliability assessment in content analysis.

The typical method of reliability assessment involves the assignment of a uniform sub-sample of cases to all coders. However, there has been some consideration of alternative models, including one that could result in *all* cases being used for reliability assessment, but without the burden of having all coders code every case. Krippendorff (2004b) argues in favor of the use of these "sequential overlapping" reliability sub-sample cases, albeit without providing a full description of how that might be handled statistically. At the same time, Potter and Levine-Donnerstein (1999) do not support such a procedure, but fail to present a statistical argument against it. It seems likely that a statistical test for this situation might readily be developed and made widely available, perhaps a variation on the venerable intraclass correlation coefficient (Haggard, 1958), or a promised future application of Krippendorff's alpha.

Blind Coding

Scholars have begun to argue for the practice of blind coding to avoid introducing potential bias in the data grounded in coder expectations or biases related to the subject matter of the investigation. There are at least two levels of "blind" status one might contemplate: (a) where the coders are unaware of the study's specific hypotheses and/or research questions; and (b) where the coders are unaware even of the study's general goals. The former is more easily achieved, and is recommended, although not currently widely reported. See Pollock and Yulis's (2004) study of newspaper coverage of physician-assisted suicide for a good example. The latter is often impractical, and may interfere with the accurate and reliable execution of the coding scheme.

Expert Coders

Any *a priori* coder qualifications may limit the validity of a coding scheme. That is, if special knowledge beyond essential coder training is required, then the coding scheme is not generalizable, and is unlikely to provide a replicable research technique. With this in mind, each researcher should think carefully before using expert coders.

In some cases, there is no question that expert coders are needed. For example, in a study of violent video game content, a modicum of gaming experience is required of coders (Haninger & Thompson, 2004; Thompson & Haninger, 2001), although this type of experience ostensibly could be part of a coder training program. If the coding scheme requires some expert status that cannot be part of coder training, it would be useful for the researchers to include such expert status as an announced, required part of their coding scheme. For example, a coding scheme might assume coder knowledge commensurate with that of a licensed pharmacist in a study evaluating physician-targeted drug advertising. This would enhance replicability.

Coder Training

It is clear that added training can increase reliability (Goetz & Stebbins, 2004; Harwell, 1999; National Center for the Analysis of Violent Crime, 1990), as can supplementary coding materials (Lievens, Sanchez, & De Corte, 2004; National Center for Education Statistics, 1982). However, sometimes no amount of training can bring a given coder into line, and a coder must be dropped from the study. This possibility of eliminating a "deviant" or "rogue" coder has only rarely been addressed in the content analysis literature (Neuendorf, 2002; Staley & Weissmuller, 1981; Wagner & Hansen, 2002). The practice of dropping coders from participation in a study seems reasonable so long as it is done either: (a) during the training process, prior to the generation of any actual data for the study, or: (b) after data collection begins, so long as all cases analyzed by the rogue coder are abandoned.

Discussion to Resolve Coder Disagreement

While discussion during training and codebook revision is quite fruitful, final coding and reliability assessment need to be conducted by coders independently. When coding actual data for a study, the practice of resolving inter-coder disagreements through discussion and consensus-seeking runs counter to the fundamental goals of content analysis. Such action moves the process away from a reliance on the coding scheme (i.e., the codebook, coding form, and coder training). Rather, it implicates a failure of some aspect of the coding scheme, and employs a tactic to try to salvage usable data. If coder responses are to be averaged, discussed with an eye to consensus, or otherwise aggregated, then the characteristics of the coders are made central to the investigation. In such a case, coders should probably be a random sample of some population of potential audience members for the message content, but the study should not be called a content analysis. Such research has moved out of the realm of content analysis and into a survey or response study mode, where the particular attributes of the coders come more prominently into play.

The Unitizing Task

Perhaps the most often ignored issue in content analysis reliability assessment is unitizing. The majority of content analyses involve breaking messages into defined, codable units. This task is variously conducted by the lead researcher, the coders themselves, or an administrative aide. The reliability of this particular task has only rarely been examined, with Bakeman (2000) and Krippendorff (2004a) among the few scholars who have directly addressed this important issue.

Consider several examples that clarify the need for such examination. First, there are instances in which unitizing is apparent and non-problematic. For example, in a study of magazine ads, the unit of analysis may simply be the ad, such as with Aiello and Larson's (2001) study of hygiene-related ads over a 60-year period. There seems no need to assess this unitizing task, as the principal cross-coder discrepancies would be clerical errors. In this case, the sampling unit is the same as the unit of analysis.

However, let's assume that we wish to examine role portrayals of human models in medical journal ads (e.g., Michelson, 1996). While this may seem straightforward, it probably will not be. Here, the unit of sampling is the ad, but the unit of analysis is the model. A coder decision must be made for each model. Will secondary models in a large group photo each count as a case? What if the model is only partially shown, or not facing the camera? In this instance, one should still conduct a unitizing reliability assessment. This would involve reporting the numbers and percentages of cases identified by one coder and not another, and the number and percentages of cases identified by both coders. Krippendorff (2004a) has proposed an adaptation of his alpha statistic (see section below) for evaluation of the unitizing task.

Even clearer is the case of a continuous flow of content, such as a television program. Some coding processes might be well served by cutting the stream of content into readily identifiable time units, as in Sprafkin, Rubinstein, and Stone's (1977) study in which they analyzed television programming in two-minute segments. At other times, consistent identification of critical discrete events such as violent acts or sexual behaviors is essential to the coding process. Good examples of research that has recognized the unitizing task as a critical reliability issue may be found in the works stemming from the National Television Violence Study (*National television violence study*, 1997; Potter et al., 1998; Wilson et al., 2002) and other, similar work on sexual messages on television (Kunkel, Cope, & Biely, 1999). These researchers' "Close Interval around the Agreement Mode" (CIAM) technique has established a two-stage process of reliability assessment that incorporates (a) unitizing reliability (i.e., agreement on recognizing the violent act or the sexual behavior) and (b) agreement on the content analytic variables measured within the units defined (see Potter et al., 1998, pp. 90–91).

Reliability Coefficient Options

The content analysis literature has only recently addressed the question of rigor with regard to reliability coefficients. In the past, a simple indicator of percent agreement was the norm. This approach is inadequate because it fails to account for the varying possibilities of chance agreement that are a function of the number of classification options available to the coder. But even though more sophisticated reliability assessment is increasingly employed, there is a lack of widely understood and accepted reliability coefficients. Similarly, there is no common, widely shared computer application that calculates high-level inter-coder reliability coefficients for more than two coders (Kang, Kara, Laskey, & Seaton, 1993; Skymeg Software, 2007). There seem to be various "folklores" with regard to accepted reliability coefficients, with different areas of study adopting different classes of favored coefficients (Bakeman, 2000). A constant stream of disagreement runs through the social science literature with regard to proper reliability measurement.

The following discussion delineates statistical options in three categories: inter-coder agreement, inter-coder agreement with correction for chance, and covariation of inter-coder scores. The first two categories generally assume nominal data; the last assumes ordinal, interval, or ratio data.

1   Inter-coder agreement. Although percentage of agreement is the simplest to calculate and historically the most popular coefficient in every area of content analysis, such analysis is quite simply not a sufficient test of inter-coder agreement (Interrater reliability, 2001; Krippendorff, 2004a; Lombard, Snyder-Duch, & Bracken, 2002). Percent agreement might provide a commonly understood "touchstone" for scholars, but is too prone to capitalization on chance to be relied upon as the sole reliability indicator. As a heuristic, there seems no harm in reporting percent agreement, one variable at a time, so long as other more rigorous coefficients are also reported.

2   Inter-coder agreement with chance-correction. Several well-used statistics take percent agreement a step further, by controlling for the impact of chance agreement. Suen and Lee (1985) provide a firm rationale for chance-correction, and they present an investigation in which previous studies were re-examined with chance-corrected reliability coefficients, resulting in rather radical differences. The main chance-corrected agreement coefficients are:

- *Scott's pi* (Scott, 1955) uses a joint marginal distribution across two coders.
- *Cohen's kappa* (Cohen, 1960) uses a multiplicative term for the coders' marginal distributions; numerous adaptations have been proposed (Banerjee, Capozzoli, McSweeney, & Sinha, 1999; Kraemer, 1980) including an extension to multiple coders (Fleiss, 1971).
- *Weighted kappa* (Cohen, 1968) disagreements of varying "gravity" are weighted accordingly. This coefficient assumes at least ordinal data, in that disagreements are given numeric weightings based on how "far" off the miss is.

Both pi and kappa are derived from the same conceptual formula:

$$\text{pi or kappa} = \frac{PA_O - PA_E}{1 - PA_E}$$

where PA_O is the observed proportion agreement and PA_E is the proportion agreement expected by chance.

One issue with regard to agreement (including agreement with correction for chance) is whether, for ordinal or higher-level measures, a near-miss is as good as a hit. This "range agreement" (Neuendorf, 2002) decision rule has been supported (Tinsley & Weiss, 1975) and used by some content analysts (Clapp, Whitney, & Shillington, 2002; Dominick, 1999).

Although a number of criticisms have been leveled at the use of kappa (Brennan & Prediger, 1981; Popping, 1988), it remains a statistically acceptable option for the assessment of inter-coder reliability, particularly for nominal data. It is the most commonly used statistic in this category.

3   Covariation. When a content analysis variable is measured at the ordinal, interval, or ratio level, the researcher may wish to look at how coders' scores co-vary, rather than only at agreement or range agreement. For example, rating the age of models in an advertisement in precise years would be a case in which exact agreement would be unlikely, but near-agreement with highly systematic covariation would meet the reliability criterion of measurement consistency among coders. Potential coefficients to assess this include:

- *Spearman's rho*   this statistic assumes rank-order ordinal data, and provides an index of the correspondence between two sets of rankings only. The values of the original scores are not taken into account.
- *Pearson's r*   this widely known bivariate statistic assumes interval/ ratio data. It is at best problematic when used to assess inter-coder reliability, due to the possibility of obtaining a very high coefficient with *no* real agreement or even near agreement. The coefficient has, however, been used widely for some inter-rater reliability tasks, as in the study of personnel selection (Salgado & Moscoso, 1996).
- *Lin's concordance correlation coefficient*   this variation on the correlation coefficient provides a type of correction for the identified flaws of the Pearson r (Lin, 1989). It constrains the correlation line to pass through the origin and have a slope of one, thus giving heavy credit for identical and near-identical scores. Although used primarily in the medical literature to date, this coefficient shows promise for future use in content analysis.

Considerations in the selection of reliability coefficients

Echoing the definitional distinctions of Nunnally (1978) and Bakeman, Quera, McArthur, and Robinson (1997), Tinsley and Weiss (2000) draw a firm line in the sand between "agreement" and "reliability," and find both types of information necessary to the evaluation of ratings such as content analysis measures. They recommend using correlational or ANOVA-type statistics for the assessment of reliability, the ratio of true score variance to total variance. They espouse the use of chance-corrected coefficients for the assessment of inter-coder agreement, including Cohen's kappa and weighted kappa for nominal data, and their own T statistic (Tinsley & Weiss, 1975), an adaptation of kappa for ordinal and interval data.

Traub (1994), in his volume devoted to the reliability assessment of a multi-measure scale for survey or experimental work, presents an intriguing statistical complement to the traditional Cohen's kappa test. He proposes a ratio of $kappa/kappa_{max}$, where $kappa_{max}$ is the largest achievable kappa with the joint distribution's marginals held constant. Given a joint distribution of marginals, the Traub ratio indicates how closely the two tests (or in this case, coder judgments) correspond, compared to the maximum possible agreement.

Some scholars have attempted to apply traditional tests of statistical significance to inter-coder reliability coefficients (Bartko & Carpenter, 1976; Gustafson, Van Koningsveld, & Peterson, 1984). However, a finding of no significant difference is not logically the same as finding evidence of consistency. Krippendorff (2004a) points this out convincingly, observing:

> A common mistake that researchers make is to accept or reject data as reliable when the null hypothesis that agreement occurs by chance can be rejected with statistical confidence. However, the whole reason for measuring the

reliability of data is to ensure that they do not deviate too much from perfect agreement, not that they deviate from chance. (p. 237)

Some proposed reliability statistics have the undesirable characteristic of inflating values simply via an increase in the number of coders. These include Rosenthal's R, which is really a reintroduction of the venerable Spearman-Brown formula with coders replacing items (Rosenthal, 1987), and Rust and Cooil's PRL indicator (Cooil & Rust, 1994; Rust & Cooil, 1994). Use of such statistics has the negative consequence of tempting researchers to increase their coder pool solely for the purpose of achieving higher reliability scores.

Recent calls for greater rigor in the application of reliability coefficients have appeared in the communication literature. Lombard, Snyder-Duch, and Bracken (2002; 2003), reviewing the sins and omissions of content analyses in communication, conclude that much rigor can be added without sacrificing expediency. Holding content analysts to higher standards than have been common in the past, these scholars emphasize the responsibility of the researcher in selecting reasonable yet appropriate methods and in fully reporting on those methods, including the application of appropriate reliability coefficients. In response, Krippendorff (2004b) argues against the use of most current reliability coefficients, and advocates for the use of his alpha set of coefficients, adapted to the four levels of measurement (Hayes & Krippendorff, 2007). With no ready method for managing the calculation of the various alpha versions with multiple coders, numerous variables, different levels of measurement, and large datasets, this recommendation leaves the reader with a specific prescription for statistical standards, but without any convenient practical means to achieve them.

Finally, when considering options for the use of reliability coefficients, one might frame a discussion in terms of an analog to the traditional "Type I" and "Type II" errors referenced in traditional hypothesis-testing. Here, "Type A" error might be the chance of concluding that a measure is reliable, when in fact it is not; "Type B" error might represent the possibility of concluding that a measure is not reliable, when in fact it is. Both types of errors are best avoided, and our aim is to find a balance that minimizes both.

A statistic such as percent agreement might be seen as potentially high on Type A error. For example, in a case where a study reports 75% agreement, a researcher might be quite satisfied, until it is pointed out that most of that agreement is likely due to chance, at least in the case of a dichotomous measure. A statistic such as Rosenthal's R might also be seen as potentially high on Type A risk, due to the fact that Rosenthal's R is inflated when many coders are used. For example, 20 coders with an average inter-coder reliability (r) of only .30 would result in a Rosenthal's R of .90 (Rosenthal, 1987), leading the researcher to believe that the measure is highly reliable when in fact it is not. Similarly, using Pearson's r might be seen as risking Type A error, in that a very high correlation may result from absolutely no agreement whatsoever.

The interpretation of a statistic such as Cohen's kappa as if it were percent agreement could be seen as an example of Type B error. For example, a kappa of .50 (seen as minimally acceptable at best by current standards) would certainly *not* be found acceptable with traditionally recommended cutoffs of .80 or .90, since those benchmarks were derived principally from percent agreement applications.

Computer Applications that Provide Reliability Coefficients

The good news is that, today, there is no need to calculate inter-coder reliability coefficients by hand. The bad news is that the variety of computer applications that support such calculations are a wide mixture, and most require that the data be formatted in a particular manner that may not match a typical data setup. Currently, the main options include statistical packages that offer only limited reliability assessment options, as well as several dedicated inter-coder reliability computer applications.

Statistical packages that provide inter-coder reliability options include:

1 SimStat: version 2.5 of this multipurpose statistical package is available from Provalis Research. The Inter-raters option under Multiple Response calculates, for two coders at a time, percent agreement, Cohen's kappa, Scott's pi, Krippendorff's r bar (an ordinal-level extension of Scott's pi), Krippendorff's R (an ordinal-level extension of Cohen's kappa), and free marginals for nominal and ordinal data (http://www.provalisresearch.com).
2 Statistical Package for the Social Sciences (SPSS): this widely-used statistical analysis program can run Cohen's kappa for two coders if one creates a mini dataset for each variable studied (http://www.spss.com).

Computer applications dedicated to the calculation of inter-coder reliability include:

1 ComKappa—Bakeman's (2007) Windows 95 application for kappa and weighted kappa is a great training exercise for understanding the application of kappa to ordinal or interval data with "weighted kappa" (i.e., it takes into account close misses vs. far misses, and the user can immediately see the results (http://www2.gsu.edu/~psyrab/BakemanPrograms.htm); see also, Robinson and Bakeman, 1998).
2 Agree 7.2: this application (Popping, 1984, 1988) can calculate a variety of agreement indicators for multiple coders, but is limited in the number of values that a variable may hold to 40 and limited to reliability coefficients that assume nominal data. Agree is available in a demo version (http://www.ppsw.rug.nl/~popping).
3 PRAM: the Program for Reliability Assessment with Multiple Coders is available in a demo version from Skymeg Software (2007). PRAM calculates percent agreement, Scott's pi, Cohen's kappa, Spearman's rho, Pearson's r, and Lin's r_c, with testing underway for the addition of the

multicoder version of kappa and Krippendorff's alpha (S. Bretmersky, Skymeg Software, personal communication, February 5, 2006). The program has the major advantage of allowing the ready analysis of an Excel or SPSS dataset containing multiple variables measured by multiple coders in a typical dataset configuration (http://www.geocities.com/skymegsoftware/pram.html; see also http://academic.csuohio.edu/kneuendorf/content/reliable/pram.htm for more documentation).

4   An SPSS/SAS macro for the calculation of Krippendorff's alpha: Andrew Hayes of Ohio State University has authored and made available online a macro that calculates Krippendorff's alpha from a single-variable dataset specifically configured such that each column represents a particular coder's score on a given variable and each row a reliability case (Hayes, 2007;   http://www.comm.ohio-state.edu/ahayes/SPSS%20programs/kalpha.htm). More information, including sample setups for many of these programs and links to relevant sites, may be found at the Lombard, Snyder-Duch, and Bracken (2005) website for practical resources related to inter-coder reliability: http://www.temple.edu/mmc/reliability.

Minimum Standards for Reliability Coefficients

There are no universally agreed-upon minimum levels for the various reliability coefficients (Krippendorff, 2004a; Neuendorf, 2002). And where recommendations have been made, they are often for percent agreement (Frey, Botan, & Kreps, 2000), which, as noted above, should not stand alone as a reliability indicator. Some recommend a minimum Pearson r (Pedhazur & Schmelkin, 1991); however, reliance on this statistic for reliability assessment is suspect. Others endorse a particular minimum cutoff, but do not identify the coefficient (Riffe, Lacy, & Fico, 1998).

Some have proposed criteria for the popular Cohen's kappa. For example, Banerjee et al. (1999) hold that a kappa of .75+ indicates excellent agreement beyond chance; .40–.75 is fair to good; and below .40 is poor agreement. Landis and Koch (1977) maintain that a kappa coefficient of .81–1.00 indicates substantial agreement; .61–.80 moderate agreement; .41–.60 fair agreement. Krippendorff (2004a) recommends relying on only those variables that achieve a Krippendorff's alpha of .80 or higher.

A variable that fails to reach a researcher's minimum standard for reliability should be dropped from further analysis (Allen, 1995; Neuendorf & Skalski, in press). This bottom-line stricture makes clear the all-important nature of reliability for human coding.

The Current State of Reliability Assessment for Health-related Content Analysis Research

Content analyses have historically not enjoyed the same rigor of reportage standards as have other quantitative methods in the study of communication-related behavior. Lombard et al. (2002) found that only 69% of content analysis studies appearing in communication journals between 1992 and 1996 contained any report of inter-coder reliability. That rate is an increase from the 49% found by Pasadeos, Huhman, Standley, and Wilson (1995) for content analyses reported in four major communication journals between 1988 and 1993. Nonetheless, the fact that nearly one in three content analysis studies fail to provide any assessment of inter-coder reliability reflects a serious methodological shortcoming. Moreover, according to Lombard et al., only 41% of the articles reported reliability coefficients for each variable separately, which is another basic aspect of evaluating the reliability of a study's measures.

To inform this chapter, a limited but systematic review was conducted to examine scholarly literature in the area of health-related media content analysis research. The review employed a search of the ISI Web of Science (including the Social Science Citation Index, the Science Citation Index, and the Arts and Humanities Citation Index) for journal articles and WordCat for book chapters that include as key terms "content analysis," "health" and "media" (or "television," "radio," "internet," "magazine," or "newspaper," each in turn). For the years 1977–2005, 133 relevant research pieces were identified. (A full list of the studies yielded by the search is available from the author on request.)

This review revealed the range of scholarly disciplines in which health media content analyses have appeared. Scholars from such diverse fields as journalism, communication, advertising, marketing, linguistics, sociology, social work, anthropology, psychology, psychiatry, medicine, public health, pharmacy, nursing, gerontology, health promotions, information technologies, and library and information sciences provided a wide range of perspectives on the study of health media content, with an occasional contribution from such fields as dietetics and nutrition, cancer research, political science, engineering, marketing, epidemiology, and geography.

Of the 133 research pieces identified, 102 presented data based upon some type of human-coded content analysis for which reporting inter-coder reliability would be appropriate.[1] Of these, 38% included no reliability assessment. This rate of omitting reliability assessment in health-related content analysis research is comparable though slightly higher than the 31% observed to occur in the field of communication broadly by Lombard et al. (2002). Although the limited numbers in this review preclude any definitive conclusions, some journals appear to be more likely to include reliability assessment for content analyses than others. For example, the following had at least two articles represented in this review, both or all of which included reliability assessment: *JAMA: Journal of the American Medical Association, Journal of Advertising, Journal of Nutrition Education, Journalism & Mass Communication Quarterly, Nursing Research,* and *Sex Roles.*

One would expect the field of communication to demonstrate stronger standards in the practice of content analysis research than other disciplines, given that the methodology originated there, as journalists and advertising scholars, media critics, and film historians attempted to quantify characteristics of the message patterns that were the focus of their scholarship. Moreover, the call for rigor in reliability assessment has emanated strongly from this field (Krippendorff, 1980; Lombard et al., 2002; Neuendorf, 2002). On the other hand, most of the other disciplines represented in this collection are ones that embrace the scientific method, so it seems reasonable to expect that the same rigorous standards should be applied to content analyses published in these realms as well.

The 63 articles that included some claim of reliability assessment represented a mixed bag with regard to reporting standards. Not a single research piece represented the "ideal" full reportage model. None indicated that the researchers had engaged in two reliability checks (i.e., pilot and final). The size of the reliability sub-sample varied from 1.6% to a full 100%. Indeed, on the positive side, 15 studies indicated a 100% reliability check. Twenty-three of the studies reported percent agreement only, and another three reported no reliability coefficients at all; thus, nearly half of the articles failed to report appropriate reliability coefficients. Only three studies reported assessment of unitizing reliability, and only 14 indicated that the reliability sub-sample was selected randomly.

Only 20 content analyses reported reliability coefficients variable-by-variable. The other studies reporting coefficients did so either by indicating an average across variables (deemed unacceptable by most methodologists; Krippendorff, 2004a; Lombard et al., 2002; Yeaton & Wortman, 1993), by reporting a minimum, or by reporting the range of low and high values. While the latter two choices are not as rigorous as reporting for each and every variable, they are obviously superior to averaging or failing to report.

Mirroring the findings of previous reviews of content analysis methodology, the most "popular" reliability coefficient among the health media content analyses was percent agreement (29 studies), followed by Cohen's kappa (21 studies). Other coefficients were reported less frequently: Scott's pi (five studies), Pearson's r (three), Rust and Cooil's PRL (two), Krippendorff's alpha (two), Holsti's reliability coefficient (1969; two), Perreault and Leigh's I (1989; one), Rosenthal's R (one), and Cronbach's alpha (one). Again, coefficients that fail to meet common standards of statistical rigor (i.e., percent agreement) or are inappropriate to the given assessment task (e.g., Pearson's r, Cronbach's alpha [Carmines & Zeller, 1979]) unfortunately are well represented in the published literature.

On the other hand, seven of the studies reported an intracoder reliability check, a proportion clearly higher than that found among most types of content analysis. This attention to another type of reliability—stability over time as opposed to the reproducibility tapped by inter-coder reliability—may signal a welcome move toward a new standard. Such intracoder checks require a re-analysis of a sub-sample of cases at a later point in time, making the coding process even more time-consuming.

The number of coders employed ranged from one (six studies) to 32, with approximately one half of the studies that reported number of coders indicating that two coders were employed. Only 10 of the studies used more than three coders. Only one study reported the implementation of blind coding, and six reported using expert coders. Seventeen of the articles reported that coding disagreements were resolved through a process of consensus establishment or "majority rule" vote, both of which run counter to the conceptual goals of reliability assessment.

This limited review seems to clarify the poor state of reliability assessment and reportage among content analyses of health messages in the media, identifying a troubling lack of rigor.

Recommended Standards for Assessing and Reporting Reliability

Summarizing points of view developed throughout this chapter, a total of 10 recommended standards are offered here for properly assessing and reporting inter-coder reliability. The recommendations presented by Lombard et al. (2002, 2005) and Neuendorf (2002) are key sources for many of these positions.

1   Reliability assessment should be conducted for (a) unitizing decisions, whenever the unit of data collection is different than the sampling unit; and (b) measurement of the content analysis variables.
2   Formal reliability assessment should be conducted (a) after coder training and prior to the commencing of coding (pilot reliability), and (b) during actual coding of data for the study (final reliability). Typically, changes may be made in the coding scheme after completing a pilot reliability test. Only the coefficients for final reliability testing are normally reported in the final research publication, although scholars who report both are to be congratulated.
3   Coders should be kept "blind" to the study's hypotheses and research questions whenever possible.
4   All final coding of data for a study should be conducted independently, without discussion among coders.
5   Reliability coefficients should be appropriately selected based upon careful consideration of the level(s) of measurement.
6   The percent agreement coefficient should be reported only as a second, supplementary indicator, if presented at all.
7   Reliability coefficients must be reported separately for each variable.
8   When more than two coders are used, a statistic that takes into account multiple coders, such as Fleiss' (1971) adaptation of Cohen's kappa, should be employed to assess reliability.
9   The researcher should consider checking intracoder reliability. While this can be burdensome, there are compelling arguments in its favor. Potter et al. (1998) recommend it as a check for coder fatigue, a real problem for large-scale, lengthy content analysis projects.

10 In addition to the above recommendations, the following information should be reported: (a) the size of the reliability sub-sample/s; (b) the selection process for reliability sub-sample/s; (c) the number of coders used, their method of recruitment, type of expertise assumed, and extent of training; and (d) where the coding scheme and training procedures might be obtained for possible replication.

New Frontiers for Statistical Quality Assurance in Reliability Assessment

In addition to these practical recommendations, there is a need for greater statistical rigor in inter-coder reliability assessment, including a more careful watch over the appropriate application of reliability coefficients (Hayes & Krippendorff, 2007; Krippendorff, 2004b; Lombard et al., 2002). Several types of initiatives are called for to accomplish progress on this front. To that end, we might consider a three-part model for the future assurance of statistical quality in the assessment of inter-coder reliability:

1 Computer applications must be developed and disseminated that provide ready calculation of multiple inter-coder reliability coefficients. It is frustrating that we have easy access to sophisticated interactive structural equation modeling in various computer software packages, while much simpler analytic tools needed to evaluate inter-coder reliability are relegated to hard-to-use peripheral sources. This difficulty has assuredly contributed to the dismal state of reliability assessment in content analysis research. The further development of new computer applications will enhance both rigor and expediency in the use of reliability coefficients, allowing for the possibility of greater standardization of the reliability assessment process.

2 There should be systematic investigations of the properties of common and potential reliability coefficients. Both the "Type A" and "Type B" problems outlined earlier in this chapter should be addressed in a comprehensive fashion. Examination of the performance of various coefficients may provide future researchers with more guidance upon which to base their selection of appropriate inter-coder reliability coefficients.

For example, the Krippendorff alpha coefficient seems to hold strong potential utility, but no independent researcher has assessed its properties, nor compared its underpinnings to those of the more common but less adaptable coefficients such as Scott's pi and Cohen's kappa. Similarly, Lin's concordance coefficient (r_c) has been used in medical diagnostic procedures, but has not been adopted for use in content analysis. It seems to answer key criticisms of other indicators of covariation such as Pearson's r. These and other aspects of the available reliability options should be evaluated more thoroughly in a manner that might lead to more systematic use of reliability coefficients in the future.

3   Content analysts should consider options for expanded methodological diagnostics (Neuendorf, 2002; 2006). These include: (a) the creation of confidence intervals for reliability coefficients (Krippendorff, 2004a; Potter et al., 1998); (b) greater sensitivity in selecting sub-samples for reliability testing that affords more strength in generalizing to the entire sample; and (c) the creation of "confusion matrices" that indicate which values of a particular variable are most often "confused" by coders, in order to pinpoint specific patterns in inter-coder disagreement (Krippendorff, 2004b). All of these techniques offer the potential to enhance the scientific rigor with which content analysis investigations are conducted.

Conclusion

Reliability is one of many standards of measurement that contribute to the rigor of a scientific investigation. In the domain of content analysis research, it holds special significance. Without it, one cannot know whether the data generated for the study are likely to be stable and replicable by others. Despite this situation, it is clear that reliability assessment in content analysis research has been treated haphazardly by many scholars who employ this method.

Strong reliability contributes to but does not guarantee a valid measure in content analysis research. Thus, reliability is seen as one essential component for a good measure. Inter-coder reliability assessment is the core method of reliability testing for content analyses using human raters. As such, it is an integral component of any credible scientific investigation involving message analysis.

This chapter offers a number of pragmatic perspectives intended to strengthen the evaluation of inter-coder reliability in content analysis research, providing a guide to methodological standards that are both rigorous and practical. The quality of content-based research can be significantly enhanced by carefully considering the optimal strategies for systematically evaluating inter-coder reliability.

Note

1 The remaining 31 included: (a) seven articles that reported solely on results obtained via CATA (computer-assisted text analysis, using such computer applications as LIWC (n = 4), Atlas.ti (n = 1; actually, principally a qualitative text analysis tool), TextAnalyst (n = 1), and VBPro (n = 1); for more information on these and other CATA programs, see the Content Analysis Guidebook Online at http://academic.csuohio.edu/kneuendorf/content), (b) eight articles that indicated that a "qualitative content analysis" had been conducted, and described a type of analysis that did not meet the definition of content analysis assumed here (Neuendorf, 2002), (c) seven articles that applied the term "content analysis" to the emergent development of a categorization scheme for open-ended questions, and (d) others that were content analysis-related, but did not report on a single full analysis (e.g., articles that reviewed content analyses, or discussed content analysis as a research technique appropriate to certain research tasks). Additionally, a number of research articles that included human-coded content analysis also included a CATA analysis—two used the CATA program Concordance, one VBPro, two LIWC, and one simple online search engines.

References

Aiello, A. E., & Larson, E. L. (2001). An analysis of 6 decades of hygiene-related advertising: 1940–2000. *American Journal of Infection Control, 29*, 383–388.

Allen, A. M. (1995). The new nutrition facts label in the print media: A content analysis. *Journal of the American Dietetic Association, 95*, 348–352.

Bakeman, R. (2000). Behavioral observation and coding. In H. T. Reis & C. M. Judge (Eds.), *Handbook of research methods in social and personality psychology* (pp. 138–159). New York: Cambridge University Press.

Bakeman, R. (2007). Computer programs written by Roger Bakeman, GSU. Retrieved on July 14, 2008, from http://www2.gsu.edu/~psyrab/BakemanPrograms.htm

Bakeman, R., Quera, V., McArthur, D., & Robinson, B. F. (1997). Detecting sequential patterns and determining their reliability with fallible observers. *Psychological Methods, 2*, 357–370.

Banerjee, M., Capozzoli, M., McSweeney, L., & Sinha, D. (1999). Beyond kappa: A review of interrater agreement measures. *The Canadian Journal of Statistics, 27*(1), 3–23.

Bartko, J. J., & Carpenter, W. T. Jr. (1976). On the methods and theory of reliability. *Journal of Nervous and Mental Disease, 163*, 307–317.

Batchelor, S. A., Kitzinger, J., & Burtney, E. (2004). Representing young people's sexuality in the "youth" media. *Health Education Research, 19*, 669–676.

Brennan, R. L., & Prediger, D. J. (1981). Coefficient kappa: Some uses, misuses, and alternatives. *Educational and Psychological Measurement, 41*, 687–699.

Carmines, E. G., & Zeller, R. A. (1979). *Reliability and validity assessment.* Beverly Hills, CA: Sage.

Chory-Assad, R. M., & Tamborini, R. (2001). Television doctors: An analysis of physicians in fictional and non-fictional television programs. *Journal of Broadcasting & Electronic Media, 45*, 499–521.

Clapp, J. D., Whitney, M., & Shillington, A. M. (2002). The reliability of environmental measures of the college alcohol environment. *Journal of Drug Education, 32*(4), 287–301.

Cohen, J. (1960). A coefficient of agreement for nominal scales. *Educational and Psychological Measurement, 20*(1), 37–46.

Cohen, J. (1968). Weighted kappa: Nominal scale agreement with provision for scaled disagreement of partial credit. *Psychological Bulletin, 70*(4), 213–220.

Commers, M. J., Visser, G., & De Leeuw, E. (2000). Representations of preconditions for and determinants of health in the Dutch press. *Health Promotion International, 15*, 321–332.

Cooil, B., & Rust, R. T. (1994). Reliability and expected loss—a unifying principle. *Psychometrika, 59*(2), 203–216.

Dominick, J. R. (1999). Who do you think you are? Personal home pages and self-presentation on the World Wide Web. *Journalism & Mass Communication Quarterly, 76*, 646–658.

Fan, X. T., & Chen, M. (2000). Published studies of interrater reliability often overestimate reliability: Computing the correct coefficient. *Educational and Psychological Measurement, 60*, 532–542.

Fleiss, J. L. (1971). Measuring nominal scale agreement among many raters. *Psychological Bulletin, 76*, 378–382.

Fouts, G., & Burggraf, K. (2000). Television situation comedies: Female weight, male negative comments, and audience reactions. *Sex Roles, 42*, 925–932.

Frey, L. R., Botan, C. H., & Kreps, G. L. (2000). *Investigating communication: An introduction to research methods* (2nd ed.). Boston, MA: Allyn and Bacon.

Goetz, C. G., & Stebbins, G. T. (2004). Assuring interrater reliability for the UPDRS motor section: Utility of the UPDRS teaching tape. *Movement Disorders, 19,* 1453–1456.

Gustafson, D. H., Van Koningsveld, R., & Peterson, R. W. (1984). *Assessment of level of care: Implications of interrater reliability on health policy.* Washington, DC: Health Care Financing Administration.

Haggard, E. A. (1958). *Intraclass correlation and the analysis of variance.* New York: The Dryden Press, Inc.

Haninger, K., & Thompson, K. M. (2004). Content and ratings of teen-rated video games. *JAMA: Journal of the American Medical Association, 291,* 856–865.

Harwell, M. (1999). Evaluating the validity of educational rating data. *Educational and Psychological Measurement, 59,* 25–37.

Hayes, A. F. (2007). SPSS and SAS macro for computing Krippendorff's alpha. Retrieved on July 14, 2008, from http://www.comm.ohio-state.edu/ahayes/ SPSS%20programs/kalpha.htm

Hayes, A. F., & Krippendorff, K. (2007). Answering the call for a standard reliability measure for coding data. *Communication Methods and Measures, 1*(1), 77–89.

Holsti, O. R. (1969). *Content analysis for the social sciences and humanities.* Reading, MA: Addison-Wesley.

Hubbell, A. P., & Dearing, J. W. (2003). Local newspapers, community partnerships, and health improvement projects: Their roles in a comprehensive community initiative. *Journal of Community Health, 28,* 363–376.

Interrater reliability. (2001). *Journal of Consumer Psychology, 10*(1&2), 71–73.

Kang, N., Kara, A., Laskey, H. A., & Seaton, F. B. (1993). A SAS MACRO for calculating intercoder agreement in content analysis. *Journal of Advertising, 23*(2), 17–28.

Kraemer, H. C. (1980). Extension of the kappa coefficient. *Biometrics, 36,* 207–216.

Krippendorff, K. (1980). *Content analysis: An introduction to its methodology.* Beverly Hills, CA: Sage.

Krippendorff, K. (2004a). *Content analysis: An introduction to its methodology* (2nd ed.). Thousand Oaks, CA: Sage.

Krippendorff, K. (2004b). Reliability in content analysis: Some common misconceptions and recommendations. *Human Communication Research, 30,* 411–433.

Kunkel, D., Cope, K. M., & Biely, E. (1999). Sexual messages on television: Comparing findings from three studies. *The Journal of Sex Research, 36*(3), 230–236.

Lacy, S., & Riffe, D. (1996). Sampling error and selecting intercoder reliability samples for nominal content categories: Sins of omission and commission in mass communication quantitative research. *Journalism & Mass Communication Quarterly, 73,* 969–973.

Landis, J. R., & Koch, G. G. (1977). The measurement of observer agreement for categorical data. *Biometrics, 33,* 159–174.

Lievens, F., Sanchez, J. I., & De Corte, W. (2004). Easing the inferential leaps in competency modeling: The effects of task-related information and subject matter expertise. *Personnel Psychology, 57,* 881–904.

Lin, L. I. (1989). A concordance correlation coefficient to evaluate reproducibility. *Biometrics, 45,* 255–268.

Lombard, M., Snyder-Duch, J., & Bracken, C. C. (2002). Content analysis in mass communication: Assessment and reporting of intercoder reliability. *Human Communication Research, 28,* 587–604.

Lombard, M., Snyder-Duch, J., & Bracken, C. C. (2003). Correction. *Human Communication Research, 29,* 469–472.

Lombard, M., Snyder-Duch, J., & Bracken, C. C. (2005, June 13). *Practical resources for assessing and reporting intercoder reliability in content analysis research projects.* Retrieved on July 14, 2008, from http://www.temple.edu/mmc/reliability

Mercado-Martinez, F. J., Robles-Silva, L., Moreno-Leal, N., & Franco-Almazan, C. (2001). Inconsistent journalism: The coverage of chronic diseases in the Mexican press. *Journal of Health Communication, 6,* 235–247.

Michelson, J. (1996). Visual imagery in medical journal advertising. M.A. thesis, Cleveland State University, Cleveland, OH.

Myhre, S. L., Saphir, M. N., Flora, J. A., Howard, K. A., & Gonzalez, E. M. (2002). Alcohol coverage in California newspapers: Frequency, prominence, and framing. *Journal of Public Health Policy, 23*(2), 172–190.

National Center for Education Statistics. (1982). *Assessment of intercoder reliability on the classification of secondary school courses.* Arlington, VA: Evaluation Technologies, Inc.

National Center for the Analysis of Violent Crime. (1990). *Criminal investigative analysis: Sexual homicide.* Washington, DC: U.S. Department of Justice.

National television violence study (Vol. 1). (1997). Thousand Oaks, CA: Sage.

Neuendorf, K. A. (2002). *The content analysis guidebook.* Thousand Oaks, CA: Sage.

Neuendorf, K. A. (2006, November 2). *Considerations and recommendations for the Annenberg Health Media Coding Project.* Retrieved on July 14, 2008, from http://www.youthmediarisk.org

Neuendorf, K. A., & Skalski, P. D. (in press). Quantitative content analysis and the measurement of collective identity. In R. Abdelal, Y. M. Herrera, A. I. Johnston, & R. McDermott (Eds.), *Identity as a variable.* Cambridge, MA: Harvard Identity Project.

Nunnally, J. C. (1978). *Psychometric theory* (2nd ed.). New York: McGraw-Hill.

Pasadeos, Y., Huhman, B., Standley, T., & Wilson, G. (1995, May). Applications of content analysis in news research: A critical examination. Paper presented to the Theory and Methodology Division of the Association for Education in Journalism and Mass Communication, Washington, DC.

Pedhazur, E., & Schmelkin, L. (1991). *Measurement, design, and analysis: An integrated approach.* Hillsdale, NJ: Lawrence Erlbaum Associates.

Perreault, W. D., & Leigh, L. E. (1989). Reliability of nominal data based on qualitative judgments. *Journal of Marketing Research, 26*(May), 135–148.

Pollock, J. C., & Yulis, S. G. (2004). Nationwide newspaper coverage of physician-assisted suicide: A community structure approach. *Journal of Health Communication, 9,* 281–307.

Popping, R. (1984). AGREE, a package for computing nominal scale agreement. *Computational Statistics and Data Analysis, 2,* 182–185.

Popping, R. (1988). On agreement indices for nominal data. In W. E. Saris & I. N. Gallhofer (Eds.), *Sociometric research* (Vol. 1): *Data collection and scaling* (pp. 90–105). New York: St. Martin's Press.

Potter, J., Linz, D., Wilson, B. J., Kunkel, D., Donnerstein, E., Smith, S. L., Blumenthal, E., & Gray, T. (1998). Content analysis of entertainment television: New methodological developments. In J. T. Hamilton (Ed.), *Television violence and public policy* (pp. 55–103). Ann Arbor: The University of Michigan Press.

Potter, W. J., & Levine-Donnerstein, D. (1999). Rethinking validity and reliability in content analysis. *Journal of Applied Communication Research, 27*(3), 258–284.

Riffe, D., Lacy, S., & Fico, F. G. (1998). *Analyzing media messages: Using quantitative content analysis in research.* Mahwah, NJ: Lawrence Erlbaum.

Robinson, B. F., & Bakeman, R. (1998). ComKappa: A Windows 95 program for calculating kappa and related statistics. *Behavior Research Methods, Instruments, and Computers, 30,* 731–732.

Rosenthal, R. (1987). *Judgment studies: Design, analysis, and meta-analysis.* New York: Cambridge University Press.

Rust, R., & Cooil, B. (1994). Reliability measures for qualitative data: Theory and implications. *Journal of Marketing Research, 31*(February), 1–14.

Salgado, J. F., & Moscoso, S. (1996). Meta-analysis of interrater reliability of job performance ratings in validity studies of personnel selection. *Perceptual and Motor Skills, 83,* 1195–1201.

Scott, W. (1955). Reliability of content analysis: The case of nominal scale coding. *Public Opinion Quarterly, 17,* 321–325.

Skymeg Software. (2007). *Program for Reliability Assessment with Multiple Coders (PRAM).* Retrieved on July 14, 2008, from http://www.geocities.com/skymeg-software/pram.html

Sprafkin, J. N., Rubinstein, E. A., & Stone, A. (1977). *A content analysis of four television diets.* Stony Brook, NY: Brookdale International Institute.

Staley, M. R., & Weissmuller, J. J. (1981). *Interrater reliability: The development of an automated analysis tool.* Brooks Air Force Base, TX: Air Force Human Resources Laboratory.

Suen, H. K., & Lee, P. S. C. (1985). Effects of the use of percentage agreement on behavioral observation reliabilities: A reassessment. *Journal of Psychopathology and Behavioral Assessment, 7,* 221–234.

Thompson, K. M., & Haninger, K. (2001). Violence in E-rated video games. *JAMA: Journal of the American Medical Association, 286,* 591–598.

Tinsley, H. E. A., & Weiss, D. J. (1975). Interrater reliability and agreement of subjective judgements. *Journal of Counseling Psychology, 22,* 358–376.

Tinsley, H. E. A., & Weiss, D. J. (2000). Interrater reliability and agreement. In H. E. A. Tinsley & S. D. Brown (Eds.), *Handbook of applied multivariate statistics and mathematical modeling* (pp. 95–124). San Diego, CA: Academic Press.

Traub, R. E. (1994). *Reliability for the social sciences: Theory and applications.* Thousand Oaks, CA: Sage.

Wagner, E. R., & Hansen, E. N. (2002). Methodology for evaluating green advertising of forest products in the United States: A content analysis. *Forest Products Journal, 52*(4), 17–23.

Wilson, B. J., Smith, S. L., Potter, W. J., Kunkel, D., Linz, D., Colvin, C. M., & Donnerstein, E. (2002). Violence in children's television programming: Assessing the risks. *Journal of Communication, 52*(1), 5–35.

Yeaton, W. H., & Wortman, P. M. (1993). On the reliability of meta-analysis reviews—the role of intercoder agreement. *Evaluation Research, 17*(3), 292–309.

6   Research Ethics in Content Analysis

Nancy Signorielli

Ethics are an important and critical component of the research process and their implementation in study design has evolved considerably during the past 40 to 50 years. Research practices that were routinely used in studies conducted during the 1960s and 1970s are now looked upon with dismay, and the research community wonders how it could have been blind to the unethical and immoral treatment of participants that often took place.

Today, textbooks on research in communication and the social sciences typically devote a chapter to ethics (see, for example, Frey, Botan, & Kreps, 2000; Hocking, Stacks, & McDermott, 2003; Wimmer & Dominick, 2006). These chapters discuss the key elements or principles of ethical research, including risks and benefits, voluntary participation, informed consent, deception and concealment, debriefing, and ethics in data gathering, analysis, reporting, and manuscript preparation. They typically examine ethics from the perspective of studies that use the participant or recipient as the unit of analysis. Surveys and experiments, for example, are designed to isolate differences between groups of respondents or between different treatment groups. The unit of analysis in these studies is the individual. Content analysis, on the other hand, is based on a research perspective in which the units of analysis are elements of message content: television programs, newspaper articles, music videos, advertisements, commercials, and the like. Consequently, ethics in content analyses must be considered from a very different perspective, one that in the past was not usually addressed. Interestingly, none of the three key texts used by content analytic researchers or in courses teaching content analysis techniques (Krippendorff, 1980, 2004; Neuendorf, 2002; Riffe, Lacy, & Fico, 1998) mentions specific or special ethical concerns in content analysis.

This chapter describes those ethical principles that are relevant to content analysis. Many of the key elements and/or principles of ethics that are discussed and documented in numerous texts on communication research are not relevant to content analysis, and thus will not be discussed in detail here. Rather, this chapter examines four ethical principles relevant to content analysis: (1) the need for appropriate debriefing and/or desensitization of coders, (2) ethics in reliability testing, (3) data fabrication and the ethical principles that come into play when reporting the results of the study, and (4) in some research scenarios, informed consent. Before exploring these topics, a review of the foundations for ethical concerns in research is in order.

Ethics from an Institutional Perspective

Ethical issues in research are so important in today's academic and research climate that rules are in place to ensure that those who participate in research studies are treated appropriately. As early as 1966, after several unethical experiments and studies were brought to public and governmental attention, the U.S. Surgeon General reviewed all studies requesting funding by the Public Health Service to make sure that participants would not be harmed and would be given adequate opportunities and sufficient information to give their informed consent to participate (Frey et al., 2000). With similar concerns arising on the country's university campuses, the National Research Act was passed by Congress in 1974. This act required any institution that conducted government sponsored research to establish an institutional review board (IRB) to examine proposed studies and give permission to researchers to proceed with data collection and analysis. Today, on most campuses, any study in which people serve as participants/respondents and/or which involves animals must be cleared by the university's IRB, whether or not the research is externally funded (Frey et al., 2000). Professional organizations such as the American Psychological Association (2002) and the American Association for Public Opinion Research (1986) also have specific codes of ethical behavior. Content analyses usually do not have to be submitted to the IRB because, as noted above, there are no participants in the classic sense. Hence, as IRB approval is not needed, it is up to the researcher to make sure that relevant ethical principles are heeded.

The National Communication Association (NCA) has a division devoted to communication ethics (www.natcom.org), and in 1999 NCA's Legislative Council approved a "Credo for Ethical Communication" (www.natcom.org/nca/Template2.asp?bid=374). This advocates "truthfulness, accuracy, honesty, and reason as essential to the integrity of communication." Similarly, NCA developed a "Code of Professional Responsibilities for the Communication Scholar/Teacher" (www.natcom.org/nca/Template2.asp?bid=509).This notes that researchers must work with integrity, maintain confidentiality and informed consent, show professional responsibility by refraining from plagiarizing, avoiding *ad hominem* attacks when criticizing or reviewing other scholars' work, and sharing credit when credit is due. Moreover, the code notes that all research should be conducted with honesty and openness, and investigators are bound to honor any commitments made to participants in research projects.

Research Ethics in Content Analysis

Content analysis is a research technique in which the units of analysis (focus of the study) are messages. These include television programs, newspaper articles, magazine advertisements, transcripts of conversations, or websites. Hence, the unit of analysis is a thing, not a human subject or a group of people. Research questions and hypotheses posit differences between sub-sets of these units. For example, a study might examine how the content of television programs on premium cable channels differs from programs on broadcast channels, how the images in advertisements in women's magazines differ from those in men's magazines, or how stories on local news programs compare to those on national news programs. Consequently, ethical elements such as risk-benefit ratios and deception and concealment, which are critical in experiments and surveys, do not translate to inanimate units such as television programs, newspaper articles, advertisements, commercials, music videos, or even websites.

Content analysis also differs from other research procedures in the way in which the data are collected. Content analysis data are generated by coders, people trained to isolate and classify the elements of content in the samples of the units of analysis according to a specified set of definitions and instructions, what Krippendorff (1980, 2004) calls the Recording Instrument. Coders may be college students or others who are hired to generate the data, or may also be students in a class that conducts a content analysis project as part of the course requirements. In addition, coding may be done by the primary investigators of a study, by a student working on a master's thesis or doctoral dissertation, or by friends, family members, or acquaintances of the primary investigator. Across all of these scenarios, a number of unique ethical issues apply to the conduct of content analysis research.

Debriefing and Desensitization of Coders

Coders who are hired or are members of a class that is conducting a content analysis for pedagogical reasons serve in the role of junior researchers, rather than study participants. They are trained in the nuances of the data collection procedures and may receive compensation for their participation in the form of money or academic credit toward their course grade. Yet, as junior researchers they have limited knowledge of the area under investigation. One could argue that continued and detailed exposure to certain types of messages, such as television programs, could be detrimental to their well-being. Alternatively, one might argue that coding television programs is nothing more than watching television, an everyday activity in which most coders have participated throughout their lives. Though we cannot be certain, it may well be the case that watching television for entertainment and for the purpose of generating scientific content analysis data are two very different processes. Watching for entertainment may be done by rote, without much thought about the images that are seen. Watching to generate data, however, involves considerable mental alertness and total involvement with the content—scenes of violence and/or sex are often viewed over and over again to determine who is involved and what has transpired. Coders are thus exposed to the potentially harmful messages in media content at a more extreme and intense level than when viewing for pleasure or to pass the time.

The 2002 ethical code of the American Psychological Association (APA) specifies that the nature of the research should be explained to participants after their participation in a study. Moreover, this code notes that if any misconceptions exist they should be corrected, and if there has been any harm to the research participant, it should be minimized (APA, 2002, section 8.08). Debriefing provides an opportunity to determine if participation in the study has generated problems other than those the investigator originally anticipated. Hocking et al. (2003) note that even though debriefing can turn participation in a research study into an educational experience, this possibility is often overlooked.

Frey et al. (2000) discuss two forms of debriefing—desensitizing and dehoaxing. They note that desensitizing is needed when participants "have acquired negative information about themselves" from participation (p. 155). For example, when a participant's self-worth/self-esteem has been manipulated as a part of the study, desensitizing is usually warranted in order to return self-worth/self-esteem to its original level. Dehoaxing is needed if the participants in the study have been deceived as part of the manipulation of the independent variables. In this type of debriefing the participants must be told of the deceit and, if necessary, its potentially harmful effects. While dehoaxing does not apply to content analysis studies, desensitizing is needed if the units of analysis contain content that may be harmful.

Debriefing of coders is critical because the research literature has shown that viewing negative images, such as television violence, may be detrimental to viewers (see, for example, Potter, 1999). Consequently, researchers who conduct analyses of media content with potentially harmful images should be prepared to desensitize the coders to their potential effects. This form of debriefing provides a way to make sure that the coders leave the study in the same physical and mental state in which they began, and, in addition, provides a way in which coders may benefit from their participation in the study. It is critical that desensitization begin in the very early stages of coder training and continue throughout the time the data are collected. In addition, there should be a final desensitization process once all the data have been collected and the coders have finished their coding tasks.

An example of how coders could be desensitized to excessive exposure to violent or sexual images comes from studies looking at the effects of violent and sexual images in films upon respondents. Although this example comes from an experimental paradigm rather than a content analysis, the procedures used for the desensitizing process provide a good model for content analysis desensitization. These procedures were part of a study of filmed violence against women in which young men were exposed to several slasher films over five days, a relatively short period of time (Linz, Donnerstein, & Penrod, 1984). The investigators in this research took considerable pains to make sure that the young men who participated would not exhibit some of the behaviors hypothesized to result from excessive viewing of movies of this type. First, the research team screened their potential respondent pool in order to eliminate those young men who might have a pre-existing psychological condition that could exacerbate the impact of these films. Second, once the data had been collected, the participants met with the investigators, who conducted a discussion about the study, its design, the stimuli, and the types of attitudes that could arise from their participation. This part of the debriefing protocol included a discussion of rape myths, and the young men were told that although they may have experienced pleasurable feelings from sexual portions of these films, the violence against women shown in the films was unjustified. Moreover, the debriefing scenario stressed that women do not want to be raped or enjoy being raped, and that when women say "no" to sexual advances their feelings should be respected. Last, after two months, the investigators contacted all of the young men who took part in this study in order to ensure that there were no long-lasting detrimental effects from their participation.

Another desensitizing scenario would be to have a series of discussions about the nature of the images the coders will see and have to analyze in the course of their coding assignments. These discussions would be an ongoing part of the coding process. They would commence at the start of coder training, when the primary investigator would tell the coders that some of the images in the materials they will code could have harmful effects. The most effective debriefing or desensitizing intervention would include several meetings or discussions during the course of the entire data collection period, with a final discussion after all the data have been collected. For example, some discussions might focus upon the negative effects of viewing violence, focusing upon violence as a negative or problematic way to solve problems. Other discussions could examine the problems inherent in seeing images that do not show the subsequent consequences of violence (see Potter, 1999).

Likewise, a coder's immersion in sexual images on television or film, particularly if the images are very explicit, risqué, or show risky sexual behavior, necessitates discussion of appropriate and less risk-laden sexual behaviors. Similar discussions might be necessary if a project isolates beauty-related images in magazine advertisements. This discussion might focus on how images of almost perfect beauty are fabricated through the use of computer simulations and airbrushing techniques and are impossible to attain in reality. Across all areas of potentially sensitive content, the primary investigator of the project should be aware of the types of images or messages that will be coded and determine what type of debriefing or desensitizing may be necessary. For a good example of coder debriefing and desensitization, see Chapter 8 by Salazar, Fleischauer, Bernhardt, & DiClemente, in this volume.

Ethics in Testing Reliability

Testing for the reliability of the data in a content analysis project is another area that may present an ethical concern. Content analysis differs from other types of studies in that coders are trained to isolate specific elements of message content. In short, the training process should ensure that all coders generate data in exactly the same way in order to come up with exactly the same observations for the same unit of analysis. The reliability analysis tests statistically the degree of trustworthiness of the data generated by the coders (Krippendorff, 2004). In other words, the reliability analysis determines whether the coders were in agreement on how they classified the message content under examination.

A preliminary reliability analysis is often conducted at the end of the training period to ensure that the coders are using the coding instructions and variable definitions in the same way and in the manner specified by the principal investigator. High levels of reliability are needed at this point in the study so that the coders can begin to analyze the actual sample of content gathered for the research. But this is not the only time in the study when reliability should be measured. It is also critical for a reliability analysis to be conducted on the data generated throughout the entire data collection period. That is, a reliability analysis should be conducted on the actual sample of units. This necessitates that two or more coders, operating independently, generate data on the entire sample or a reasonable sub-set of the sample of the units of analysis. These independent datasets should be generated throughout the entire data collection period and analyzed for reliability once all the data have been collected and prior to the statistical analyses that will answer the study's research questions and test its hypotheses.

Certain situations may occur during data collection that may raise ethical concerns. First, during training coders routinely ask questions about the coding process. This is a critical component of training because it is by asking questions that possible inconsistencies in the operational or coding definitions may be uncovered and addressed. During training, questions are often asked when the coders meet for instruction and clarification. In this case all coders have access to the same information. Coders may also ask questions individually during the training period and the trainer typically has opportunities to relay any additional pertinent information to the entire group of coders. This process, however, may be more difficult to continue once the coders are immersed in coding the actual sample of materials. In this case, the trainer may inadvertently give pertinent information to some but not all of the coders. This may raise ethical concerns in the sense that the principal investigator may be offering "coaching" or hints to individual coders in order to increase the prospects for obtaining acceptable levels of reliability. However, such individual communications may in practice have a detrimental effect on reliability coefficients, as different coders will then perform their work based on a differing foundation of information and instructions. It is important that all coding rules, instructions, and clarifications be shared fully and in timely fashion with all coders during the data collection phase of any content analysis project.

Ethics in Data Analysis and Reporting

As well as treating participants with dignity and protecting them from harm, research investigators have an equal ethical obligation to colleagues and the academy to analyze their data and report their findings in an appropriate manner (Babbie, 2001). Researchers are also morally obligated not to fabricate or falsify their data in order to find support for their hypotheses.

Consistent with this obligation, the investigator should take precautions to ensure that coders actually review and analyze their assigned sample of content and do not make up or falsify the data (e.g., because it would take less time and/or work). Coders should also work independently in generating their data. In short, data should not be fabricated, changed, or tampered with. The results should be reported honestly. Fraud is such an important ethical consideration that in the fall of 1988 the Association of American Universities (AAU) in conjunction with the National Association of State Universities and Land-Grant Colleges and the Council of Graduate Schools developed a "Framework for Institutional Policies and Procedures to Deal with Fraud in Research" (AAU, 1988). This framework was developed taking into consideration guidelines previously developed by the Public Health Service (PHS) and the National Science Foundation in dealing with misconduct in conducting research.

The AAU (1988) framework defines research fraud as "scientific misconduct involving deception," where misconduct refers to "fabrication, falsification, plagiarism, or other serious deviation from accepted practices in proposing, carrying out, or reporting results from research" as well as "failure to comply with Federal requirements for protection of researchers, human subjects, or the public ..." The AAU and PHS also note that individual institutions should develop specific policies for dealing with research fraud efficiently and in a timely fashion. At the same time, the framework, the AAU, and the PHS all note that it is important to distinguish fraud from honest error or honest differences among researchers in how data should be interpreted.

The National Communication Association in its "Code of Professional Responsibilities for the Communication Scholar/Teacher" (www.natcom.org/nca/Template2.asp? bid=509) also notes that integrity is a critical component of the publication/writing process and that authors should properly acknowledge previous and/or current work that has contributed to this research and that the publication/presentation process should proceed with honesty and openness.

Moreover, as noted above, the results of the data analysis and statistical tests should be reported honestly. The results reported should be those that are fully supported by the data analysis. Half-truths should be avoided. Care must be taken to make appropriate attributions throughout the research report or manuscript that will be submitted for presentation at a conference or for publication in a journal. Finally, those who have made substantial contributions to the research should be suitably acknowledged. For example, students or research assistants who have helped gather the data, interpret the results, and write the manuscript should be acknowledged and, when appropriate, given authorship credit.

Informed Consent

Informed consent is not usually an issue in content analysis research, because media content, rather than human subjects, is the focus of research. And although, as pointed out above, there is an ethical responsibility to protect coders from potential adverse effects of coding, coders are not research participants but are essentially hired or voluntary junior researchers. In most large, long-term projects, coders are hired and work in return for payment. In other cases, the data are collected by the principal investigator along with help from classmates, friends or family. Moreover, when a project is conducted as part of a class, coding becomes a class activity and/or assignment and serves an educational or pedagogical purpose. Students often collect the data that they then use to complete other class assignments such as writing a final research report. As long as coding is a paid activity or is done voluntarily, informed consent is not an issue.

Informed consent, however, may be needed when coding units such as conversations, group interactions, chat room or Instant Messenger (IM) interactions. Participants in a conversation or group situation must give the researcher permission to tape, record, or digitally capture their conversations or interactions. Not surprisingly, friends or acquaintances using IM may be reticent to have their conversations recorded. Consequently the participants in these discussions must be given sufficient information about the study so that they can make informed decisions about their participation.

The situation is somewhat different in studies of chat room interactions and the contents of message boards. While some message boards and chat rooms do not require a log-in and are readily available to the public, others require you to register in order to access what is on the site. While informed consent is not necessary in the former case, there are, as yet, no clear guidelines for the latter situation. In either case, however, it may prove difficult to get consent because chat room and message board participants are often unknown to each other and want to maintain their anonymity. Facebook provides yet another situation in which it may be difficult to give study-related details to enable the researcher to get informed consent from participants.

Clearly, the possibility exists that by asking for permission to capture the interactions the entire nature of the interchange will be altered by the fact that someone is "listening" and paying close attention to what is being said. Participants might feel that they are being "spied upon" and may choose to withdraw from the study rather than give their permission for the research to be carried out. Or, more problematically, most of the participants may refuse to agree to have their interactions captured, thus making it impossible to do the research.

Conclusion

Ethics is a critical, often neglected component of the research process in content analysis research. Ethics should be part of both the undergraduate and graduate school curriculum, particularly in teaching research methods. Students should be expected to understand the ethical principles of research and be able to defend their research designs from an ethical as well as a methodological perspective. Content analysis studies need only be concerned with the principle of informed consent if the units of analysis involve conversations or other messages (e.g., chat rooms, IM) where participants can be clearly identified. It is critical, however, that coders who generate the data be protected. If the study deals with a topic that might have a negative impact, such as isolating violence and/or sexual behaviors in the media, sufficient time and energy must be spent desensitizing the coders. Those who have collected the data should not be negatively influenced by the images they have had to examine in the course of the coding process. Last, but certainly not least, findings should be reported accurately and honestly, and conclusions should not go beyond what the data indicate, so that the findings will be beneficial to the discipline and society.

References

American Association for Public Opinion Research (1986). *Code of professional ethics and practices.* Available at http://www.aapor.org/default.asp?page=survey_methods/ standards_and_best_practices/code_for_professional_ethics_and_practices

American Psychological Association (2002). *Ethical principles of psychologists and code of conduct.* Available at http://www2.apa.org/ethics/code2002.doc

Association of American Universities (1988). *Framework for institutional policies and procedures to deal with fraud in research.* Available at http://www.aau.edu/reports/ FrwkRschFraud.html

Babbie, E. (2001). *The practice of social research* (9th ed.). Belmont, CA: Wadsworth/ Thompson Learning.

Frey, L. R., Botan, C. H., & Kreps, G. L. (2000). *Investigating communication: An introduction to research* (2nd ed.). Boston, MA: Allyn and Bacon.

Hocking, J. E., Stacks, D. W., & McDermott, S. T. (2003). *Communication research* (3rd ed.). Boston, MA: Allyn and Bacon.

Krippendorff, K. (1980). *Content analysis.* Thousands Oaks, CA: Sage Publications.

Krippendorff, K. (2004). *Content analysis: An introduction to its methodology* (2nd ed.). Thousand Oaks, CA: Sage Publications.

Linz, D. G., Donnerstein, E., & Penrod, S. (1984). The effects of multiple exposures to filmed violence against women. *Journal of Communication, 34*(3), 130–177.

Neuendorf, K. A. (2002). *The content analysis guidebook.* Thousand Oaks, CA: Sage Publications.

Potter, W. J. (1999). *On media violence.* Thousand Oaks, CA: Sage Publications.

Riffe, D., Lacy, S., & Fico, F. G. (1998). *Analyzing media messages: Using quantitative content analysis in research.* Mahwah, NJ: Lawrence Erlbaum.

Wimmer, R. D., & Dominick, J. R. (2006). *Mass media research: An introduction* (8th ed.). Belmont, CA: Thomson Higher Education.

Part 3
Case Studies

7 Teens and the New Media Environment

Challenges and Opportunities

*Srividya Ramasubramanian and
Suzanne M. Martin*

Researchers interested in the impact of media on the adolescent audience often use content analysis as a first step in assessing the kinds of messages available in mainstream media. These content analytical studies typically sample from prime-time television programs, blockbuster movies, or top-selling video games. But do these samples accurately reflect the media content to which teens are exposed? The sheer increase in the number of media types and information sources available to teen audiences has opened up a wide variety of options to choose from. This proliferation of media technologies has brought about dramatic changes to when, where, and how adolescents access media content.

In this chapter, we provide an overview of our efforts to assess teens' exposure to media content and the challenges we have encountered in developing our measures. Specifically, we present data from an exploratory study which illustrates that adolescents are growing up in a multiple-media environment, much of adolescent media use is idiosyncratic, and their media encounters are increasingly "interactive." Content analysis methodology needs to adapt and adjust to these revolutionary changes in the media ecology. We propose an audience-centered, media-ecological approach to content analytical research in response to this emerging interactive new media scenario.

A Media-ecological Approach to Content Analysis

There is no doubt that the media environment today's teens experience is very different from that of any past generation. With the rapid explosion of media technologies, virtually limitless media sources are available to audiences. Given the availability of a variety of media choices, it is not surprising that teens are spending more time with the media in general, often engaging with more than one medium simultaneously (Roberts, Foehr, & Rideout, 2005). According to research conducted by the Kaiser Family Foundation in 2005, among 8–18-year-olds, average daily media use is almost six hours when single medium use is considered. The average exposure time increases to eight hours per day when more than one medium is taken into account (Roberts et al., 2005).

The convenience of wireless, portable, miniaturized media gadgets has made it easier for adolescents to access information outside conventional media access venues such as homes and schools. Because of increased niche marketing, customization, and interactivity, we can no longer talk about adolescents as one "mass audience" that shares similar media experiences. In many senses, distinctions between print media such as magazines and newspapers, audio-visual media such as television and movies, and interactive "new" media such as video games, computers, and the internet have become less meaningful because of the growing convergence of media types.

The changing media landscape brings into question traditional conceptualizations of terms such as "content," "exposure," and "audience" from a media-centric, technology-focused approach to content analysis. In response, we argue that content analysis needs to shift to a more audience-focused, ecological approach. Such a media-ecological approach to content analysis takes into consideration the complex relationships between media *content* and media *environments.*

In our own research, conducted at the Annenberg Public Policy Center, on assessing sexual content across various teen media, we find that media consumption patterns of teens have changed dramatically in recent years. Below, we present findings from a preliminary study that was conducted among adolescents to understand what types of media teens are exposed to, how they typically engage with media, and what types of formats they use to access media content.

A Preliminary Study on Media Consumption Patterns Among Teens

Participants

We conducted 19 focus groups (n = 196 participants) in 2003 and 2004 with teens in a metropolitan Northeastern city to explore issues related to sexual behavior and sex in the media. The study surveyed a convenience sample of 196 12–19-year-olds. The sample was diverse (by gender and race). Of the 191 respondents for whom demographic information was available, 118 were females and 73 were males. While most of the participants were Black (n = 98), there were a considerable number of Hispanics (n = 45) and Whites as well (n = 33).

Methods

Upon arrival and completion of general instructions, youth were given a background questionnaire and media diary form. First, youth were given a paper and pencil measure to collect demographic information, as well as length of time and type of media youth used the previous day. Next, youth were shown one of two five-minute media clips from *The OC* or *Boston Public* and given a checklist of behaviors with instructions to put a check next to each item on the list that they thought was present in the scene. Then the youth listened to and read lyrics to a song by the artist Fabolous and were given the same behavior checklist they completed after the media clip. Upon completion of the behavior checklist there was a brief open-ended question-naire covering beliefs about sex, followed by a group discussion about sexual behavior and sex in the media. Youth were then asked to complete a media log of their media use on the previous day in half-hour increments between 6:00 and 10:00 p.m. in a closed-ended format. They were asked: "What was your main media activity? (Fill in at least one)" and given the following choices: reading magazines, listening to music (radio/CD player), using computer chat room/instant messenger, playing computer games/video games, surfing the web, other computer (excluding word processing), watching television, watching videotaped TV program, going to the movies (in theater), watching a video or DVD, or no media. If participants indicated media use, they were then asked the name or title of the media. Following the media log, youth rated 11 behaviors to indicate how sexual and intimate they were and the different dating contexts in which they were likely to occur. Participants were then asked to "highlight the shows they watched for at least ten minutes yesterday" on an actual copy of a TV guide for that day. They were also asked to list the programs that were sexy or sexual and to rate the "sexiness" of each show listed.

Results

This study surveyed 196 12–19-year-olds about their average weekday and weekend day use of a variety of media, as well as their favorite media titles and their typical consumption patterns (e.g., whether they read magazines "cover to cover" or whether they "flip through" for interesting articles). Participants indicated their media use patterns for six media types that are popular amongst teens: television, music, movies, internet, video games, and magazines.

The lack of consensus among respondents on their favorite media titles was evidence for the growing fragmentation of "mass" audiences and the increase in customization of media selection. Even the most popular media titles were not reported as favorites by more than 15–20% of the participants. For instance, *The Simpsons* and *Friends* were mentioned as one of the top three favorite television shows by only 39 and 30 respondents respectively. Similarly, magazines such as *Seventeen* and *Vibe*, which are typically known to be very popular with teens, were not seen as favorites by very many respond-ents (only n = 23 each). Music artists and favorite music videos showed a high degree of diversity in what were considered favorites by listeners, with each given music video being mentioned by only a handful of respondents at best.

More than half (53%) of teens indicated they had downloaded music from the internet, which may be important as teens may be exposed to different content depending on where they obtain their music and how they listen to music (internet vs. radio vs. CD purchased in a store). Teens varied in the sources from which they downloaded music lyrics as well. A majority say they used the internet (65%) but CD covers were only slightly less popular as a source for lyrics (50%).

Respondents showed significant variations in the time spent with various media types. For instance, average time spent per week on listening to CDs (M = 28.5 hours) and watching television (M = 27.8 hours) was more than twice the time spent with video games (M = 11.8 hours) and on the web (M = 10.8 hours). Reading magazines took up the least amount of time (M = 4.9 hours) per week.

Moreover, the way in which magazines were "read" differed significantly within this seemingly homogeneous group of teen magazine readers. Almost equal numbers of respondents indicated that they typically read certain sections of the magazines (38%), flipped through the magazine (36%), and read it from cover to cover (23%). Therefore, it seems that while some teens might pay careful attention to printed materials in magazines, others simply browse through quickly, stopping to read only what really catches their attention.

Another notable observation that emerged during the course of conducting this preliminary survey was that adolescents in this sample often listed TV channels instead of specific TV shows, search engines (such as Google.com) for favorite websites, and music artists instead of the CD titles when asked to indicate their favorite CD. These details provided insights about the ways in which teen audiences categorize their media exposure. It seemed that they often classified media content information in terms of generalized media units (such as TV channels and music artists) rather than specific units (such as scenes from a TV episode or songs from a particular CD). Such information is helpful in making decisions related to unitization of media content, especially when we need to make comparisons across various types of media.

Overall, the findings from this preliminary study showed that teens accessed a variety of media sources in many different ways that in turn influenced the manner in which they experienced media content. There was very little overlap in the media channels and media titles considered favorites in this group, acting as further evidence for the increase in customization in media selection. This study illustrates that teens are living in a dynamic multiple-media, niche media marketing environment where media use is fairly idiosyncratic. The implications of these dramatic changes in teen media environment for the media-ecological approach to content analysis are discussed below.

Interactivity in Media Encounters: Implications for Content Analysis

Interactivity can be conceptualized as a process-related variable that describes the iterative, dialogical manner in which meanings are created in communication contexts. It is defined as "the extent to which communication reflects back on itself" (Newhagen & Rafaeli, 1996, p. 2). In the new media context, conceptualization of "audiences" in the traditional uni-directional linear information flow from source to destination is now being replaced by terms such as "users" to indicate their more active participatory role in producing media content. As a variable, interactivity can range on a spectrum from one-way mass-mediated communication to "simultaneous and continuous exchanges" resembling face-to-face conversations involving complex forms of interruptions and turn-taking, as seen in web environments (Rafaeli & Sudweeks, 1997). Media interactivity has been classified into three types: user to system, user to document, and user to user (McMillan, 2002). Each of these types of interactivity has different implications for content analytical research.

User-to-system Interactivity

This type of interactivity involves human–computer interaction such as that found in video games and search engines. Because digital data are represented numerically, it becomes easily possible for researchers to input mathematical formulas to search for specific types of data within a larger pool of available information. Internet search engines such as Yahoo, newspaper databases such as *LexisNexis*, and online versions of the *TV Guide* have greatly reduced the time it takes to identify media units of relevance to a given study. Indeed, defining the sampling frame for a study based on media units generated from "keyword searches" is becoming a popular sampling technique within content analysis (Weare & Lin, 2005). An audience-centered approach to sampling would recommend that a preliminary observational study be conducted to understand the "routes" that users are most likely to take while navigating a webpage, followed by analyses of these identified access patterns.

For example, Keller and colleagues (2002) used an audience-oriented sampling technique for studying health messages online where they asked young people to report the search terms that they would use while looking up sexual health information online. These researchers later analyzed the top 100 hits that came up in three popular search engines upon entering the search terms provided by participants. They used the "one-click rule" by including the homepage and links available directly from the homepage that lead to unique content (and not just to another external site). Other researchers such as Hong and Cody (2002), who studied pro-social websites online, have used the entire website as the unit of analysis by examining all the pages linked to a given domain name.

Taking the highly interactive world of video games as an example, situations experienced during gameplay could vary vastly from one gamer to another within the same media unit. The way a game proceeds may be contingent upon the type of game being played, the skill level of the player, the type of platform, and familiarity with the game. Decisions regarding units of analysis are also complicated when it comes to interactive media. For example, while studying video games, researchers have to decide if they will analyze each level of the game, every encounter that the player has with a character, or a time-bound segment within the game.

Content analyses of video games are often based on arbitrarily determined durations of play as coding units, making it difficult to compare findings across studies. For example, Beasley and Standley (2002) analyze characters from the first 20 minutes of gameplay, Haninger and Thompson (2004) indicate that at least one hour of play was coded, while Dietz (1998) does not mention the duration of the analyzed segments.

To further complicate matters, many action games have several "avatars" of the same character. Researchers have to decide whether to code these as distinct characters or the same character. In the context of first-person shooter games, the character is the player himself/herself. To deal with this challenge, Smith, Lachlan, and Tamborini (2003) define an interaction as the number of times a player starts over within the first 10 minutes of gameplay. Under such circumstances, it might be helpful to take a user-oriented approach in determining the ways in which the audiences themselves categorize content, which could then guide researchers in deciding what units would be most meaningful to study.

User-to-document Interactivity

Non-linear access to information is another unique characteristic of new media (Newhagen & Rafaeli, 1996; Weare & Yin, 2005). This non-linear access is typical of user-to-document interactivity experienced while navigating hypertextual content on the internet. User-to-document interactivity in new media allows for inclusion of variables such as navigability, download speed, and availability of non-English-language translation, which are not meaningful in the context of traditional media (Bucy, Lang, Potter, & Grabe, 1999; Musso, Weare, & Hale, 2000).

Unlike television programs, magazines, and movies that have a definite beginning and a definite end, media such as internet and video games do not have rigid fixed boundaries, thus creating problems in defining the population of interest in content analyses. This endless web of interconnected sites with no identifiable beginning or end becomes extremely tedious to analyze (Mitra & Cohen, 1999). Defining a sampling frame to choose from in this ever-growing, non-linear repository of information becomes tough. Although it has been estimated that the world wide web has over 800 million websites (Lawrence & Giles, 1999), this figure is increasing exponentially, making it is impossible to know exactly how many sites are available on the internet at any given point in time (Stempel & Stewart, 2000; Weare & Lin, 2005). Whereas the Audit Bureau of Circulation keeps track of all the newspapers available, there is no such entity that keeps a catalog of all of the websites available on the internet. According to Lawrence and Giles (1999), only 42% of available sites are catalogued and any given search engine indexes only 16% of the sites found in the web. Moreover, every minute new material is being added, deleted, and edited from various websites all across the world by millions of users.

These aspects of new media have several implications for content analytical research. It becomes important for content researchers to keep track of when they retrieved information from a given website, because website content can change rapidly. Researchers should ensure that all coders have access to the same content using similar monitors, internet connections, and browsers in order to improve inter-coder reliability (Bucy et al., 1999). Archiving the contents of the websites being analyzed allows for researchers to save the contents for future reference (Weare & Yin, 2005).

From an audience-centric perspective, search engine-based sampling is emerging as a useful tool in new media content analysis because it provides information on the sites that a typical teen user is likely to encounter on the web. By using meta-search engines or multiple search engines, researchers can hope to map a larger portion of the web than through a single search engine. While some researchers have explored other sampling techniques such as selecting a random sample of most popular sites online (Bucy et al., 1999), this approach is not helpful for public health scholars interested in a specific audience segment such as adolescents.

User-to-user Interactivity

E-mail, Instant Messaging, web logs (blogs), peer-to-peer file sharing networks, and chat spaces are examples of locations where user-to-user interactivity can be observed. Teens are especially likely to engage in such user-to-user interactive content, using social networking sites such as MySpace.com and Facebook.com. More than half of teens (51%) aged 13 to 18 report visiting a social networking site in the past week compared to only 6% of tweens aged 8 to 12 (Harris-Interactive, 2006). Thirty-four percent of teens and seven percent of tweens report spending more than a half an hour on a typical day sending and receiving messages on a social networking site (HarrisInteractive, 2006). Consumer-generated media consist of blogs, discussions, recommendations, and word of mouth online. It is providing a new avenue of media to sample and companies such as Nielsen Buzzmetrics are doing just that to gather current information, referred to as "buzz" regarding a given company, brand, or trend.

In such avenues, communication is typically conversational in tone, resembling face-to-face interactions in social settings. Thus, analyzing user-to-user interactive new media might be closer to conversational analysis than analysis of "mass-mediated" texts. Shank (1993) categorizes conversation into monologue, dialogue, discussion, and multilogue. Monologue is the one-way communication typical of mass media, dialogue is a more reactive stimulus-response type of communication, discussion involves one-to-many communication where the initiator continues to maintain control as a moderator, and finally multilogue is similar to discussion except that the initiator does not retain control over the conversation. E-mail and Instant Messaging often involve dialogical conversations. Blogs tend to be discussion-oriented, where the primary blogger initiates conversations on a given topic of interest. Chat rooms are typically multilogue-oriented, with multiple participants expressing their thoughts and opinions, often challenging traditional notions of turn-taking in dialogical conversations. Therefore, depending on the type of user-to-user interactivity, the techniques of content analysis will also vary considerably.

Media Proliferation: Implications for Content Analysis

The proliferation of media technologies has brought about dramatic changes to when, where, how much, and to what types of media adolescents have access. The sheer increase in the number of media types and information sources available to audiences has opened up a wide variety of options from which to choose. It is not just that the proliferation of media technologies has changed *what* media content teens are consuming, but *how* and *where* these audiences are receiving such content. It is important for researchers to apply a media-ecological approach in analyzing teen media content by considering how these various new media formats and multiple access locations affect media content.

Younger audiences have been known to be early adopters of new and interactive technologies and are often more media-savvy than adults. In fact, children start learning to use the computer mouse, video game consoles, and television remote at a very young age, making it easy for them to operate media equipment without assistance from older family members. A little more than half (55%) of tweens and teens see their computer knowledge as better than most people or at an expert level (HarrisInteractive, 2006). Often, youth take the role as the experts in the household in regards to technology, with 41% of teens aged 13–18 reporting that their parents have gone to them for help with the internet (HarrisInteractive, 2006).

The multiplication of media technologies has implications for content analysis because content can be accessed in multiple media formats at different times and various locations. In such instances, the content itself could vary slightly from one media source to another. Even if the content is the same across media formats, the meanings derived can vary depending on the physical and social environment in which content is accessed.

While analyzing movies, for example, content analysts should be conscious that movies might be modified when they are broadcast for general television audiences. Similarly, people who watch movies on DVD might have a chance to view additional materials beyond just the movie itself. Extra-featured content could include previously unseen footage, interviews with crew members and cast, commentary from experts, and behind-the-scene perspectives on the efforts which went into the making of the film. Along the same lines, when it comes to analyzing songs listed to by adolescents, crucial decisions have to be made regarding whether to sample from radio stations that typically carry "cleaner" versions of songs, or from unedited versions of the songs from CDs, or use both versions of the song lyrics from iTunes.

In the context of public health messages, such decisions become even more

Table 7.1 Media in the home of 8–18-year-olds

Does anyone in your home own ...?	% Yes
TV	92
Computer	92
DVD player	91
Computer printer	87
VCR	86
Cell phone	86
Cordless telephone	83
Digital camera	75
Video game system	74
Stereo system	72
Portable CD player	72
CD burner	69
Scanner	59
Camcorder or video camera	56
Digital music player(portable MP3 player, iPod)	45
DVD burner	40
Fax machine	37
Digital photo printer	26
Digital TV/video recorder (TiVo, Replay)	20
Personal digital assistant	16
Digital/satellite radio	14
Pager	9
E-book	5

Source: HarrisInteractive YouthPulse[SM], July 7–29, 2006; n = 1,693 8–18-year-olds.

important when the object of the study is to examine sensitive topics (such as sexuality, violence, or illicit drugs), whose prevalence could vary greatly from one media format to another. Exposure to such topics may depend on the explicit and implicit access restrictions that are inherent to the media formats through which teens access information. For instance, accessing the internet at a public library versus a coffee shop, in solitude versus while hanging out with friends, outdoors or indoors, may have profound effects on what type of content will be viewed, the duration of exposure, the frequency of access, and the level of attention paid to the content.

Multiple Media Environment: Implications for Content Analysis

With the steady drop in prices of digital technologies, more and more sophisticated media equipment is finding its way into the homes of average Americans (Roberts et al., 2005). Not only are people willing to buy the latest media gadgets, but they are also likely to own multiple units within the same household. Youth aged 8–18 report that their bedrooms contain the following media: a television set (69%), a DVD player (42%), a video game system (40%), a VCR (38%), a computer connected to the internet (24%), a telephone (29%), a computer not connected to the internet (12%) (*see Table 7.2*).

The ready availability of multiple media units under the same roof suggests that media exposure has likely become a personalized rather than a family activity. In general, greater personalized time for children with media might imply that there is less parental supervision. The lack of parental monitoring of children's media habits could mean that children are more likely to be exposed to topics that are typically restricted by parents, such as sexuality, violence, and substance abuse depicted in the media. Exposure to such topics has been shown to affect children by increasing aggressive behaviors (Anderson & Dill, 2000), sexist thoughts (Dorr & Rabin, 1995), smoking (Strasburger & Donnerstein, 1999), and drinking alcohol (Austin, Pinkleton, & Fujioka, 2000). For example, Ybarra and Mitchell (2004) found that among otherwise similar youth internet users' infrequent parental monitoring was associated with 54% higher odds of being a harasser of others online.

While conducting content analyses, researchers have to take into account the discrepancies between intended and actual audiences. Although adolescents are not the intended audiences for shows and games rated for mature audiences, in reality they often have access to such content, especially when adolescent media use is not closely monitored by parents. While studying public health messages in the context of adolescents, it becomes crucial to use an audience-centered approach to document the types of content that media users are being exposed to, including content not intended for their consumption. Parents are often unaware or confused about media ratings such as the V-chip or video game ratings, thus allowing their children to play games or see television shows meant for older audiences (Walsh & Gentile, 2001). Forty-five percent of youth aged 8–12 have no parental limits put on the shows they watch (HarrisInteractive, 2006). Parental supervision of online activity falls

Table 7.2 Media in the bedrooms of 8–18-year-olds

Which are in your bedroom ...?	8–12-year-olds % Yes	13–18-year-olds % Yes	Total 8–18-year-olds % Yes
TV	70	68	69
Video game system	42	38	40
DVD player	40	44	42
VCR	40	35	38
Telephone	18	38	29
Computer with internet access	12	35	24
Computer without internet access	10	13	12
Answering machine	2	6	4

Source: HarrisInteractive YouthPulse[SM], July 7–29, 2006; n = 831 8–12-year-olds; n = 802 13–18-year-olds.

precipitously after the age of 12 *(see Figure 7.1)*. Youth aged 13–18 and older report that fewer parents know or care what sites they visit online.

Multi-tasking and Multiple Media Use: Implications for Content Analysis

Multi-tasking has become the norm rather than the exception, with count-less media messages vying for the attention of teenagers. Multi-tasking may include the use of a medium along with a non-media activity such as eating or hanging out with friends. Or it could involve multiple media use where the user is interacting with more than one medium at a time. In response to increasing multi-tasking and multiple media exposure, content analyses should shift from a media-centric approach of examining a single medium in

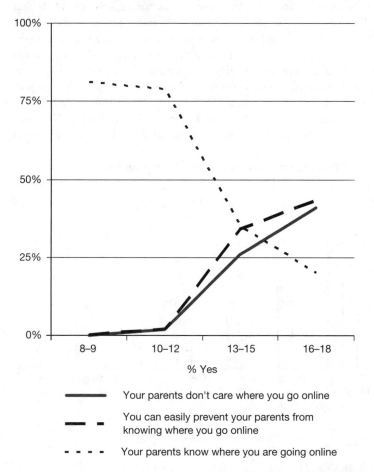

Figure 7.1 Parental involvement in 8–18-year-olds' online media consumption

Source: HarrisInteractive YouthPulse^{SM}, July 7–29, 2006; n = 1,766 8–18-year-olds.

isolation towards an ecological approach by examining the entire multiple-media environment experienced by audiences.

While watching television, for instance, youth can be experiencing a multi-tude of other media (*see Figure 7.2*). The same phenomenon can be seen online, as most young people engage in a number of activities, from reading and homework to eating and listening to music. Older youth are more adept at multi-tasking, with only 12% saying they do nothing else while online compared with over half of 8–12-year-olds (HarrisInteractive, 2006). The most common time for multi-tasking to occur in those aged 8–18 is after dinner and before bedtime (HarrisInteractive, 2006).

As human beings, we have a limited capacity for processing multiple sources of information concurrently (Lang & Basil, 1998). With a significant amount of time being spent with more than one medium, the ability to attend to each individual source is reduced. Under these circumstances, it is very likely that during multi-tasking, one medium becomes the primary activity and the other is pushed to the background as the secondary activity. Whereas old media such as television, magazines, and music are often pushed to the background for passive, habitual consumption alongside non-media activities, when new media are introduced in a household, they are consumed in a more involved, instrumental fashion (Livingstone, 2002; Neuman, 1991, Rubin, 2002).

While conducting content analytical research, the distinctions between habitual and instrumental media use might mean that differential emphases

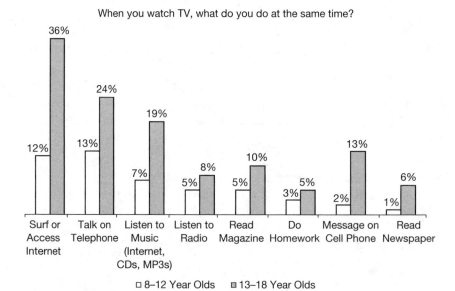

Figure 7.2 8–18-year-olds' media use while watching television

Source: HarrisInteractive YouthPulse[SM], July 7–29, 2006; n = 741 8–12-year-olds; n = 671 13–18-year-olds.

have to be placed on different types of content such as text, images, audio, and video. For instance, if magazines are browsed in a habitual fashion, then it might mean placing greater emphasis on visual content such as photographs and graphics rather than on textual information. Even though self-reports of media exposure might indicate that there is an overlap between old media use and new media use, further investigations are often required to understand the variations in the level of attention paid to each medium in comparison to the other.

Niche Segmentation and Customization: Implications for Content Analysis

Media scholars suggest that new media rarely displace old. Relatively well-established media such as music and television typically continue to be popular among audiences despite the presence of new media such as computers and video games, suggesting that audiences find new ways to fit in old media into their everyday life. Traditional media typically reinvent themselves by offering more customized and specialized content rather than mass audience generalist content (Livingstone, 2002; Neuman, 1991). Interactive television, TiVo systems, and direct-to-home television provide an increased level of customization such that viewers have the freedom to decide when they would like to view their favorite programs instead of being constrained by the prime-time slots defined by television channels. From the perspective of a media-ecological approach to content analysis, media exposure is no longer confined to a uniform "prime-time" period where everyone watches the same content at the same time in their living-room.

Upon examination of tween media behavior from 2000–6 we see that traditional media use has not declined significantly with the increase of media choices *(see Figure 7.3)*. In the case of television watching, media consumption is not in a major decline. In fact, new ways to consume television are entering the media landscape. Youth are now able to view full episodes of network shows on their computers; indeed, one quarter of tweens aged 8–12 report watching television shows on the internet (Davis, 2006; Siebert, 2006).

In response to niche segmentation and personalization, we recommend more genre-based, audience-oriented sampling techniques while conducting content analyses. Considering the high degree of fragmentation in teen media content, it may not be realistic to expect a great degree of overlap in media exposure amongst the seemingly homogeneous adolescent group of viewers. Despite the presence of adolescent-oriented niche magazines, video games aimed at teenagers, and television channels focused on youth, there is a marked lack of uniformity in the types of content that are popular within this set of people. Research indicates that older adolescents especially have a more varied, fragmented media diet in comparison to their younger counterparts. This is evident in their consumption of online media. When looking at the types of websites visited in the last week we see that tweens visit websites less often, with a much smaller variety of websites, than do teens *(see Table 7.3)*.

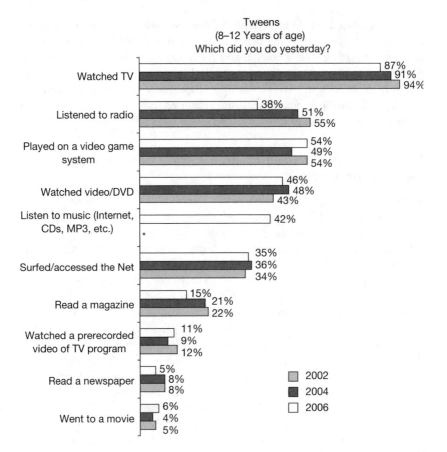

Figure 7.3 Media consumption of 8–12-year-olds in the previous day 2002, 2004 and 2006

Source: HarrisInteractive YouthPulseSM, July 18–31, 2002; n = 842 8–12-year-olds, June 4–17, 2004; n = 849 8–12-year-olds, July 7–29, 2006; n = 877 8–12-year-olds.

Note: * Did not ask the question in 2002 or 2004.

This is especially crucial when analysis of teen media content is considered. Instead of sampling from the most popular, top-selling media content viewed by this entire group, as is traditionally the case, we recommend using an audience-centered approach to content analysis such that this mass audience is further categorized into narrowly defined sub-groups. Typically these niche segments are defined demographically, based on factors such as gender, race, and social class. However, some researchers have also used media-related variables to classify youth into categories such as traditional media users, audio-visual media users, low media users, computer-savvy, music fans, and book enthusiasts (Livingstone, 2002). Once the adolescent audience has been thus segmented, a stratified sampling approach representing content popular within each of the

Table 7.3 Types of websites visited last week by 8–18-year-olds

Last week, which types of sites did you visit?	*8–12-year-olds % Yes*	*13–18-year-olds % Yes*
Kid sites	63	13
Interactive game sites	48	45
Video or computer game sites	23	30
Music sites	18	41
Search engines	13	50
Entertainment sites (to look up information, show times, etc.)	9	32
Sports sites	7	16
Community sites/Social networking sites	5	48
Celebrity websites	4	13
Library sites	4	11
School or university site	2	26
News	2	22
Car sites	2	8
eCommerce sites	2	8
Financial services	<1	7
Health sites	<1	7

Source: HarrisInteractive YouthPulseSM, July 7–29, 2006; n = 877 8–12-year–olds; n = 889 13–18-year-olds.

audience sub-categories might be more representative of media exposure as compared to simple random sampling of general teen media content. Another strategy that might be useful is to use genre-based sampling. For example, while studying teen movies, researchers could sample from genres such as action or horror that are particularly popular within this given section of the audience.

Conclusion

In summary, there has been a tremendous increase in the number of media types and the range of entertainment options available in every given medium in the last decade. In the multi-media environment, adolescents are extending media use to locations beyond the home and are learning to multi-task with more than one medium at a time. Audiences have tremendous freedom in deciding what types of content they would like to view, what times they would like to interact, and in what environments. Niche media segments focusing on small sections of the population imply that we cannot envision the audiences as one mass but have to account for differences in media choices. Technology such as on-demand TV, video games, and the internet have increased interactivity such that users of the same medium encounter totally different scenarios depending on their choices and preferences. It is against this changing, dynamic new media environment that effective strategies related to sampling, unitizing, and conceptualizations of variables in content analyses have to be developed to overcome the challenges and utilize the opportunities that such media present to researchers.

Preliminary findings from the exploratory studies presented in this chapter suggest that researchers who wish to link content with potential effects must consider audiences as differentially constructed. They must sample content accordingly (e.g., by including content that might be more heavily used by one gender or by minority teens), and orient content analytic strategies to the audiences they assume will be affected. We conclude by arguing that content analysis remains a useful tool for those interested in tracking media messages received by teens, but that researchers must nuance their methodological strategies in order to give greater recognition to the audiences' ability to shape their media environment.

References

Anderson, C. A., & Dill, K. E. (2000). Video games and aggressive thoughts, feelings, and behavior in the laboratory and life. *Journal of Personality and Social Psychology, 78*, 772–790.

Andsager, J. L., & Powers, A. (1999). Social or economic concerns: How news and women's magazines framed breast cancer in the 1990s. *Journalism & Mass Communication Quarterly, 76*(3), 531–550.

Austin, E. W., Pinkleton, B. E., & Fujioka, Y. (2000). The role of interpretation processes and parental discussion in the media's effects on adolescents' use of alcohol. *Pediatrics, 105*, 343–349.

Beasley, B., & Standley, T. C. (2002). Shirts vs. Skins: Clothing as an indicator of gender role stereotyping in video games. *Mass Communication & Society, 5*(3), 279–293.

Bucy, E. P., Lang, A., Potter, R. F., & Grabe, M. E. (1999). Formal features of cyberspace: Relationships between web page complexity and site traffic. *Journal of the American Society for Information Science, 50*(13), 1246–1256.

Cohn, L. B. (1995). Violent video games: Aggression, arousal and desensitization in young adolescent boys. *Dissertation Abstracts International, 57*, 2-B (UMI No. 9616947).

Davis, W. (2006). Fox streams prime-time shows on MySpace.com. *Media News Daily*. Retrieved October 5, 2006, from http://publications.mediapost.com/index.cfm?fuseaction=Articles.showArticleHomePage&art_aid=49119

Dietz, T. L. (1998). An examination of violence and gender role portrayals in video games: Implications for gender socialization and aggressive behavior. *Sex Roles, 38*, 425–442.

Dorr, A., & Rabin, B. E. (1995). Parents, children, and television. In M. Bornstein (Ed.), *Handbook of parenting* (Vol. 4, pp. 323–351). Mahwah, NJ: Lawrence Erlbaum.

Haninger, K., & Thompson, K. M. (2004). Content and ratings of teen-rated video games. *JAMA, 291*, 856–865.

HarrisInteractive (2006) *YouthPulse*. New York: Author.

Hong, T., & Cody, M. J. (2002). Presence of pro-tobacco messages on the Web. *Journal of Health Communication, 7*, 273–307.

Keller, S. H., Labelle, H., Karimi, N., & Gupta, S. (2002). STD/HIV prevention for teenagers: A look at the Internet universe. *Journal of Health Communication, 7*, 341–353.

Lang, A. & Basil, M. D. (1998). Attention, resource allocation, and communication research: What do secondary task reaction times measure, anyway? In M. Roloff (Ed.), *Mass communication yearbook* (pp. 443–473). Beverly Hills, CA: Sage Publications.

Lawrence, S., & Giles, C. L. (1999). Accessibility of information on the Web. *Nature, 400*, 107–109.

Livingstone, S. (2002). *Young people and new media.* London: Sage Publications.

McMillan, S. J. (2002). Exploring models of interactivity from multiple research traditions. In L. Lievrouw & S. Livingstone (Eds.), *Handbook of new media: Social shaping and social consequences* (pp. 205–229). London: Sage Publications.

Mitra, A., & Cohen, E. (1999). Analyzing the web: Directions and challenges. In S. Jones (Ed.), *Doing internet research: Critical issues and methods for examining the net* (pp. 179–202). Thousand Oaks, CA: Sage Publications.

Musso, J. A., Weare, C., & Hale, M. (2000). Designing Web technologies for local governance reform: Good management or good democracy? *Political Communication, 17*, 1–19.

Neuman, W. R. (1991). *The future of the mass audience.* Cambridge: Cambridge University Press.

Newhagen, J., & Rafaeli, S. (1996). Why communication researchers should study the Internet: A dialogue [Electronic version]. *Journal of Computer-Mediated Communication, 1.* Retrieved September 29, 2006, from http://jcmc.indiana.edu/vol1/issue4/rafaeli.html

Rafaeli, S., & Sudweeks, F. (1997). Networked interactivity [Electronic version]. *Journal of Computer-Mediated Communication, 2.* Retrieved October 5, 2006, from http://jcmc.indiana.edu/vol2/issue4/rafaeli.sudweeks.html.

Roberts, D. F., Foehr, U. G., & Rideout, V. (2005). *Generation M: Media in the lives of 8–18 year olds.* Menlo Park, CA: Kaiser Family Foundation.

Rubin, A. M. (2002). The uses-and-gratifications perspective of media effects. In J. Bryant & D. Zillmann (Eds.), *Media effects: Advances in theory and research* (2nd ed., pp. 525–548). Mahwah, NJ: Lawrence Erlbaum.

Shank, G. (1993). Abductive multiloguing: The semiotic dynamics of navigating the net [Electronic version]. *The Arachnet Electronic Journal on Virtual Culture, 1.* Retrieved October 5, 2006, from www.ibiblio.org/pub/academic/communications/papers/ejvc/SHANK.V1N1

Siebert, T. (2006). MindShare finds many kids watch TV via web [Electronic version]. *Media News Daily.* Retrieved October 5, 2006 from http://publications.mediapost.com/index.cfm fuseaction=Articles.showArticleHomePage&art_aid=49173

Smith, S. L., Lachlan, K., & Tamborini, R. (2003). Popular video games: Quantifying the presence of violence and its context. *Journal of Broadcasting & Electronic Media, 47*(1), 58–76.

Stempel, G. H., & Stewart, R. K. (2000). The Internet provides both opportunities and challenges for mass communication researchers. *Journalism & Mass Communication Quarterly, 77*, 541–548.

Strasburger, V. C., & Donnerstein, E. (1999). Children, adolescents, and the media: Issues and solutions. *Pediatrics, 103*, 129–139.

Walsh, D. A., & Gentile, D. A. (2001). A validity test of movie, television, and video game ratings. *Pediatrics, 107*, 1302–1308.

Weare, C., & Lin, W.-Y. (2005). Content analysis of the world wide web: Opportunities and challenges. *Social Science Computer Review, 18*(3), 272–292.

Ybarra, M., & Mitchell, K. (2004). Youth engaging in online harassment: Associations with caregiver-child relationships, Internet use, and personal characteristics. *Journal of Adolescence, 27*(3), 19–36.

8 Sexually Explicit Content Viewed by Teens on the Internet

Laura F. Salazar, Pamela J. Fleischauer, Jay M. Bernhardt, and Ralph J. DiClemente

Introduction

With home internet access more affordable and commonplace, coupled with the ubiquity of pornography on the web, many adolescents have easy access to content that heretofore was inaccessible. Much of this content has been deemed illegal and inappropriate to be viewed by persons under the age of 18. Not surprisingly, there has been a growing concern among health practitioners, parents, researchers, and policymakers over the potential deleterious effects that exposure to sexually explicit content can have upon the psychological and physical well-being of adolescents.

One particularly important concern is that viewing sexually explicit content frequently and repeatedly may be associated with negative outcomes related to adolescents' sexual attitudes, beliefs, and behaviors. Before relationships between exposure to sexual content over the web and outcomes can be determined, however, a clearer understanding of the nature of this content is warranted. Pornography or explicit sexual content is not monolithic in nature, but rather is multifaceted, ranging from partial nudity, to soft-core porn, to hard-core porn, and may include other qualitative characteristics such as violence, fetishes, group sex, and the use of real or implied children. Thus, it is important to identify the range of characteristics found in sexually explicit internet material and, furthermore, to classify this material into degrees of explicitness so that a sensitive and precise assessment of content-specific effects can be made.

In this chapter we present a case study of a content analysis of web pages containing sexually explicit and sexually oriented content. The case to be presented is from the Tracking Teen Trends (T3) project, a federally funded panel study of a nationally representative sample of teen internet users. As part of our case study, we will provide an overview of the decision-making process we used to construct and conduct the content analysis, and we will illustrate our rationale and method employed in identifying and categorizing the relevant content. Our procedures are outlined to assist other researchers who use content analysis to understand better the myriad facets underlying sexual content available on the web. First, we provide some background on the internet, pornography, and adolescents.

The Internet, Adolescents, and Pornography

As of February 2004, the online population in the U.S. passed the 200 million mark (Nielsen//NetRatings, 2004). Nearly 75% of the total U.S. population now has home internet access. Among the U.S. population aged 2 to 17, the access penetration rate is 78%, which represents the largest proportion of web surfers, accounting for nearly 49 million of the total 204 million U.S. web users. Survey data also indicate that in addition to the large number of teens (aged 12 to 17) online, almost half indicate that they go online every day (Pew Internet & American Life Project, 2001), and the amount of time they spend in a typical day (approximately 46 minutes) rivals the amount of time they spend playing video games (55 minutes), talking on the telephone (60 minutes), or reading books (49 minutes) (Annenberg Public Policy Center, 2000). Among older teens (aged 15 to 17), the amount of time per week spent online ranges from one hour to as much as six hours or more (Kaiser Family Foundation, 2002).

With internet use becoming an increasingly common daily activity for teens, there has been a heightened interest regarding the possible exposure to unsafe or inappropriate content online. Some estimates have suggested that there may be as many as 1.3 million pornographic websites containing some 260 million porn web pages (N2H2, 2003). Although few studies have explored adolescents' exposure to pornographic websites, some data indicate that such sites are regularly accessed by teens. One survey of a national sample of 1,500 teens 10 to 17 years of age found that 25% of the web users experienced an unwanted exposure to pictures of naked people and/or people having sex during the past year (Finkelhor, Mitchell, & Wolak, 2000). Of these exposures, 71% occurred while searching for something else and 28% occurred when opening an e-mail message; therefore, it is not uncommon for teens to inadvertently encounter pornography on the web. Of the teens surveyed, only 8% admitted to intentionally accessing sexually explicit websites but the real percentage has been estimated to be considerably higher. A study by National Public Radio, the Kaiser Family Foundation, and the Harvard Kennedy School found that 31% of teens 10 to 17 years old and 45% of 14- to 17-year-olds from households with computers report seeing a pornographic site, even if by accident (National Public Radio, 2005).

To ascertain the degree to which adolescents are exposed to sexually explicit material, the manner in which they are exposed and the types of content to which they are exposed, Cameron et al. (2005) conducted four online focus groups with teens aged 14 to 16. Boys indicated voluntary exposure, while girls indicated only involuntary exposure (e.g., mistyping a web address or clicking an e-mail link). Almost all indicated that they did not believe the content to have had any effect on them. Together, the findings from these studies indicate that many teens come across sexually explicit web content, either intentionally or inadvertently, and few believe it affects them.

The Nature of Pornography

Regardless of the channel of exposure, teens are exposed to content that holds the potential to have serious effects on psychological, psychosocial, and health-related outcomes (Harris & Scott, 2002). One major limitation of the previously mentioned research conducted with adolescents is that although the studies captured teens' exposure to sexually explicit content, they failed to identify the nature of the content or its effects. People have different ideas and opinions regarding what constitutes pornography (Thornburgh & Lin, 2002). Defining pornography would ostensibly seem to be a simple task, but definitions can be culturally, politically, or socially specific. Thus, there is no consensus. Consider that Supreme Court Justice Potter Stewart stated that he was unable to define pornography, but, to paraphrase, he "knew it when he saw it" (Thornburgh & Lin, 2002, p. 21). Also, certain researchers define pornography simply as "any sexually explicit representation" (Lillie, 2002, p. 43). Even among teens there is considerable variation when identifying what constitutes pornography (Thornburgh & Lin, 2002). Thus, instead of trying to define pornography, it may be more fruitful to characterize the many facets of sexually explicit content as objectively and accurately as possible.

Research on Sexually Explicit Content

Many researchers have attempted to characterize aspects of complex and varied sexual content through content analysis, with several content analyses specific to pornographic websites. Some of these studies have built upon earlier content analyses of sexually explicit content found in magazines, movies, comics, and television (e.g., Bogaert, Turkovich, & Hafer, 1993; Cowan & Campbell, 1994; Palmer, 1979; Scott & Cuvelier, 1987; Winick, 1985) in which images and/or text have been coded for a spectrum of sexual characteristics, including degree of nudity, homosexuality, bondage and discipline, supersexed males, nymphomaniac females, incest, and fetishes. For example, Mehta and Plaza (1997) content analyzed 150 pornographic images found via the internet on Usenet or User's Network, a collection of electronic bulletin boards (called newsgroups) organized by subject matter. The authors found that among 150 images posted to Usenet, prevalent themes emerged such as images with erect penises, fetishes, bestiality, urination, group sex, bondage, and masturbation. In addition, 15% of the sample included images with children. Expanding upon his previous study, Mehta (2001) conducted another study of 9,800 randomly selected images found on Usenet. Categories were more inclusive and identified the number of participants interacting sexually, the type of sexual penetration, oral sex, masturbation, ejaculation, homosexual sex, bondage and discipline, and the use of children. Fewer bondage and discipline images were found than in the 1997 study, but more children and adolescents were depicted. Decreases were also found for images of homosexual sex and bestiality. Similarly, Harmon and Boeringer (1997) performed a content analysis of 196 stories posted to a Usenet newsgroup and found similar results, but also found a large prevalence (41%) of the theme of non-consensual sex, which involved stories of rape, child molestation, forced slavery, and mind control.

Although detailed and informative, some of these studies have been criticized for failing to capture the different levels of explicitness and reducing a constellation of material to one overarching category, "pornography" (Sanders, Deal, & Myers-Bowman, 1999). Other researchers have suggested that sexually explicit material be placed along a continuum that comprises gradually increasing levels or degrees of sexual explicitness. For example, Sanders, Deal, & Myers-Bowman (1999) created seven categories to reflect more accurately the degrees of sexual content ranging from low (i.e., no actual nudity, with images of men and women in bathing suits or underwear) to high (i.e., images depicting unconventional sexual practices such as multiple partners).

Still other researchers assert the importance of distinguishing sexual content by the presence or absence of violence. This distinction is important because of the disturbing results from sexual violence research that have found exposure to violent pornography to be associated with desensitization toward violence against women in general, greater acceptance of rape myths, and, in some instances, sexual arousal of young men when viewing women portrayed as being aroused by an assault (Harris & Scott, 2002). Thus, it is extremely important to classify images or text depicting rape, bondage, etc. as violent sexual content and to further distinguish this content from nonviolent content.

The studies thus far that have content analyzed sexually explicit material accessible on the internet have identified various themes indicating a wide range of available sexual content. Conducting a content analysis of this material necessitates a coding scheme that is detailed and inclusive of numerous characteristics such as fetishes, bondage and discipline, homosexuality, children, and violence. Content should be analyzed with as much specificity as possible and by degrees, so that effects of the content can be more readily measured and identified.

Case Study: Tracking Teen Trends (T3)

To determine definitively the nature of the sexually explicit content being viewed by adolescents, in 2004 we began a panel study of 530 teens aged 14 to 17 who regularly access the internet from home. The goals of the Tracking Teen Trends (T3) study were to examine the associations between exposure to sexual content via the internet and health-related attitudes, beliefs, and behaviors. For obvious ethical reasons, we used an observational design rather than intentionally expose participants to sexual content over the web. To capture their *actual* web usage, we employed specialized proprietary software.

Panel Recruitment

Adolescents were recruited using a two-tier approach involving random digit dialing procedures followed by subsequent mailings of a recruitment packet. Via our telephone screening procedure, we identified 1,253 households that met study inclusion criteria. Parents or legal guardians who indicated interest in receiving more information about the study were mailed a recruitment packet (n = 1,243). To be enrolled in T3, we required both parental consent and adolescent assent and installation of the T3 tracking software. At the end of the recruitment period, we enrolled 530 teen panelists.

Content Sampling

The main goal of T3 was to first determine whether teens had viewed or had been exposed to sexual content, and if so, the level of exposure to different categories of sexual content. Only after identifying teens' exposure could we determine whether exposure was related to health-related outcomes. Before associations could be examined, however, we first needed to identify the specific web pages containing sexual content that were viewed by the teen panelists.

Previous content analyses of web pages have created sampling frames by randomly or deliberately selecting web pages identified through internet search engines (e.g., Gossett & Byrne, 2002; Ribisl, Lee, Henriksen, & Haladjian, 2003). Although this sampling approach can provide a representative sample of *available* and *accessible* web pages on the internet, a significant limitation of this sampling strategy is that it does not produce a *valid* sample of web pages viewed by an intended audience and it does not capture the frequency or level of exposure of the selected and coded web pages by the intended audience for the research. In our study, the universe of web pages from which our sample was drawn included all web pages viewed by our teen panelists from their home computer during the 30-day time period prior to the administration of an online survey. Using proprietary software from our commercial subcontractor, all of the web traffic from study panelists was routed through proxy web servers and stored. Because it would not be feasible to visually code every page viewed by the panelists, we developed a multi-stage sampling strategy to identify web pages that contained sexual content while screening out those pages that did not.

Our sampling strategy involved generating a queue of web pages that were filtered from the entire universe of web pages. Web pages were checked to determine if the web page address or Universal Resource Locator (URL) was on a list of "adult" web pages or if the URL or web page programming code contained sexually oriented words. If either of these filter checks were positive, then the web page was added to the coding queue. The decision to implement this sampling strategy was made after weighing the advantages and disadvantages pertaining to the use of sexually oriented words matched to the URL or programming code. The main advantage of this strategy was that we enhanced the sensitivity of our data capture system so that we could capture pages containing sexual content that had not been categorized previously. In this way, we were able to increase the likelihood that we did not miss or exclude pages containing sexual content. The disadvantage was that we decreased our specificity; we added a large number of pages in our coding queue that did not contain sexual content. Once we generated the sexual content queue, we implemented the second phase of our sampling strategy, which involved trained coders viewing each page in the queue to code for the presence of sexually oriented and sexually explicit content and sexual-health content as well. Essentially, this phase constituted the in-depth content analysis. The following sections describe the mechanism we used to accomplish this task and the codebook that was derived to code each web page.

Coding Interface

Given the extraordinary number of web pages that constituted our sample, a system was needed to facilitate the coding process. Our commercial subcontractor constructed a process by which all stored web pages and data could be accessed, viewed, and coded via a secure web-based interface. Each stored web page is viewable through a browser-like window that displayed embedded images retrieved in real-time over the internet as the page was displayed when the teen viewed it. Furthermore, this interface allows human coders to enter data directly into a secure database. This setup facilitates rapid coding of a large number of web pages without having to change programs or to toggle back and forth between pages.

Initial Coding Scheme

Before we began to conceptualize our coding scheme, we chose web pages as our unit of analysis mainly because we were able to capture the URL for each web page that teens viewed and we had a large number of web pages to code. Web pages are the ideal unit of analysis because in this instance we were certain that they were accessed, they can be rapidly stored and coded, and they are clear, discrete units. A methodological review of web-based content analysis recommends that researchers can and should employ individual pages as the unit of analysis whenever possible (Weare & Lin, 2000). Other possible units of analysis could be the entire website, individual images contained on a web page, or smaller chunks of text found on the web page. Coding the entire website (i.e., all pages contained within the website) was unnecessary because we wanted only pages visited by teens. Another reason we chose the web page as the unit of analysis versus using individual images or chunks of text was the question of the implications for our findings. For example, using individual images as the unit would result in having equal weights for 20 rather large detailed and graphic sexual images generated by 20 different web pages and for

20 small thumbnail images generated by only one web page. The assumption was that the former may have more of an effect than the latter.

The main research question in this study was to examine the associations between exposure to sexual content and teens' sexual attitudes, beliefs, and behaviors. To answer this question we needed to identify and categorize a wide range of sexual content. We were also interested in knowing whether panelists viewed any material containing health information and the relation between this exposure and study outcomes. Thus, we identified two overarching variables for the content analysis: health-related and sexually related web content. Once analyzed, the data from the content analysis would subsequently be linked to data collected from several online surveys that measured the teens' sexual attitudes, beliefs, and behaviors.

Coding Variables

Using previous research findings as a guide, we decided that the sexual variable should be ordinal and reflect different levels of explicitness. This decision was based on the hypothesis that as content becomes more explicit, it may have a greater impact on the attitudes, beliefs, and behaviors of adolescents who are exposed. The health variable had only two nominal levels, general health (Health 1) and sexual health (Health 2), because we did not anticipate differences in exposure to the two types of information. We defined Health 1 as any text that describes or image that depicts information on any health-related topic other than sexual health. For coding purposes, health information was defined as one or more sentences on any topic designed to educate, inform, or instruct that is related directly or indirectly to physical, mental, social, emotional, or spiritual health and well-being. We defined Health 2 as any text that describes or any image that depicts information on any sexual-health-related topic. Sexual health information included one or more sentences on any topic designed to educate, inform, or instruct that is related to reproduction, anatomy, pregnancy, safer sexual behaviors, sexually transmitted infections or diseases, etc.

It proved to be more of a challenge to decide the number of levels for the sexual variable and then to operationally define those levels. Given that we decided the content should be classified on a continuum ranging from low to high degrees of sexual explicitness, we needed to identify the optimal number of categories to reflect the varying degrees of explicitness. We were also concerned that too many categories would make the process of accurately distinguishing between levels of explicitness difficult for coders, a challenge which could compromise the accuracy and consistency of assigned codes. On the other hand, we did not want to diminish sensitivity through having too few categories.

Because we had conducted a small pilot study prior to beginning the main study, we were able to test the validity of our preliminary codebook. Initially, we began with eight levels of the sexual variable and attempted to define them so that the variable was represented by exhaustive and mutually exclusive categories. We initially created two categories for the sexual variable: Sexually Oriented (3 levels) and Sexually Explicit (5 levels). Unfortunately, during the coder training for the pilot study, it became apparent that it would be too difficult to code with this many levels and also too difficult to distinguish between contiguous levels. For example, the category we initially labeled as Oriented 2 for text was defined as having "any text that provides general advice on how to perform non-penetrative sexual activities or provides a general story or description of people engaged in non-penetrative sexual activities (e.g., flirting)." Distinguishing between Oriented 2 and the next level, Oriented 3, proved to be difficult, however. Oriented 3 was defined as "text that provides detailed advice on how to perform non-penetrative sexual activities or provides a detailed story or description of people engaged in non-penetrative sexual activities (e.g., kissing)." Furthermore, it was also difficult to distinguish Oriented 3 from Explicit 1, which was defined as "any text that describes vague or implied descriptions of the breast, buttocks, vagina, or penis of one or more person intended to arouse or excite." Thus, to increase validity and enhance inter-coder reliability, we reduced the coding scheme to six levels such that there were 3 levels for both Oriented and Explicit categories.

We operationally defined each of the six categories for both text and images. Our unit of analysis was the web page rather than each image or chunk of text found on each page. The definitions for each of the categories matched our conceptualizations of the range of material and were also conceptualized to reflect mutually exclusive categorizations to provide clear distinctions between the levels.

Previous content analyses of sexual content have included other critical aspects of sexual content (e.g., violence) that we considered. Moreover, previous media effects research has identified that some of these aspects of the content may have significant negative effects on persons viewing such content (Harris & Scott, 2002). Thus, in addition to categorizing level of explicitness, we decided to code for several of these critical aspects. We felt it important to denote the type or nature of the sexual behavior. Thus, we created an additional five categories: (1) sexual violent behavior (i.e., real or implied violence, rape, sadomasochism, etc.); (2) dehumanizing behavior (i.e., person or persons are being intentionally dehumanized, exploited, or humiliated); (3) bestiality (i.e., sexual act between a person and an actual or simulated animal); (4) group sexual behavior (i.e., three or more people engaged in simultaneous sexual activity); and (5) extreme types of sexual behavior (i.e., sexual activities including "scat," defecation, urination/water sports/golden showers, necrophilia, auto-eroticism, pregnant sex, hermaphrodites, transsexuals, or others). These five categories were not mutually exclusive and were to be used in conjunction with the six coding categories related to sexual explicitness. Therefore, depending on the web page, all five codes could potentially be checked or none at all.

Because previous content analyses also gathered information regarding the *type* of people being depicted in the images and described in the text, we felt that this information was pertinent to our study and would provide more detail. After reviewing myriad sexually explicit web pages and using previous research as a guide, we constructed the following four categories: (1) child porn—real (i.e., at least one of the participants is **clearly or explicitly** stated to be under 18 years of age); (2) child porn—simulated (i.e., at least one of the participants is **implied or pretending** to be under 18): (3) same sex (i.e., two or more people of the same gender engaged in sexual activity with each other); and (4) diversity (i.e., two or more people engaged in sexual activity with one or more of the participants being of a race or ethnicity other than Caucasian). As with the type of sexual activity, these four categories were not mutually exclusive and, if relevant, were used in conjunction with all of the other categories.

One of the main study outcomes of T3 was sexual risk behavior. Thus, we were interested in determining whether any web pages portrayed the use of condoms either in images or in text, described or promoted abstinence in messages or images, or depicted or described alcohol, drugs, or tobacco within a sexual context. We created additional codes designed to capture this type of information. Finally, we thought it would be interesting to note whether any web pages were retail sites that offered goods for sale or of if they provided opportunities for downloading or viewing video clips. Two additional codes were created for this information.

Codebook Refinements for Main Study

We used this codebook in our pilot study. Using four trained coders, we found that our definitions failed to provide clear and mutually exclusive distinctions between the contiguous categories. Thus, we decided that the coding scheme needed further simplification before beginning our main study.

Final Codebook and Codes

The challenge in refining our codebook was to assure that the range of content was captured in the coding scheme while also maintaining distinct code definitions such that there was no ambiguity in assigning codes. One major decision we made in refining the codebook for the main study was to change the category *labels* from "Sexually Oriented" and "Sexually Explicit" to the better-known ratings used by the Motion Picture Association of America (MPAA) (i.e., PG-13, R, and X). We also used the rating G to indicate no sexual content. We felt these ratings satisfied the components of a fine coding scheme, were intuitive, and could be easily adapted for our purposes but still retain basic properties that would translate well to coders' conceptualizations of the web content. Although we used the MPAA ratings as labels for our categories, we operationally defined each to capture sexually oriented and explicit content on web pages. For example, the MPAA considers many factors such as violence, language, and drug use to determine movie ratings, whereas our categorizations were defined on the basis of the presence or absence of sexual text and images and the context in which this material was displayed. For instance, despite the explicit cruelty and violence conveyed on a web page depicting Ku Klux Klan members carrying out a lynching, because this page does not match our operational definitions for PG-13, R, or X, this page would be rated G for text and G for images by virtue of the fact that there is no sexual content present.

Text Code Definitions

We defined operationally each of the codes used to categorize the text of web pages found in our queue. These new definitions were modifications from the previous codebook where we essentially collapsed the three sexually oriented categories into one (PG-13) and condensed the three sexually explicit categories into two (R and X). As previously stated, we added the code G to indicate nonsexual content. The following codes were to be assigned to the most extreme text on each web page.

A G code was defined as text that is devoid of anything related to sex either directly or indirectly (e.g., "A favorite ice cream among college students is Rocky Road"). A PG-13 code was defined as text that contains suggestive sexual references or innuendo stated in general terms (e.g., "hooking up") or words that are sexual in nature (e.g., "horny" or "check out that rack") but do not describe sexual acts or use explicit or graphic terminology. An R code was defined as text that includes general descriptions of sex acts (e.g., "oral sex" or "ejaculation") or sexual situations (e.g., "she was on the bed with her legs spread") but without provision of explicit details. An X code was defined as text that contains explicit and detailed descriptions of sex acts or body parts (e.g., "She felt the tip of his penis rubbing over her hard clitoris."). A code of "none" was also created and was defined as web pages that contained no text (i.e., page contained only images or was blank).

A major goal of creating an effective codebook is to draw distinct lines between mutually exclusive code categories. In the stages of refining our new codebook, we were confronted with challenging semantic nuances that required us to establish further guidelines to provide additional clarification in the codebook definitions so that coders could make consistent and accurate decisions. Some of these guiding principles are presented in the following section.

When it came to words associated with sex, we decided that words containing "sex" in the root of the word would be coded PG-13 because "sex" does not always refer to the act. Likewise, words surrounding the notion of having sex (e.g., "condoms") or words that represent potential outcomes of sex (e.g., "pregnancy") but do not describe a sex act would be coded PG-13. The word "porn" is short for pornography and means sexually explicit content; however, the word would be coded PG-13 if it was used by itself or without additional phrases.

Coding of terminology referring to body parts was clarified by differentiating biological descriptions and sexually explicit representations. Biological uses of the words "penis," "breast," or "vagina" that in no way refer to sexual activity would be coded G. The proper way to code "breasts" also depends on context. "Breastfeeding" and "breast cancer" would warrant a G rating, whereas a statement like "she is stacked" referring to a woman's breasts would be coded PG-13.

When words like "gay" or "lesbian" are used to describe a person in general terms but do not allude to their sexual behavior text would be deemed G. On the other hand, "gay teens get it on" uses the word "gay" in a sexual context and would warrant a PG-13 rating. Even though certain vernacular terms or derogatory obscene terms are often not intended to be oriented toward sex, the words do have a sexual derivation. Therefore, when the context was not sexual, these words and phrases would still be coded as PG-13. When the word "adult" is used in the context of "adult materials" or "adult movies" on a web page, even if those materials are not presented on the web page, it would be coded as PG-13. Similarly, "You must be 18 years or older to enter this website" would be coded PG-13 because it indicates the presence of sexually explicit material further inside the website.

With the growing number of websites dedicated to online dating (e.g., Match.com), we had to consider how to code the text of web pages related to relationships. We decided that text surrounding personals or dating would be coded PG-13 because it implies the search for an intimate partner or romantic relationship. Even though sexual intimacy is an important part of marriage, unless text described sexual aspects of married life, words like "marriage" would be coded G. The following text is an excerpt from an online journal posting found on a web page in the queue. Because this text describes the romantic feelings a person has for someone, it was coded as PG-13.

> To be blunt, I really like her. And not just in a normal way. I mean ... look at me, I can't even sleep ... I feel like if I don't do something about this girl now ... I'd live my days in complete regret. She's so beautiful. I saw a picture of her but ... that picture doesn't hold a candle to making her smile in person. I feel like such a complete faggot. I've always looked at girls as sexual targets only because I got crushed by a chick really hard a while back (on my birthday no less).

Establishing these additional guidelines for the idiosyncrasies often found in textual information was essential in aiding the coders through their coding decisions.

Image Code Definitions

Images were defined as all illustrations, animations, photos, video screen-shots, and streaming video on a web page, including those in advertisements.

As with the coding of text, we defined operationally each of the codes used to categorize the web pages based on the images found in our queue. A G code was defined as material having images not sexual in nature, context that was nonsexual, and full clothing coverage (e.g., an image of the Eiffel Tower in Paris, man in business suit reading paper). For PG-13, R, and X codes, we created definitions for both solo images (images of one person) and contact images (images of two or more people). A PG-13 code for solo images was defined as images showing partial nudity without explicit depictions of body parts such as penises, vaginas, or female breasts or nipples, and the partial or full depiction of buttocks in a nonsexual context. A PG-13 code for contact images was defined as images being suggestive of sexual acts (e.g., images of people kissing on a bed) without explicit depictions of body parts. An R code for solo images was defined as images that include non-close-up images of nudity including bare breasts, non-erect penises, and female pubic regions depicted in a sexual context and non-graphic or non-close-up self-stimulation. An R code for contact images was defined as images that include implied sexual acts between nude or partially clothed people without a graphic depiction of penetration. X codes for solo images were defined as images depicting or containing graphic or close-up images of nudity. X codes for contact images were defined as images containing graphic or close-up images of sex, including oral sex, anal sex, and manual sex including penetration with objects. A code of "none" was also created and was defined as web pages that contained no images (i.e., page contained only text or was blank).

Context

Because we do not purport to know the intention behind every image or whether a viewer would be aroused by certain images, coders were instructed to consider the level of clothing coverage (i.e., full clothing to completely nude) in addition to the context. We hypothesized that given very similar images, the context surrounding those images was important to consider when determining effects on teens. Images meeting the definition of R or X but placed in a nonsexual context may not have the same effect as the same level of images placed in a sexual context. For example, the internet site for *Playboy* magazine (www.playboy.com) contains images of completely nude women that intend to arouse and titillate its subscribers; thus, the intention is clear and the context surrounding the images is sexual. On the other hand, the website www.nationalgeographic.com may contain images of partially or completely nude people, including bare breasts and/or non-erect penises, which would warrant a code of R, but the intention is to educate and convey knowledge. Clearly, the context surrounding the images found on this particular website is nonsexual. Of course, one could imagine that some viewers could become aroused by some of the images despite the context. Indeed, before the onset of the internet, viewing *National Geographic* magazine was considered a "rite of passage" for many adolescent boys (Thornburgh & Lin, 2002). Nevertheless, images placed in a nonsexual context, although exemplifying PG-13, R, or X definitions, were coded as one level lower to account for the nonsexual context and the possibility that the effect would be attenuated.

Health and Sexual Health Definitions

All text and images on a page were assessed for health content and we hypothesized that exposure to sexual health content may have an effect on teens' sexual beliefs, attitudes, and behavior. Health content included all text and images surrounding any general-health- or sexual-health-related topics. We defined general health content as one or more sentences addressing or images depicting any topic designed to educate, inform, or instruct that is related directly or indirectly to physical, mental, social, emotional, or spiritual health and well-being (e.g., "vegetables, fruits, grains, and legumes constitute a rich source of dietary fiber"). We defined sexual health content as one or more sentences addressing or images depicting any topic designed to educate, inform, or instruct that is related to reproduction, anatomy, pregnancy, safe sexual behaviors, and sexually transmitted infections or diseases (e.g., "condoms act as a protective barrier against transmission of sexually transmitted infections").

To be coded as having health or sexual health content, web pages would contain a take-home message. For example, the text "Trojan brand condoms—why wear anything else?" does not indicate to the reader the benefits of the protective aspects of wearing a condom and consequently the page would not be coded as having health content. Conversely, if the text read "Wear condoms during sex to protect yourself from STDs and AIDS," then it would qualify for a sexual health code because it provides a higher level of knowledge related to safer sex.

Web pages with text addressing the emotional aspects of a healthy sex life would not be considered as having sexual health content. To qualify as sexual health information web content had to relate directly to disease prevention, health promotion, or reproduction.

Chat Rooms and Message Boards

Many popular websites contain chat rooms and message boards where people can post comments. Medical websites are no exception. For example, web chat rooms allow people to post health information that may or may not be accurate. Regardless of the accuracy of the information, because panelists could potentially view this information, we decided to code these pages as health.

Sexual Characteristics Definitions

In addition to assigning each web page a code for sexual content and health, pages were examined further for the presence and context of several sexual characteristics that, if present on the page, may be important to consider when examining the effects. Though many of the definitions were similar to those of the pilot study, some were modified for the final codebook and a few characteristics were added.

Sexual Violence

As a result of previous research that indicates that exposure to violent pornography has been associated with negative effects (Harris & Scott, 2002), we felt that it was important to classify whether the web page had visual or textual depictions of violence. We decided that pages coded as being R or X coupled with sexual violence would represent the highest degree of sexual explicitness and we further hypothesized that exposure to these pages may be associated with greater negative effects. Sexual violence was defined as *contact images* that depict or text that describes real or implied violence, rape, bondage, discipline, sadomasochism, or other acts intended to inflict pain or injury, with or without the consent of all participants. It is important to note that solo images would not warrant this code regardless of how victimized a person looked.

Sexual Fetish

One of three criteria used to decide obscenity cases that are brought before the courts is "prurient interest." That is, when deciding whether content is obscene and thus would not be protected under the First Amendment, judges must determine whether the content reflects a morbid, degrading, and unhealthy interest in sex, as distinguished from a mere candid interest in sex. Although the purpose of this content analysis was not to determine whether the pages viewed met the criteria for obscenity, we decided to code for sexual fetishes, as these characteristics, which may be deemed "unhealthy," could have the potential for negative effects. We defined sexual fetish as images that depict or text that describes sexual activity outside the "mainstream" (mainstream defined here as sexual activity by one person or between two consenting partners in a private location), which can include emphasis on specific acts (e.g., lactation, urination), body parts (e.g., feet), or participants (e.g., group sex, bestiality), but not include same-sex partners.

"Anthro" (Anthropomorphic) Sex or Animated Cartoons

Animated cartoons have been widely popular ever since Walt Disney created the first cartoon in 1922. We did not hypothesize that pages containing animated cartoons coded as R or X would affect teens in a different way from similarly coded pages containing actual humans; however, we felt it was important to capture this characteristic from a descriptive perspective. Anthro sex was defined as images that depict sexual activity of human-like characters or human-like characters without clothing. Images include hand-drawn or computer-generated images or other objects in human form (e.g., dolls, figurines) regardless of the resolution or degree of realism depicted.

Child Sex (Real or Simulated)

Given that our sample comprised teens aged 14 to 17, we felt that sexually explicit content containing images of teens or children may have a significant effect over and above similar images using adults because the teens in our sample may more readily identify with images of other teens. We hypothesized that viewing these images would strongly shape their beliefs and conceptions of reality. Thus, we decided to characterize whether or not the images were of teens or children. We defined child pornography as images that depict or text that describes one or more people without clothes (including both partial and complete nudity) or engaged in sexual activity where at least one of the participants is explicitly stated to be or implied to be less than 18 years of age. Use of terms like "teen," "teenybopper," "young," and "barely legal" would not be sufficient to warrant this code, as people depicted may be teenagers but of legal age (18 years old), whereas words like "child," "pre-pubescent," and "pre-teen" clearly refer to people under legal age and would warrant this code. Some pages contained text stating that "persons are 18 years old"; however, if the image suggests a minor then it would be coded as child sex. In this situation, coding decisions would be based upon examining the sexual characteristics of the person in question. For example, undeveloped female breasts could be used as a prompt for identifying pages warranting a child sex code. Because of the ethical and legal concerns regarding child pornography, we established a protocol for handling web pages that were coded as such. Each time child pornography was encountered, the website and date of coding was documented in a log and reported to the National Center for Missing and Exploited Children (NCMEC) website, http://www.missingkids.org.

MSM (Men Having Sex with Men)

We modified our original category, which was labeled "same sex," to MSM because our interest was in identifying sexual orientations other than heterosexual. Pages depicting MSM may affect teens' sexual beliefs and attitudes, especially from a developmental perspective, as these years represent a time when adolescents are forming their sexual identities. Moreover, for teens whose sexual orientations may be homosexual or gay, this type of content could have an effect on their sexual behavior. Thus, we felt it important to capture this content. Because images of two women engaged in sexual activity (WSW) does not necessarily imply a lesbian sexual orientation and because of the ubiquity of WSW images or text on most pornographic websites, we felt that coding these pages would not be an accurate representation of lesbian orientation nor would it offer additional details of interest. MSM was defined as images that depict or text that describes two or more males engaged in sexual activity with each other.

Training of Coders and Reliability Testing

Web pages in the baseline queue were coded by 11 female graduate research assistants (GRAs) aged 22 to 28. Prior to coding study pages, they were trained extensively on the codebook and the secure web-based coding interface. We trained two cohorts of coders for the baseline queue (cohort 1, n = 7, and cohort 2, n = 4). Training comprised approximately 50 hours per coder (550 person-hours) and concluded with a final coding evaluation to assess inter-rater reliability (IRR). Members of cohort 1 coded a final training queue of 500 pages; cohort 2 coders completed a 100-page queue. Responses for both queues were scored against a standard. We used the results to calculate Krippendorff's alphas for the T3 codebook's main text and image categories. The average text alpha for cohort 1 (n = 7) was .93 with a range of .90–.95. For image codes, this group's average alpha was .98 with a range of .97–.99. Within cohort 2 (n = 4) text alphas ranged from .85–.91 yielding an average of .88. Image alphas for this group ranged from .93–.98 with an average of .95.

As indicated above, the interface created by our subcontractor enables coders to view actual web pages from the queue while assigning codes. A screenshot of the coding interface can be seen in Figure 8.1. Because we wanted to ensure that coders were able to assign a code for text without the profound, often subconscious influence of images, they were instructed to read the text first without the presence of images. The coding interface enabled us to eliminate images and view only the text. Coders were instructed to scroll all the way to the bottom of the page. Although we cannot be certain that the teen panelists scrolled all the way down on every page, our experience with sexual web content suggested that the more extreme sexual text is located further down the page. Thus, to capture potential exposure, we decided to take a more inclusive approach. After coding text, images were displayed and coded. We noted early on that many pages with very explicit text often had no images or had nonsexual images and that many pages containing very explicit images often contained no text or very benign text. Thus, our decision to code each web page for both text and images versus providing only one monolithic code for each web page allows us to differentially weight web pages. For instance, we may want to give more weight to a web page containing both X-coded text and images than a page containing X-coded text but no image or a G-coded image. The rationale for this is that when adolescents view sexually explicit content, interpretation of images is more or less immediate, whereas reading text requires different processing that is more involved. One weakness in content analysis is not knowing to what degree the adolescents are reading and interpreting the text on the page. Thus, we can adjust for this with a weighted approach. Using this dual approach to coding also has implications for future analyses that will examine the effects of this content. If we coded certain pages

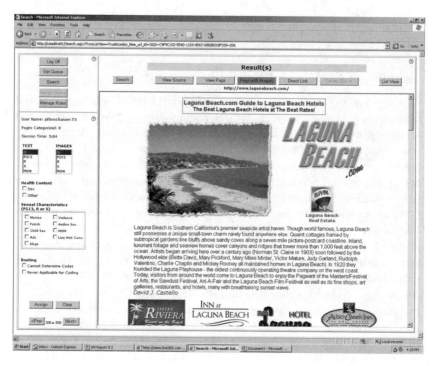

Figure 8.1 Screenshot of an actual web page in the queue

containing extreme *textual* content with G or no images as X, then we may not find statistical associations between exposure and outcomes because exposure may be attenuated.

Preliminary Results

The nature of the sexual content for web pages that were coded is presented in Table 8.1. At the writing of this chapter, we have not yet linked the web pages to teen panelists; thus, we cannot say exactly how many teens contributed to the number of sexually explicit pages in our queue. Regardless of this, in a rather short period we found that over 10,000 of viewed web pages were coded as X for either text or image. This appears to be an alarming number given the modest size of our sample. Essentially, if spread out over the full period, this number equates to over 300 X-rated web pages accessed and viewed per day by the more than 500 panelists in the study.

Our results also indicate that although proportionately not a large number of pages contained sexual characteristics that are considered outside the mainstream (e.g., fetishes, violence), it is still worth noting that in this sample, the number viewed in such a short period is still rather large. For example, over 9,000 were viewed that were classified as depicting fetishes and over 3,000 were viewed that depicted graphic sexual violence. These results suggest that

Table 8.1 The nature of sexual content in web pages viewed by T3 panelists

All coded web pages	n = 120,765	
"G" or "None"	n = 58,452	(48%)
PG-13, R, or X	n = 62,313	(52%)
Sexual content only[a]	n = 62,313	
PG-13	n = 20,572	(33%)
R	n = 13,041	(21%)
X	n = 10,337	(17%)
Fetish	n = 9,060	(15%)
Sexual violence	n = 3,465	(6%)
Anthro sex	n = 4,123	(7%)
MSM	n = 2,216	(4%)
Child	n = 536	(<1%)

Note

a Percentages do not add up to 100 (n = 62,313) because codes were assigned to both text and image and these numbers reflect the number of pages with the presence of codes in either text or image.

teens are viewing content that may hold the potential to affect their views regarding the types of sexual behavior deemed as normative.

Lessons Learned

In preparing this content analysis and determining our methodology, it was important to conceptualize sexual content as a matter of degree. If we had reduced the number of levels of sexual content and/or limited the number of additional sexual characteristics, then we would have lost a great deal of specificity and richness in describing this content. Furthermore, although we cannot say at this point whether the levels of sexual content are associated with differential effects as we have not yet linked these data to participants, we nonetheless feel strongly that measuring sexual content in this way gives us much more information and the option of performing more sophisticated analyses.

We learned through trial and error and several iterations of our codebook, however, that trying to balance degree of explicitness with an appropriate number of reliable, mutually exclusive levels was a challenge, especially given the large number of pages we were coding. Unfortunately, to enhance precision and insure reliability in our codes, we had to condense several codes and drop others that were of interest. In the end, we used only three main categories but retained many of the sexual characteristics. Even so, coding all the pages in our queue proved to be quite ambitious in terms of time and the potential effect on our graduate student coders.

Future studies could expand our categorizations and examine additional details. For example, a more manageable sample could be generated (e.g., a random sample of 400 pages from the queue) and human coders could conduct a much more in-depth content analysis that captured each instance of group sex, perceived age differences between sexual participants, the racial or ethnic characteristics of the participants, dehumanizing images or disparaging text, the presence of condoms, abstinence messages, alcohol use, substance use, the presence of age-restricted warnings, and more detail regarding the actual sex act (e.g., anal, oral, or vaginal). We acknowledge that this type of in-depth content analysis is warranted and would provide valuable insight.

One very interesting area of research that stems directly from our coding process is the phenomenon of blogs. We found that teens are generating their own content to a large degree and are putting themselves out in cyberspace: many teens are expressing their creativity and revealing their thoughts, opinions, and experiences. Based on many of the blogs viewed in our analysis, we suggest that future research examine teen blogs in greater detail. Such research could provide valuable insight into this new generation of heavy and savvy internet users.

An issue directly related to the conducting of this type of research and one that must be considered is the potential harmful effects on the coders. Our study's adult coders, despite their extensive training, were not exempt from potential psychological effects. Because we were sensitive to and cognizant of the potential effects, we took several measures to mitigate any issues that arose from working on this project.

First, initial trainings contained several team-building exercises designed to "break the ice" and familiarize coders with the extreme nature of the content so that they could begin to become more desensitized. This would allow them to perform their job comfortably and with less visceral reaction. Second, a licensed clinical psychologist was also made available to our coders, so that they could, if they chose, work through any adverse effects they were experiencing as a result of coding. The psychologist also conducted several group sessions to determine qualitatively the effects. In fact, several issues were voiced in these sessions. The main issue was that viewing sexual violence (e.g., rape) and child pornography in particular was extremely disturbing and evoked a wide range of feelings including anger, sadness, helplessness, and a sense of injustice. Coders also reported that study goals were often obscured by the overwhelming amount and nature of the content. Some coders reported shame and guilt when viewing material that inadvertently aroused them when they were coding alone. Coders who had relationship partners also revealed that these individuals could sometimes recognize changes in their behavior on days they coded (e.g., that they were more sad). Coders also expressed the fact that viewing the objectification or degradation of women caused them to question societal norms and how they, as women, were viewed by the world.

In order to mitigate potential deleterious effects on coders, additional steps were taken. Coders were not scheduled to work alone, so that in the event they viewed something extreme there would be someone else there with whom they could discuss the content. They did not code for more than 20 hours per week. Frequent breaks during shifts were encouraged and additional non-coding tasks were assigned.

Conclusion

In implementing this study, we discovered that conducting content analyses of sexually explicit content is not for the faint of heart. Nevertheless, we felt that this research was vitally important and urgently needed to address the glaring empirical gap in our understanding of teens' exposure to sexually explicit material and its impact on their sexual health. Because of recent advances in computer and web-based technologies we were able to capture and view actual web pages visited by a representative sample of teens residing in the U.S. Moreover, our categorizations and the level of detail recorded by our team of trained human coders will enable us to eventually determine with precision the effects of viewing this content. Thus, the results from this content analysis will provide much-needed information regarding the nature of sexually explicit content that is available and is being seen by teens. More important, we can then begin the task of ascertaining with confidence whether this content shapes their sexual attitudes, beliefs, and behaviors.

References

Annenberg Public Policy Center of the University of Pennsylvania. (2000, June). *Media in the home 2000: The fifth annual survey of parents and children.* Philadelphia, PA: Author.

Bogaert, A. F., Turkovich, D. A., & Hafer, C. L. (1993). A content analysis of *Playboy* centerfolds from 1953 through 1990: Changes in explicitness, objectification, and model's age. *Journal of Sex Research, 30*(2), 135–139.

Cameron, K. L., Salazar, L. F., Bernhardt, J. M., Burgess-Whitman, N., Wingood, G. M., & DiClemente, R. J. (2005). Adolescents' experience with sex on the web: Results from online focus groups. *Journal of Adolescence, 28*(4), 535–540.

Cowan, G., & Campbell, R. R. (1994). Racism and sexism in interracial pornography. A content analysis. *Psychology of Women Quarterly, 18*, 323–338.

Finkelhor, D., Mitchell, K. J., & Wolak, J. (2000). *Online victimization: A report on the nation's youth.* Alexandria, VA: Crimes Against Children Research Center. National Center for Missing and Exploited Children. Available at http://www.unh.edu/ccrc/pdf/Victimization_Online_Survey.pdf

Gossett, J. L., & Byrne, S. (2002). "CLICK HERE": A content analysis of Internet rape sites. *Gender & Society, 16I*(5), 689–709.

Harmon, D., & Boerginger, S. B. (1997). A content analysis of Internet-accessible written pornographic depictions. *Electronic Journal of Sociology, 3*(1). Available online at http://www.sociology.org/archive.html

Harris, R. J., & Scott, C. L. (2002). Effects of sex in the media. In J. Bryant & D. Zillmann (Eds.), *Media effects: Advances in theory and research* (pp. 307–332). Mahwah, NJ: Lawrence Erlbaum Associates.

Kaiser Family Foundation. (2002). *Key facts: Teens online.* Menlo Park, CA: Author. Available online at http://www.kff.org/entmedia/loader.cfm?url=/commonspot/security/getfile.cfm&PageID=14095

Lillie, J. J. M. (2002). Sexuality and cyberporn: Towards a new agenda for research. *Sexuality & Culture: An Interdisciplinary Quarterly, 6*(2), 25–47.

Mehta, M. D. (2001). Pornography in Usenet: A study of 9,800 randomly selected images. *Cyberpsychology & Behavior,4*(6), 695–703.

Mehta, M. D., & Plaza, D. E. (1997). Pornography in cyberspace: an exploration of what's in Usenet. In S. Kielser (Ed.), *Culture of the internet* (pp. 53–67). Mahwah, NJ: Lawrence Erlbaum Associates.

N2H2. (2003). N2H2 reports number of pornographic web pages now tops 260 million and growing at an unprecedented rate. Available online at http://www.prnewswire.com/cgi-bin/stories.pl?ACCT=105&STORY=/www/story/09-23-2003/0002022223

National Public Radio. (2005). Survey shows widespread enthusiasm for high technology. Available at: http://www.npr.org/programs/specials/poll/technology/

Nielsen//NetRatings. (2004, March). Nielsen//NetRatings enumeration study, February 2004. Available online at: http://direct.www.nielsen-netratings.com/pr/pr_040318.pdf

Palmer, C. E. (1979). Pornographic comics: A content analysis. *Journal of Sex Research, 15*(4), 285–298.

Pew Internet & American Life Project. (2001, June). Teenage life online. The rise of the instant-message generation and the Internet's impact on friendships and family relationships. Washington, DC: Author.

Ribisl, K. M., Lee, R. E., Henriksen, L., & Haladjian, H. H. (2003). A content analysis of web sites promoting smoking culture and lifestyle. *Health Education & Behavior, 30*(1), 64–78.

Sanders, G., Deal, J., & Myers-Bowman, K. (1999). Sexually explicit material on the Internet: Implications for family life educators. *Journal of Family and Consumer Sciences, 91*(3), 112–115.

Scott, J. E., & Cuvelier, S. J. (1987). Sexual violence in *Playboy* magazine: A longitudinal content analysis. *Journal of Sex Research, 23*(4), 534–539.

Stahl, C., & Fritz, N. (2002). Internet safety: Participants' self-report. *Journal of Adolescent Health, 31*, 7–10.

Thornburgh, D., & Lin, H. S. (Eds.). (2002). *Youth, pornography, and the Internet.* Washington, DC: National Academy Press.

Weare, C., & Lin, W. Y. (2000). Content analysis of the World Wide Web: Opportunities and challenges. *Social Science Computer Review, 18*, 272–292.

Winick, C. (1985). A content analysis of sexually explicit magazines sold in an adult bookstore. *Journal of Sex Research, 21*(2), 206–210.

9 (De)coding Television's Representation of Sexuality
Beyond Behaviors and Dialogue

Lynn Sorsoli, L. Monique Ward, and Deborah. L. Tolman

The popular notion that the provocative images of sexuality saturating television programming could push adolescents prematurely into sexual encounters is well entrenched in our society. Indeed, over the last few decades the sexual content of television has increased substantially (Kunkel, Cope-Farrar, Biely, Farinola, & Donnerstein, 2001; Kunkel et al., 2003), and adolescents are consuming media in ever larger doses (Rideout, Roberts, & Foehr, 2005). Hence, it is not surprising that understanding how television may influence adolescent sexual behavior has been identified as an important research objective. However, in order to assess the impact of television on adolescents' sexual choices, it is necessary to first analyze the programming that adolescents watch to determine the salient dimensions of its sexual content.

Historically, researchers engaging in content analyses have focused primarily on the manifest (i.e., clear and observable) content of communication exchanges, in other words, "the attributes of what we read, watch and listen to" (Anderson, 1987, p. 8). In terms of television, the primary purpose of content analyses has traditionally been to identify, document, and trace some major characteristics of the programming, from the demographics of television characters (Greenberg, 1980), to the frequencies of violent acts (National Television Violence Study, 1998), or sexual talk and behaviors (Kunkel et al., 2003).

Some researchers have used such content analysis in combination with survey data to relate content viewed to individual outcomes. This approach has been highly successful in demonstrating predictive and causal connections between viewing violence and violent behavior among adults, children, and adolescents (e.g., Huesmann, Moise, & Podolski, 1997). Recently, inroads have been made concerning the association and predictive value of viewing sexual content on sexual behaviors and attitudes—with greater exposure to sexual content predicting earlier initiation of intercourse (e.g., Brown et al., 2006; Collins et al., 2004).

However, shifting to behavior prediction from message production and processing has created complications for media studies. Attempting to relate content exposure to behaviors such as violence or sexuality demands a different approach to study design—it becomes more important to consider not only what acts or behaviors are present and who consumes them, but what the actions mean to a particular audience and how that audience is likely to engage in them. Building on Gerbner (1958), Hsia (1988) outlines the difference between macro- and micro-content analyses by noting that "micro" analysts are interested in gathering information about people so that they can make predictions about their behaviors, while "macro" analysts are looking for ways cultures manifest laws and behaviors of societies in artifacts (e.g., in mass media). In this paper, we will describe our approach to content analysis, which is designed to extend and bridge such "micro" and "macro" analytic approaches, both by documenting cultural norms and the contextual meaning of behaviors manifested in media messages *and* by using this information to make predictions about the sexual behaviors of individuals.

This chapter describes two separate projects involving analyses that code gendered themes surrounding sexual content in the media. These two projects are integrally related, largely because one project (Tolman and Sorsoli's) was designed to extend the prior work initiated during the other (Ward's), but also because we share a feminist, constructivist perspective that guides our research questions and analyses. In particular, we take a feminist constructivist approach to media analysis which challenges traditional understandings of sexuality and its connections to media consumption *and thus* the manner in which these dynamics are assessed or captured. Because we put sexual and gender norms at the center of our explorations, our approach involves a new set of questions and decisions about what and how to code television programming, including how to incorporate messages about the gendered nature of sexuality as well as the meanings of sexual behaviors and the relational contexts in which they emerge.

Past Content Analyses: Learning from Prior Research

Building on studies of media violence, many analyses of the sexual content on prime-time television have been conducted over the past several decades. Typically, television content is considered to be sexual "if it contained a depiction of sexual behavior, seductive display of the body, or an explicit or implied reference to intimate sexual behavior, sexual organs, or sex-related activities" (Sapolsky, 1982, p. 216). These studies often analyze the content of one week of prime-time network television programming (e.g., Sapolsky, 1982), counting visual (and sometimes verbal) references to various categories of physical intimacy. The current standard approach to coding and tracking sexual content includes categories designed to capture concrete physical behaviors, such as kissing or passionate embraces, as well as categories that capture broader aspects of sexuality, such as depictions of sexually transmitted diseases, pregnancy, and birth control (Kunkel et al., 2001, 2003).

Because past analyses suggested that depictions of sexuality tended to be subtle or understated (e.g., Greenberg, Graef, Fernandez-Collado, Korzenny, & Atkin, 1980), content analyses during the 90s began to explore more of the nuances in depictions of sexual situations, such as contextual elements. Several contextual elements of sexual content have been studied, including participants' marital status, the degree of explicitness of the sexual behavior, and the gender of the instigator (Kunkel et al., 2001, 2003). Although gender differences in portrayals of sexual roles, dress, or conduct have been noted (e.g., Aubrey & Harrison, 2004), few content analyses have been anchored in a perspective that explicitly privileges gender. We agree that it is important to include some of the factors that surround sexual behaviors in the media, as context offers viewers cues about how to interpret what they see. Drawing explicitly from feminist theory, we suggest that gender—including messages about the ways men/boys and women/girls should feel and act in romantic relationships—is an essential contextual factor to consider. Given the limited ways gender has been explored, we see a need for media research to focus on gender, particularly as it relates to sexuality, and to begin to incorporate the cultural meanings associated with sexual behaviors as an intrinsic part of the investigation.

Indeed, a feminist perspective highlights differences in the social conditioning men and women receive in relation to their sexuality (Castañeda & Burns-Glover, 2004), noting, for example, how sexuality is assumed and encouraged in boys and men regardless of their context, but is highly constrained for girls and women (Tolman, 2002). Both women and men receive messages that men are more sexual (Rich, 1983). Thus men are trained, even pressured (Connell, 1995), to be more active in their pursuit of (hetero)sexual experiences. As women learn to think of men as constantly motivated by their sexual drive, women are urged to be more passive and reserved. Men learn that they should want to avoid commitment, whereas women are supposed to seek it (see, e.g., O'Sullivan & Byers, 1993). These social differences are accompanied by value judgments. The double standard, which traditionally suggests that men should be rewarded for sexual exploits, while women should be reviled, if not punished, continues to be perceived among adolescents and is also present in television programming (Aubrey, 2004). Keeping track only of the number of verbal and behavioral references fails to address and may even obscure the gendered meanings of sexuality being conveyed. Outside of communication studies, the sexual socialization literature focuses on the transmission of values and other meanings that can be transmitted by parents, peers, or social institutions (e.g., Kim, 2005). These observations validate efforts to incorporate the specific and gendered messages associated with sexuality into analyses of media's sexual content. Specifically, we argue that messages about gender roles, sexual roles, and power are particularly salient in media representations of sexual behaviors, and, because they reflect societal or cultural norms, may be a new and significant approach to understanding associations between what adolescents view and how they behave.

Thematic Analyses of Television: Coding Messages About Gender and Power

From a feminist perspective, sexual content is not equivalent in what it depicts nor is it likely to be neutral. Coding television for gendered themes and values involves a directed effort to identify and analyze the presence of closely connected and theoretically salient concepts that suffuse sexual portrayals with gendered meanings. Because thematic codes rely on features that may be distributed throughout or across a television program, like other forms of contextual analysis, this type of coding can involve judgments and interpretations that should be anchored in a firm understanding of the theoretical frameworks guiding the study (in our case, this involves the gendered meanings of sexuality). Although potentially more challenging than other forms of content analysis, a more complex and meaning-focused assessment of sexual content may enhance our ability to account for adolescents' sexual choices and behavior. Accordingly, in addition to coding for sexual behaviors and talk, we evaluate the presence of a particular set of gender rules or "scripts" (Gagnon & Simon, 1973; Simon & Gagnon, 1986) that govern relationships and sexual encounters in order to include the meanings associated with sexual behaviors in such analyses.

Sexual scripts reflect the underlying social structures and conventions organizing (heterosexual) romantic relationships in our culture. Scripting theorists (e.g., Abelson, 1976) suggest that we organize the information we take in about the world into sequences of events and actions, and plan our behaviors in accordance with these prescribed hierarchies of sequences. Our specific knowledge and experiences map on to these cognitive sequences. In brief, sexual scripting theory promotes the idea that sexuality is learned from culturally available messages that define what counts as sex, how to recognize sexual situations, and what to do in sexual encounters (Gagnon & Simon, 1973); it represents a turn toward the social nature of sexuality, suggesting that it is socially constructed rather than being a rigid set of biological drives determining specific, hard-wired (heterosexual) behaviors. As Frith and Kitzinger (2001) note, "The directions aren't in DNA, but culture," (p. 210). These directions—the norms governing sexual relationships—are also present in cultural artifacts, such as the media.

In the following sections of the chapter, we first talk separately about our individual approaches to coding gendered messages in the media as two case studies. In these case studies, we illustrate our distinct theoretical and analytical approaches to content analysis. Then, we reunite our voices in a discussion designed to introduce other shared elements in our work with youth and the media that we have found to be critical for studies attempting to understand adolescent behavior in relation to content analyses. These elements include the specific ways adolescents engage with the media (i.e., viewing context and involvement) and developmental and gendered patterns in adolescent viewing choices.

Case Study 1: Analysis of Sexual Messages in Youth-oriented Programming (Ward)

Drawing from a socialization and feminist, constructivist framework, my goal (Ward, 1995) was to conduct a comprehensive, empirical coding of specific sexual themes and scripts appearing in popular prime-time programming heavily consumed by children and adolescents. Driving this study were concerns about the *types* of sexual messages dominating this programming, messages that seemed more complex than pro and con statements about premarital sex. The goal, here, was to obtain a richer understanding of the *specific* messages conveyed about sexuality, sexual roles, and sexual relationships. I chose to focus on sexuality in its broadest definition, encompassing aspects of sexual attraction, courtship, physical intimacy, and the maintenance of heterosexual relationships. In addition, I placed gender and sexual role norms at the center of my analysis, acknowledging that many societal messages about sexuality are gender-specific. My interest was in documenting both the prevalence of sexual content and the types of messages appearing most frequently.

A threefold process was enacted to accomplish this goal. First, using ratings information obtained from network officials, I recorded 3 episodes of the top 10 programs watched most by children and the top 10 programs watched most by adolescents. Second, because my interest was in the sexual messages and discourses conveyed, I chose to focus on the sexual content of the dialogue instead of the behaviors (e.g., kissing). For each episode, sexual content was extracted interaction by interaction, defined as exchanges occurring in a single location with one set of participants present without interruption by time, changes in participants or locations, or commercial breaks. Following paradigms used in linguistics and other analyses of dialogue, the units for analyzing the content of interactions were segments of dialogue presented during conversational turns. Finally, each segment of dialogue extracted for coding was transcribed and then coded for sexual content using a set of themes that I had identified as dominant sexual scripts.

The main challenge for this project was developing this coding system. I began by reading broadly to become familiar with the nature and content of dominant sexual scripts. Here, I drew heavily from social psychological literature on sexual scripts, including work by Colwill and Lips (1981), DeLamater (1987), and Marsiglio (1988), among many. From this material, I began to develop a list of messages about sexuality present in our culture. To keep this list pertinent to television content, I also watched TV programs and documented the kinds of messages about sexual roles and relationships present. Once the list began to take shape, I presented it to colleagues, who helped add to and shape the group of messages. Resulting from all of these efforts was a list of 108 messages about sexuality that are common in our culture. I then used paradigms from the psychological literature to help organize these individual messages into overarching categories. This re-organization produced 17 categories that consisted of 5 scripts specific to the female sexual role, 5 scripts specific to the male sexual role, and 7 scripts that crossed gender lines and described the following general orientations to sexuality, as defined by DeLamater (1989) and others: recreational, procreational, and relationship/marital. For example, one of the 17 categories is the centrality of sexuality to masculinity. Coding manuals included this category label as well as examples of how this larger theme is manifested in everyday interactions. These examples were designed to aid coders in identifying this larger cultural message. Such examples included the following messages and stereotypes:

- Men obtain approval from other men for sexual achievement. They boast of their sexual conquests and gain respect for sexual exploits. Men who have had multiple partners or who are "good with the ladies" are looked up to as "players" and "studs."
- Men are always ready and willing for sex. They never give up a chance to have sex. They have to work hard to keep their strong animal urges in check. Something is wrong with a man who turns down a chance to have sex.
- Men fantasize about sex and women and think about it all the time.
- Men like to make jokes about sex, dirty jokes. Men like to tease each other about sexual performance, sexual partners (or the lack thereof), and skills in attracting women.
- It's difficult for men to resist their sexual urges and to remain faithful. Young men shouldn't be expected to stay with one partner for too long; they need to "sow their wild oats" and "play the field."

Once the system had been established, I worked with two undergraduate coders to help them become familiar with the categories. We discussed the categories and their examples extensively. As part of the training, each coder was given a scrambled list of the 108 messages or examples and was asked to place them within the appropriate 17 categories. As part of the training, we also tested the system and established reliability using an unrelated set of recorded programs. Like Durkin (1985), we also coded for the presence of "counterscripts," segments that seemed to run "counter" to the categories being coded, such as the presence of female activity (versus passivity) in the sexual role. By utilizing a system of categories reflecting male and female sexual roles and/or a variety of orientations toward sexuality, this study illustrates one way of capturing the role of gender in negotiations of romantic relationships.

Although a decade has passed since this project was initiated, I can still see its merits. However, I also acknowledge its limitations, and have noticed both that some cultural sexual scripts were not included, such as messages about homosexuality, and that some categories are a bit murky, having been defined too broadly (e.g., Women are Attracted to Specific Types of Men). Still, I believe that any empirical analyses of thematic content would carry similar limitations, and offer a richness that is difficult to obtain otherwise.

Case Study 2: Adolescent Sexuality and the Media (Tolman and Sorsoli)

The Television Consumption and Adolescent Sexual Activity project, led by Tolman, is one of the first studies to investigate whether and how early and middle adolescents' viewing of sexual content in television programming is related to or predictive of their sexual beliefs and behavior. This study builds on and extends Ward's innovative work (1995; see also Ward, Gorvine, & Cytron, 2001) with the coding of gendered messages about sexuality. A central question of this study is whether using a broader and feminist conception of sexuality in coding sexual content could yield more powerful predictions of viewers' sexual behavior. This approach is based on the theory of compulsory heterosexuality (Rich, 1983) that identifies the invisible but powerful interplays between institutions (social and political) that produce and uphold male power and suppress and oppress women, in particular through regulating their sexuality. To identify how this process plays out at the individual level, we utilize the concept of sexual scripts to identify a dominant cultural (White, middle class) set of norms about (adolescent) male and female sexuality, social regulation of romantic and sexual encounters between men and women, and especially how this "heterosexual script" gives more sexual agency to men than to women (Gagnon & Simon, 1973; Hyde & Oliver, 2000).

There are separate but related scripts that guide what is appropriate feminine behavior for girls and women and appropriate masculine behavior for boys and men that constitute one integrated heterosexual script (Tolman, 2006). These scripts are defined and recognizable as deliberate verbal or nonverbal expressions of beliefs about how males and females should act in romantic or sexual situations. This set of rules for negotiating romantic and sexual relationships involves well-defined roles for players of both genders and is organized around the double standard. A young man who reveals repeated sexual encounters or conquests may be seen as quite desirable or "studly," but a young woman who has many sexual encounters may be deemed a "slut." Thematically, these scripts outline a variety of behaviors and reveal beliefs about how boys and men should act, including being actors or initiators in sexual relationships, seeing women as sexual objects, enhancing masculinity by pursuing sexual relationships, experiencing sexual feelings as uncontrollable, being demanding in sexual situations, denying any feelings or experiences that could be associated with homosexuality, and not becoming emotionally attached to women. The complementary beliefs about how females should act include being sexually passive, attracting male interest by being physically attractive, being manipulative rather than direct, setting sexual limits, appearing sexually chaste, and not having sexual desires. Clearly, taking this specific perspective shifts what we attend to as being sexual content in coding television programs.

Therefore, in addition to coding for the presence of sexual talk and behaviors based on the work of Kunkel and his colleagues (e.g., Kunkel et al., 2003), we code for the presence of messages about sexuality and gender on primetime television that are illuminated by our understanding of this "heterosexual script." Our coding system operationalizes the conception that relational and sexual thoughts, feelings, beliefs, and behaviors are scripted in ways that press boys and men to be (hetero)sexually aggressive and to objectify women and sex, and that position girls and women as being sexual gatekeepers who are interested in sexuality only insofar as it enables romantic relationships. Thus, this coding system goes beyond tracking physical sexual interactions or the sequence in which they are conducted. To develop this coding scheme, we followed Ward's lead (1995) and leverage a broader conceptualization of sexuality to encompass the contexts in which sexuality emerges, such as romance and dating. Most importantly, when we focus on the heterosexual script, the intersection between gender and power is at the center of these behaviors.

While the heterosexual script as we describe and evaluate it is what Gagnon and Simon (1973) would deem a "cultural level" script, in television programming it is in the portrayal of what they would call "interpersonal interactions" that the cultural level script becomes visible. That is, the interpersonal interactions of television characters do not involve real people but instantiations of the cultural script, the characters serving as "straw people" for portraying the script, reflecting and reinscribing it. Television programming is one of the purveyors of this dominant heterosexual script, against which individuals may compare themselves to "check" on their compliance with or on their deviation from (or resistance to) the prescribed norms.

In order to code for the presence of this "heterosexual script," we rely on an approach set forth by Gagnon and Simon (1973). If we assume that a script defines "the proper elements" for something sexual to happen and the appropriate sequencing of those elements (including what is to be done, and with whom, and under what circumstances, and at what times, as well as what feelings and motives are appropriate), specific behaviors, thoughts, feelings, and reactions are codeable aspects of the heterosexual script. We disaggregate the larger sequence of events to identify discrete messages about how to enact, manage, and negotiate romantic relationships and sexual experiences, with particular attention to the heterosexual script's sanctioned pattern for who does what and when. This approach incorporates the justification or explanation for such patterns in relation to power and gender in particular elements that illustrate the complementary roles in courtship and relationships taken by each gender.

After extensive attention to code development (see Kim et al., 2007 for more detail), our final codebook included eight complementary codes reflecting four specific elements of the heterosexual script. This set of codes reflect: (1) the sexual double standard (in which men are sexual initiators who are inherently preoccupied with sex, while women are passive sexual partners or chaste gatekeepers); (2) gender differences in courtship strategies (men are protectors and providers while women court indirectly); (3) attitudes toward commitment (men avoid commitment, while women prioritize relationships above all else); and (4) attitudes toward homosexuality (men must reject and distance themselves from any suggestion of homosexuality, while women's being sexual with other women is arousing for men). Once our codebook was finalized, our coders were trained on episodes of shows not contained in our sample. During the training process, each episode was coded independently by multiple coders. Coders met, discussed, and resolved any discrepancies. At each meeting, coders calculated the percentage of agreement in order to assess reliability. Coding of the sample was conducted only after all coders had established reliability averaging greater than 80% agreement for all codes. Because of the complexity of the coding scheme, this process took several months; also because of this complexity, we decided that the codes in every show should be verified by a second coder to ensure against coder "drift" and to enhance the credibility of our findings.

Based on surveys of 273 eighth grade, 144 ninth grade, and 430 tenth grade students in two diverse school districts in the northeastern United States, we selected the top 25 programs in the 2001–2 season that participants reported watching regularly (i.e., at least a few times per month) and coded three episodes of each program. Like Ward (1995), our unit of analysis is the interaction. Within interactions we coded for either dialogue or behaviors that reflected the presence of one of these eight codes. This coding system reveals the pervasiveness of the dominant cultural heterosexual script in prime-time network programming viewed by adolescents. Because our work developing our codebook for the heterosexual script highlighted the presence of certain kinds of "counterscripted" behaviors and dialogue, we have developed a second codebook that will allow us to explore the ways that this programming may portray alternatives to the heterosexual script.

As is evident, many of the specifics of the heterosexual script overlap with the sexual themes and scripts identified by Ward (1995), and to a certain extent with the sequence identified by Pardun (2002) in her qualitative analysis of the rules for romance present in movies popular with teens. Our focus, however, is on the systemic nature of the overall dominant cultural script that makes it difficult for girls and women to assert their feelings and desires (Thompson, 1995; Tolman, 2002) and also for boys to express fears, reservations, or desires about their sexuality that do not conform (Kimmel, 2005). In our project, we use standard coding principles developed by Kunkel and his colleagues, counting instances in which specific elements of the heterosexual script are invoked, enacted, followed, or triggered. In coding programs for the presence of elements of the heterosexual script, we are coding the *meaning* of sexual and relational behavior, not just that the behavior occurred. This system of coding necessarily includes context of such behaviors (or cognitions or emotions), because meaning is infused by contexts.

Documenting the extent to which the heterosexual script infuses sexual content in the media is particularly important when studying a population of adolescents. For adolescents, gender ideologies—beliefs about good, normal, and appropriate behaviors for males and females—play an important role in shaping behaviors and attitudes (Impett, Schooler & Tolman, 2006; Sorsoli, Porche & Tolman, 2005; Tolman, 2002, 1999; Tolman, Impett, Tracy & Michael, 2006; Tolman & Porche, 2000). For example, the more strongly a young girl endorses conventional femininity ideology, the less likely she is to believe she can be efficacious in her use of contraception (Impett, Schooler, &

Tolman, 2006). It is likely that evaluating sexual content through this uniquely gendered lens will be useful, particularly given the fact that television rarely emphasizes sexual risks and responsibilities (Kunkel et al., 2003). Including these kinds of approaches to coding in a content analysis could be critical because they include information about context and capture the unifying structure of the messages rather than merely the existence of particular sexual behaviors. Indeed, it may be the ways these behaviors are prescribed that makes them meaningful or relevant.

Relating to the Media: Understanding Viewing Context and Involvement

Not only does our feminist approach to media analysis shift our attention to gendered messages in television content, it also encourages us to foreground the relational contexts in which viewers exist, including who viewers watch with and the relationships they form with the media itself. Indeed, we argue that exposure level is only one avenue through which media use may shape the behaviors of individual viewers, and that content analysis alone does not account for viewing context or viewer engagement. Although cultivation theory (Gerbner, Gross, Morgan, & Signorielli, 1986) posits that attitudes and expectations about the world are gradually derived from the media as viewing time accumulates, certain aspects of the experience of viewing may not be related to the sheer amount of exposure, or even to the frequency of viewing particular content, but to the way that content is received and "digested." That is, it may be more than a simple matter of "how much" and "how often" viewers are exposed to sexual behaviors on television, but instead may be a consequence of who adolescents watch with, where, and why.

Adolescents frequently watch TV with friends or significant others (Greenberg & Linsangan, 1993). As adolescents mature, the influence of peers may begin to outstrip that of parents; watching with peers and romantic partners has been shown to influence both the amount of television watched by adolescents and the sexual content of what is watched (Greenberg & Linsangan, 1993). Understanding these kinds of developmental differences in media use is important because the context in which media exposure occurs may shape the way in which the content is received; similarly, viewing context may mediate or moderate the associations between exposure and subsequent behaviors or attitudes. Thus, on our surveys, we have included questions about who adolescents watched and talked with before, during, and after watching television. Our examination of relational viewing contexts has revealed that girls who watch with boyfriends report more sexual experience (Sorsoli, Porche, Collins, & Tolman, 2003), and that adolescents whose parents watched or talked with them about television had both greater self-esteem and less sexual experience (Schooler, Kim, & Sorsoli, in press). Understanding viewing context can thus help researchers make better decisions about what content to analyze and how to examine its impact for various groups of adolescents.

In addition to thinking about viewers in a relational context of viewing, our constructivist perspective highlights the active, sense-making role of the viewer in general (Ward, 2002), encouraging us to consider diverse ways in which one can engage portrayals of sexuality. Children and teenagers often get conflicting information about sexuality from the sources around them. Indeed, some teens might approach the media deliberately as a source of information about sexuality to fill this void; for others, exposure to sexual content may be purely incidental. Because of these complexities in viewing motivations, associations between sexual content viewed and teens' subsequent sexual attitudes and behavior may vary according to the initial reasons for choosing to view that content. Prior research on media effects has explored the importance of the motivation underlying media use (e.g., Haridakis & Rubin, 2003) and the ways these differing strategies for use may be related to individual outcomes.

We conceptualize viewing involvement as a broad construct that includes a viewer's motivation or expected uses of television (i.e., whether it is for entertainment, education, or company); how actively he or she attends to the media; how accurate he or she perceives the media's portrayal of reality to be; and how closely he or she identifies with what is seen. Previous research has suggested that more actively involved viewers—those who view television with specific motives and intentions, who identify more strongly with what they see, and believe these portrayals are more realistic—are more likely to be affected by its content (e.g., Potter, 1986; Rubin, 2002). Ward's past studies provide solid support for this assumption, finding that dimensions of viewer involvement are more strongly related to sexual behaviors than is strict measurement of viewing amounts (e.g., Ward, 2002; Ward & Friedman, 2006). Although performing content analysis provides essential information about the precise nature of the media content to which adolescents are exposed, attending to the context in which the content is viewed and variances in the ways of engaging with media add another important layer of information.

Clusters of Viewers: Analyzing Adolescent Media Use Patterns

There is a vast array of media to which adolescents are exposed on a daily basis. Some media usage is fairly common among all teens, such as exposure to popular songs, television programs, and movies. Other media use is more specialized, reflecting a developing sense of identity and a desire to be unique (Brown, 2000). Brown refers to these differing consumption patterns as a "media diet," which is a reference to the choices adolescents make about what media they will "consume" (Brown, 2000). We know that some of these program preferences clearly differ by gender as well as race (Brown & Pardun, 2004; Brown, Steele, & Walsh-Childers, 2002; Greenberg & Linsangan, 1993). The few studies that have examined whether gender differences in viewing preferences are associated with attitudes and behaviors have produced mixed results:

while some find no differences (Collins et al., 2004), other studies find that breaking adolescents into groups by gender and examining the exposure to different genres of programming can yield stronger or different results (Ward, 2003). Because our theoretical framework recognizes that sexual content carries different meanings and consequences for girls and boys, we examine all associations separately for girls and boys when exploring links between media content and behavior.

Examining gender differences is particularly crucial in developmental studies because differences in viewing patterns may be even stronger in adolescence than in adulthood. Not only is adolescence the time when biological changes are creating wide separations between boys and girls, it is at this time when adolescents are most likely to hold most stringently to behavioral rules or norms. Because media use can vary by location, gender, and race, a content analysis that does not pay attention to these variables in their study population may miss important nuances of the viewing behaviors specific to that population. Overall, although examining associations separately by gender is a good initial solution, the differences in media diets among groupings of adolescents illustrate that media exposure is likely to vary tremendously across individuals. In essence, rather than exploring the influence of media as a whole, as if all individuals consume the same programs, and as if the effects of media use are monolithic, we feel that researchers who utilize content in their analyses should attend to *differences* in media use and *preferences* in particular study populations, as well as clusters of viewers that may exist, as this will more accurately represent the reality of these particular adolescent experiences.

The existence of particular groupings of adolescents (i.e., clusters or cliques of teens with the same viewing habits) can be explored statistically through the use of person-centered statistical methods such as cluster analysis or latent variable mixture modeling (Muthén, 2001) that allow nuances beyond gender groupings to materialize. The strength of a latent variable mixture modeling approach is that it can be used to infer the presence of hidden subpopulations for whom the elements of a model are differentially interrelated, thus preserving essential qualitative differences in experience while still utilizing the statistical power available in a large sample. For feminist researchers, this technique is especially beneficial: experiential disparities, both *within* as well as *across* demographic groups that have traditionally been of interest (i.e., race/ ethnicity, gender, social class) can be examined (see Tracy & Sorsoli, 2004). Clusters have been found among adolescents that illustrate the importance of both age and gender in viewing decisions (see Schooler, Sorsoli, Kim, & Tolman, 2006 for more detail). Empirical evidence also suggests that because the effect of media use on adolescent sexual behavior may be either mediated or moderated by other factors (Brown & Newcomer, 1991; Peterson, Moore, & Furstenberg, 1991; Schooler, Ward, Merriwether, & Caruthers, 2004; Ward, 2002), it seems likely that not only will different groups of adolescents have different media "diets" but also that sexual content will affect different groups of adolescents in different ways; these important differences deserve continued examination.

Conclusion

Building on a rich history of content analysis, media studies have slowly begun to expand their ways of thinking about and analyzing content exposure. Although it is possible to conduct successful studies by simply categorizing and counting portrayals of discrete behaviors and relating them to real-world behaviors, many studies are now exploring the nuances of media content in an effort to unravel, for example, the ways the association between content and behavior may be moderated or mediated by certain contextual elements in media content, certain motives for viewing, particular viewing contexts, or engagement or identification with individual characters. Paying close attention to the nuances in content seems particularly necessary when attempting to link viewing practices to complex social behaviors such as sexuality.

The goal of this chapter was to present a theoretical perspective for content analysis research and to illustrate how our perspective affected what we examined and how we examined it. The particular choices we have made about interpreting content stem from our backgrounds as feminist constructivist researchers. This background has influenced every step of our research: from what we consider salient content for coding and the ways we interpret that content, to the other factors we have chosen to consider alongside our content analyses and the ways we conduct our statistical analyses. As developmental psychologists, we view adolescence as a critical time for understanding the potential effects of media use; our choice to incorporate viewing contexts and involvement and to explore viewing patterns in our studies results from considering media in the specific context of adolescent development. We use information about these aspects of media use to inform our work with content analyses and have found that they can provide critical insight into understandings of adolescent viewing and sexual behaviors.

From our perspective, it has been particularly informative to think about sexual content from a perspective that incorporates understandings of gender and power. However, further research is needed to establish how watching sexual portrayals on television may also shape girls' and boys' understandings of their roles in romantic relationships (Ward, 2003) and how identification with these roles may relate differentially to health-related outcomes. As the sexual content on television and other forms of media continues to increase, it is also necessary for us to think about the ways younger and more ethnically diverse audiences relate to the gendered and sexual content they consume, and to conduct more broad longitudinal studies of media use. Finally, although it is difficult for media researchers to "keep up" with the pace at which media use changes, we must follow the lead of those considering sexual content across many different types of media (Brown et al., 2006).

References

Abelson, R. P. (1976). Script processing in attitude formation and decision making. In J. Carroll and J.W. Payne (Eds.), *Cognition and social behavior* (pp. 33–46). Hillsdale, NJ: Lawrence Erlbaum.

Anderson, J. A. (1987). *Communication research: Issues and methods.* New York: McGraw-Hill Book Company.

Aubrey, J. S. (2004). Sex and punishment: An examination of sexual consequences and the sexual double standard in teen programming. *Sex Roles, 50*(7–8), 505–514.

Aubrey, J., & Harrison, K. (2004). The gender-role content of children's favorite television programs and its links to their gender-related perceptions. *Media Psychology, 6*, 111–146.

Brown, J. D. (2000). Adolescents' sexual media diets. *Journal of Adolescent Health, 27*, 35–40.

Brown, J. D., L'Engle, K. L., Pardun, C. J., Guo, G., Kenneavy, K., & Jackson, C. (2006). Sexy media matter: Exposure to sexual content in music, movies, television, and magazines predicts black and white adolescents' sexual behavior. *Pediatrics, 117*(4), 1018–1027.

Brown, J. D., & Newcomer, S. F. (1991). Television viewing and adolescents' sexual behavior. *Journal of Homosexuality, 21*(1/2), 77–91.

Brown, J. D., & Pardun, C. J. (2004). Little in common: Racial and gender differences in adolescents' television diets. *Journal of Broadcasting & Electronic Media*, 48, 266–279.

Brown, J. D., Steele, J. R., & Walsh-Childers, K. (2002). *Sexual teens, sexual media: Investigating media's influence on adolescent sexuality.* Mahwah, NJ: Lawrence Erlbaum Associates.

Castañeda, D. & Burns-Glover, A. (2004). Gender, sexuality, and intimate relationships. In M. A. Paludi (Ed.), *Praeger guide to the psychology of gender* (pp. 69–91). Westport, CT: Praeger Publishers/Greenwood Publishing Group, Inc.

Collins, R. L., Elliot, M. N., Berry, S. H., Kanouse, D. E., Kunkel, D. K., Hunter, S. B., & Miu, A. (2004). Watching sex on TV predicts adolescent initiation of sexual behavior. *Pediatrics, 114*(3), e280–e289.

Colwill, N., & Lips, H. M. (1981). Power and sexuality. In H. Lips (Ed.), *Women, men, and the psychology of power* (pp. 109–130). Englewood Cliffs, NJ: Prentice Hall.

Connell, R. W. (1995). *Masculinities.* Berkeley: University of California Press.

DeLamater, J. (1987). Gender differences in sexual scenarios. In K. Kelley (Ed.), *Females, males, and sexuality: Theories and research* (pp. 127–139). Albany, NY: SUNY Press.

DeLamater, J. (1989). The social control of human sexuality. In K. McKinney & S. Sprecher (Eds.), *Human sexuality: The societal and interpersonal context* (pp. 30–62). Norwood, NJ: Ablex.

Durkin, K. (1985). *Television, sex roles, and children: A developmental social psychological account.* Philadelphia, PA: Open University Press.

Frith, H. & Kitzinger, C. (2001). Reformulating sexual script theory: Developing a discursive psychology of sexual negotiation. *Theory & Psychology*, 11(2), 209–232.

Gagnon, J. H. & Simon, W. (Eds.). (1973). *Sexual conduct: The social sources of human sexuality.* Chicago, IL: Aldine Publishing Co.

Gerbner, G. (1958). On content analysis and critical research in mass communications. *Audiovisual Communication Review, 6*(3), 85–108.

Gerbner, G., Gross, L., Morgan, M., & Signorielli, N. (1986). Living with television: The dynamics of the cultivation process. In J. Bryant & D. Zillman (Eds.), *Perspectives on media effects* (pp. 17–40). Hillsdale, NJ: Lawrence Erlbaum Associates.

Greenberg, B. S. (1980). *Life on television: A content analysis of U.S. TV drama.* Norwood, NJ: Ablex.

Greenberg, B., Graef, D., Fernandez-Collado, C., Korzenny, F., & Atkin, C. (1980). Sexual intimacy on commercial TV during prime time. *Journalism Quarterly, 57,* 211–216.

Greenberg, B. S., & Linsangan, R. (1993). Gender differences in adolescents' media use, exposure to sexual content and parental mediation. In B. S. Greenberg, J. D. Brown & N. L. Buerkel-Rothfuss (Eds.), *Media, sex and the adolescent* (pp. 134–144). Cresskill, NJ: Hampton Press, Inc.

Haridakis, P. M., & Rubin, A. M. (2003). Motivation for watching television violence and viewer aggression. *Mass Communication & Society, 6*(1), 29–56.

Hsia, H. J. (1988). *Mass communications research methods: A step-by-step approach.* Hillsdale, NJ: Lawrence Erlbaum Associates.

Huesmann, L. R., Moise, J. F., & Podolski, C. (1997). The effects of media violence on the development of antisocial behavior. In D. Stoff, J. Breiling & J. D. Maser (Eds.), *Handbook of antisocial behavior* (pp. 181–193). New York: John Wiley & Sons.

Hyde, J. S. & Oliver, M. B. (2000). Gender differences in sexuality: Results from meta-analysis. In C. B. Travis & J. W. White (Eds.), *Sexuality, society, and feminism* (pp. 57–77). Washington, DC: American Psychological Association.

Impett, E. A., Schooler, D., & Tolman, D. L. (2006). To be seen and not heard: Femininity ideology and girls' sexual health. *Archives of Sexual Behavior, 35*(2), 131–144.

Kim, J. L. (2005). Sexual socialization among Asian Americans: A multi-method examination of cultural influences. Unpublished doctoral dissertation, University of Michigan, Ann Arbor.

Kim, J. L., Sorsoli, [C.] L., Collins, K., Zybergold, B., Schooler, D., & Tolman, D. L. (2007). From sex to sexuality: Exposing the heterosexual script on primetime network television. *Journal of Sex Research, 44*(2), 145–157.

Kimmel, M. (2005). What about the boys? In H. S. Shapiro and D. E. Purpel (Eds.), *Critical social issues in American education: Democracy and meaning in a globalizing world* (3rd ed., pp. 219–225). Mahwah, NJ: Lawrence Erlbaum Associates.

Kunkel, D., Cope-Farrar, K., Biely, E., Farinola, W., & Donnerstein, E. (2001). *Sex on TV: II. A biennial report to the Kaiser Family Foundation.* Menlo Park, CA: Kaiser Family Foundation.

Kunkel, D., Biely, E., Eyal, K., Cope-Farrar, K., Donnerstein, E., & Fandrich, R. (2003). *Sex on TV: III. A biennial report to the Kaiser Family Foundation.* Menlo Park, CA: Kaiser Family Foundation.

Marsiglio, W. (1988). Adolescent male sexuality and heterosexual masculinity: A conceptual model and review. *Journal of Adolescent Research, 3,* 85–103.

Muthén, B. (2001). Latent variable mixture modeling. In G.A. Marcoulides & R.E. Schumaker (Eds.), *New developments and techniques in structural equation modeling* (pp. 1–33). Mahwah, NJ: Lawrence Erlbaum Associates.

National television violence study (Vol. 3). (1998). Thousand Oaks: Sage Publications.

O'Sullivan, L. F., & Byers, E. S. (1993). Eroding stereotypes: College women's attempts to influence reluctant male sexual partners. *Journal of Sex Research, 30*(3), 270–282.

Pardun, C. J. (2002). Romancing the script: Identifying the romantic agenda in top-grossing movies. In J. D. Brown, J. R. Steele, & K. Walsh-Childers (Eds.), *Sexual teens, sexual media: Investigating media's influence on adolescent sexuality* (pp. 211–225). Mahwah, NJ: Lawrence Erlbaum Associates.

Pardun, C. J., L'Engle, K. L., & Brown, J. D. (2005). Linking exposure to outcomes: Early adolescents' consumption of sexual content in six media. *Mass Communication and Society, 8*(2), 75–91.

Peterson, J., Moore, K., & Furstenberg, F. (1991). Television viewing and early initiation of sexual intercourse: Is there a link? *Journal of Homosexuality, 21*(1–2), 93–118.

Potter, W. J. (1986). Perceived reality and the cultivation hypothesis. *Journal of Broadcasting and Electronic Media, 30,* 159–174.

Potter, W. J., & Smith, S. (2000). The context of graphic portrayals of television violence. *Journal of Broadcasting & Electronic Media, 44*(2), 301–323.

Rich, A. (1983). Compulsory heterosexuality and lesbian existence. In A. Snitow, C. Stansell, & S. Thompson (Eds.), *Powers of desire: The politics of sexuality* (pp. 177–205). New York: Monthly Review Press.

Rideout, V., Roberts, D. F., & Foehr, U. G. (2005). *Generation M: Media in the lives of 8- to 18-year-olds.* Menlo Park, CA: Kaiser Family Foundation.

Rubin, A. M. (2002). Media uses and effects: A uses-and-gratifications perspective. In J. Bryant & D. Zillman (Eds.), *Media effects: Advances in theory and research* (2nd ed., pp. 525–548). Mahwah, NJ: Lawrence Erlbaum Associates.

Sapolsky, B. S. (1982). Sexual acts and references on prime-time TV: A two-year look. *Southern Speech Communication Journal, 47,* 212–227.

Schooler, D., Kim, J. L., & Sorsoli, L. (in press). Setting rules or sitting down: Parental mediation of television consumption and adolescent self and sexuality. *Sexuality Research and Social Policy.*

Schooler, D., Sorsoli, L., Kim, J. L., & Tolman, D. (2006). Beyond exposure: A person-oriented approach to adolescent media diets. Manuscript in preparation.

Schooler, D., Ward, L. M., Merriwether, A., & Caruthers, A. (2004). Who's that girl: Television's role in the body image development of young White and Black women. *Psychology of Women Quarterly, 28,* 38–47.

Simon, W., & Gagnon, J. H. (1986). Sexual scripts: Permanence and change. *Archives of Sexual Behavior, 15*(2), 97–120.

Sorsoli, L., Porche, M., Collins, K., & Tolman, D. L. (2003). The one about sexual content and relational context. Paper presented at the Society for Research on Adolescence, Tampa, FL, April, 2003.

Sorsoli, [C.] L., Porche, M. V., & Tolman, D. L. (2005). "He left her for the alien." Girls, television and sex. In E. Cole & J. Daniel (Eds.), *Featuring females: Feminist analyses of the media.* Washington, DC: APA Press.

Thompson, S. (1995). *Going all the way: Teenage girls' tales of sex, romance and pregnancy.* New York: Hill and Wang.

Tolman, D. L. (1999). Femininity as a barrier to positive sexual health for adolescent girls. *Journal of the American Medical Women's Association, 54*(3), 133–138.

Tolman, D. L. (2002). *Dilemmas of desire: Teenage girls talk about sexuality.* Cambridge, MA: Harvard University Press.

Tolman, D. L. (2006). In a different position: Conceptualizing female adolescent sexuality development within compulsory heterosexuality. In L. M. Diamond (Ed.), *Rethinking positive adolescent female sexual development: New directions for child and adolescent development, 112* (pp. 71–89). San Francisco: John Wiley & Sons, Inc.

Tolman, D. L., Impett, E. A., Tracy, A. J., & Michael, A. (2006). Looking good, sounding good: Femininity ideology and girls' mental health. *Psychology of Women Quarterly, 30*(1), 85–95.

Tolman, D. L., & Porche, M. V. (2000). The adolescent femininity ideology scale: Development and validation of a new measure for girls. *Psychology of Women Quarterly, 24*(4), 365–376.

Tracy, A. J., & Sorsoli, L. (2004). *A quantitative analysis method for feminist researchers: A gentle introduction.* Wellesley Centers for Women Working Paper no. 414. Wellesley, MA: Wellesley Centers for Women.

Ward, L. M. (1995). Talking about sex: Common themes about sexuality in the prime-time television programs children and adolescents view most. *Journal of Youth and Adolescence, 24*(5), 595–615.

Ward, L. M. (2002). Does television exposure affect emerging adults' attitudes and assumptions about sexual relationships? Correlational and experimental confirmation. *Journal of Youth and Adolescence, 31*, 1–15.

Ward, L. M. (2003). Understanding the role of entertainment media in the sexual socialization of American youth: A review of empirical research. *Developmental Review, 23*, 347–388.

Ward, L. M., & Friedman, K. (2006). Using TV as a guide: Associations between television viewing and adolescents' sexual attitudes and behavior. *Journal of Research on Adolescence, 16*, 133–156.

Ward, L. M., Gorvine, B., & Cytron, A. (2001). Would that really happen? Adolescents' perceptions of sexual relationships according to prime-time television. In J. Brown, K. Walsh-Childers, & J. Steele (Eds.), *Sexual teens, sexual media: Investigating media's influence on adolescent sexuality* (pp. 95–124). Mahwah, NJ: Lawrence Erlbaum Associates.

10 Linking Media Content to Media Effects

The RAND Television and Adolescent Sexuality Study

Rebecca L. Collins, Marc N. Elliott, and Angela Miu

Introduction

Media effects research has the goal of linking exposure to media with changes in attitudes, beliefs, or behavior. In some cases, effects may be thought to stem directly from the use of a medium, rather than its content. For example, television viewing may substitute for more physically active pursuits, leading to weight problems among children who are heavier viewers (Andersen, Crespo, Bartlett, Cheskin, & Pratt, 1998; Hancox, Milne, & Poulton, 2004). For the most part, however, research on media effects has focused on the effects of message content. The most studied example of this is the proposed effect of viewing television- or film-based violence on aggression. Through hundreds of studies and decades of work, it is now well established that, under certain conditions, exposure to violent content can lead to greater acceptance of violence and increased aggressive behavior (American Psychological Association, 1993; Paik & Comstock, 1994). The hypotheses tested by the RAND Television and Adolescent Sexuality (TAS) study are of a similar nature, examining whether exposure to television portrayals of sexual content influences adolescents' sexual attitudes and behavior.

A key period of sexual exploration and development occurs during adolescence, as youth begin to consider which sexual behaviors are enjoyable, moral, and appropriate for their age group. Many will become sexually active during this period of life; currently, 47% of high school students in the U.S. have had sexual intercourse (CDC, 2006). There are good scientific reasons to believe that television may be a key contributor to this developmental process. The average youth watches about three hours of television daily (Roberts, Foehr, Rideout, & Brodie, 2003), and most programs (other than sports and news) are laden with sexual content (Kunkel, Eyal, Finnerty, Biely, & Donnerstein, 2005). Entertainment programs typically portray sex as casual and risk free (Kunkel et al., 2005). Theories of media effects predict that under such conditions, youth who view more sexual content will perceive sexual activity more positively and casual sex as more appropriate, and may become sexually active sooner.

Social learning theory (Bandura, 1986), in particular, argues that people learn how to behave through observation of others. According to the theory, observation of others' actions and beliefs can be mediated through television (Bandura, 1986). Through social learning, television viewers acquire information about possible actions, about who engages in them, and about the contexts in which they are appropriate. This information is applied to oneself when the characters observed resemble the viewer, or they possess valued characteristics such as attractiveness or social status. The "lessons" observed are put into practice when they are triggered by situational cues in everyday life, that is, when viewers encounter situations similar to those they have seen on television. Finally, socially learned behaviors are acted upon only if observation has taught the viewer that he or she will be rewarded for the behavior. Thus, specific aspects of media content, not just whether it is sexual or violent, determine its effects. For example, watching violent television is most likely to produce aggressive behavior among viewers when the portrayed violence is enacted by a similar or attractive person, and when it is portrayed without punishment of the perpetrator or serious injury to the victim (see Bushman & Huesmann, 2001, for a review).

Applying social learning to the effects of sexual content exposure suggests that adolescents who see more portrayals in which sex (1) is normative among individuals in the kinds of relationships that youth typically have (e.g., short-term, casual dating relationships), and (2) seldom results in negative outcomes (e.g., unplanned pregnancies or sexually transmitted diseases) will have sex sooner. In contrast, youth who see very little casual sex on television, or who most often see it portrayed as having negative consequences, should in fact be less likely to engage in sexual activity. However, the general preoccupation with sex among television characters, together with the dearth of negative consequences portrayed, led TAS researchers to the general prediction that earlier initiation of sexual intercourse would occur among youth with greater exposure to sex on television.

The TAS study used field methods of data collection in order to test this hypothesis. More specifically, TAS researchers used survey techniques in conjunction with content analysis to test for effects of television sexual content on sexual behavior. While most survey-based research on television effects has looked only at the overall amount of television viewed (e.g., average hours per week) as a predictor of behavior change, we went a step beyond this by determining the actual content of youths' television diets. We asked about the specific programs that each TAS participant watched and how frequently they watched them. Using content analysis, we then quantified the average amount of sexual content in an episode of each of those programs. By multiplying the viewing-frequency for each program by the amount of sexual content in that program and summing across all programs, we produced a measure of sexual content exposure reflecting the unique viewing pattern of each of our participants. This approach allowed us to distinguish, for example, between a youth who was a frequent viewer of a number of particularly sex-laden sitcoms like *Friends* and another whose viewing included a lighter dose of such programs, mixed with child-oriented cartoons. Although these two teens might watch the same number of hours of television, they would certainly differ in the amount of sexual content to which they were exposed, and our viewing measure was able to detect and quantify this difference. We used this measure to predict sexual behavior change across the study period, and found that adolescents whose television diets included more sexual content were more likely to initiate sexual intercourse over the year subsequent to viewing. This relationship remained significant even after controlling for characteristics of participants that might affect both television viewing patterns and sexual behavior, such as age and parenting practices in participants' families (Collins et al., 2004).

The purpose of this chapter is to illustrate this method in detail, using TAS data to demonstrate how to effectively combine survey data and content analysis to estimate exposure to media content and to test for exposure effects. We will discuss some of the challenges posed by this approach to testing media effects, identify various options for dealing with these challenges, and suggest methods of choosing among them. We begin with an overview of the previously published TAS methods and results (Collins et al., 2004). Following this overview, we identify some general methodological issues in the measurement of content exposure in the context of TAS. Finally, the bulk of the chapter examines TAS methods in detail, describing choices made at each research phase from survey development through data analysis, and discussing the implications of these decisions. We begin that section with a description of how to measure viewing habits in a way that will best differentiate heavier viewers of a particular kind of content from lighter viewers. Next, we consider various approaches to quantifying content in light of the goal of testing media effects, rather than simply describing content. We discuss data analysis, focusing in particular on intercorrelation among exposure measures and the effect of this on results and their interpretation. In the conclusion of the chapter we present some examples of how these methods might be applied to other research questions, and discuss how our methodological approach enhanced the validity of our results and illuminated our understanding of how adolescents use, process, and react to television.

TAS Methods and Results

As noted earlier, one of the key hypotheses tested by TAS was that youth exposed to greater amounts of televised sexual content would initiate intercourse earlier than those exposed to lesser amounts of such content. In the article testing this hypothesis (Collins et al., 2004), we also examined two additional research questions, examining (1) whether the effects of exposure to sexual behavior are different from those of exposure to talk about sex, and (2) whether exposure to sexual content that includes a depiction of the risks and responsibilities associated with sexual activity (e.g., unintended pregnancy or sexually transmitted disease) makes youth more likely to delay sexual intercourse.

To test these research questions, Collins et al. (2004) focused on the first two waves of data from a national telephone survey of 12–17-year-olds. At baseline and one-year follow-up, 1,762 participants reported their television viewing habits and sexual experience, and responded to measures of more than a dozen factors known to be associated with adolescent sexual initiation. At baseline, the television viewing data included self-reported frequency of viewing for 23 television series. Methods developed by Kunkel and colleagues as part of their much larger study of television sexual content were used to determine the sexual content of these programs (see Kunkel et al., 2005, for details). The content analysis was performed in Kunkel's lab, using experienced coders who had been highly trained as part of that larger study. We combined the content data with reports of viewing frequency from the survey to derive three measures that we employed for analyses: exposure to sexual content, exposure to relatively more depictions of sexual behavior (versus talk about sex), and exposure to depictions of sexual risk or responsibility concerns.

Multivariate logistic regression analysis predicted initiation of intercourse by the second survey wave among the 1,292 youth who were virgins when they completed the baseline survey. The candidate predictors were the three measures indicating exposure to various forms of sexual content at baseline. The analyses also included statistical controls for numerous factors shown to predict intercourse initiation in other studies, such as religiosity and parental monitoring, as well as a control for the average amount of television adolescents viewed, regardless of its content. Results are shown in Table 10.1. As indicated by the coefficient for sexual content exposure, adolescents who viewed more such content at baseline were substantially more likely to initiate intercourse over the subsequent year. Exposure to television that included only talk about sex was associated with the same outcomes as exposure to television that depicted sexual behavior. However, youth who watched more depictions of sexual risks were no more or less likely to initiate intercourse over the subsequent year (Collins et al., 2004).

General Issues in Measuring Exposure to Specific Content

To link sexual content exposure and sexual behavior, Collins et al. (2004) created something analogous to a content analysis of the television watched by each individual participating in the study. To reliably test TAS hypotheses, that measure needed to differentiate between youth in the study whose television choices, environment, and viewing hours resulted in more exposure to sexual content and those with less exposure. This is important because linking media content to changes in individuals' beliefs and behavior requires an analysis that can specify the characteristics of *individual* television diets.

In the past, this was not always necessary to the testing of television effects. Indeed, a prominent early theory of media effects, cultivation theory (Gerbner, Gross, Morgan, & Signorielli, 1994), is based on the premise that the content

Table 10.1 Multivariate regression equations predicting sexual initiation

Baseline predictor	Standardized coefficient
TV exposure to:	
Sexual content	.32*
Sexual risk or need for safety	−.18
Sexual behavior vs. talk	.11
Average hours TV viewing	.04
Covariates:	
Age in years[1]	.42**
Female gender[1]	−.16
Hispanic[1,2]	−.50
African American[1,2]	.40
Has mostly older friends[1]	.69*
Lives with both parents[1]	−.58*
High parent education	−.31**
Parental monitoring	−.25*
Parent disapproval of sex[1]	−.37
Low school grades	.27*
Religious	−.27*
Good mental health	−.24*
Sensation seeking	.39**
Deviant behavior	.25*

Source: Based on data and analyses originally reported in Collins et al., 2004.

Notes
* $p < .05$.
** $p < .01$.
1 Age and dichotomous variables were not standardized because their scales are interpretable in unstandardized form.
2 The comparison group was non-Hispanic Whites and races other than Hispanics and African Americans.

of television is largely uniform across programs, genres, and channels. Gerbner and colleagues argue that this homogeneity in content created a mediated social environment that communicated distorted social norms. This uniform content might suggest, for example, that sex is a primary preoccupation among most people, if everywhere one looks in the television universe sex is referenced or portrayed. Cultivation theory was developed at a time when three broadcast networks dominated most viewing choices, among just a handful of competing channels. Given that those networks carried similar programming, it was possible at that time to test for content-based media effects by simply measuring the number of hours that an individual spent watching TV. Simply knowing that someone watched television gave you a good idea of the content that they viewed. As such, variations in total consumption were quite likely to be a close proxy for variations in consumption of sexual, violent, or other kinds of content.

In recent years, however, television programming has diversified dramatically, with hundreds of channels now available to the 80% of U.S. households with cable or similar access (Nielsen Media Research, 2007) and even more choices available by purchasing access to premium channels and pay-per-view programming. Even basic broadcast television service has expanded. This diversity makes it possible for different viewers to watch equally large amounts of television each day, but be exposed to entirely different kinds of content. One person may watch only daytime soap operas and made-for-TV movies, while another might select only sports programming, and a third may focus on the Cartoon Network or Nickelodeon. The impact of three hours of television viewing per day is likely to be quite different for these three viewers.

An additional complicating factor is the proliferation of multiple-set households. While in the 1960s the average household had only one television, the typical number is now three (Roberts, Foehr, Rideout, & Brodie, 2003). Indeed, many adolescents now have a television set in their bedrooms (Roberts et al., 2003), reducing any effects on their viewing of either parental oversight or of the competing program preferences of other viewers. This makes it more likely that any given teen's television diet will be maximally different from every other teen's. In spite of this increasing "privatization" of viewing, many youth still watch television with their parents, other family members, or friends for some part of the day (Nathanson, 2001). This co-viewing can make measuring viewing habits complicated, since it becomes important to capture exposure to programs that youth watch regularly because someone else chooses them, as well as those that they choose and view of their own accord. Asking about program preferences or favorite programs (in addition to introducing other biases) would fail to tap exposure to content that occurs through co-viewing of others' choices (Peterson, Moore, & Furstenberg, 1991).

In summary, television diversification, co-viewing, and privatization all complicate measurement of the content of individuals' television diets. Diversification and privatization render measures such as viewing hours insufficient, and co-viewing undermines the validity of favorite programs or program types as measures. An alternative is to capture the complete television universe as experienced by a given individual: all of the television content that a person encounters during a specified period. One might do so by employing a recording device attached to a television that this individual, and only this individual, watches. However, the person in question would also have to watch only that one television, so that programs seen on other sets are not missed. This is, of course, unrealistic and might even undermine the measure's validity by altering individuals' viewing habits from their usual pattern. Nor is it feasible, given limits on time and money, for researchers to conduct an analysis of all of the content watched by each individual in a large study. Recall that our study surveyed more than a thousand youths and measured exposure over most of a television season.

An alternative is to create an indicator of exposure to sexual content. Such a measure can, ideally, differentiate relatively high and low viewers of sex on television, even though it does not quantify the actual amount of such content viewed by any given individual (i.e., 20 minutes per day, 100 scenes per week, etc.). Like other research techniques, this method relies on sampling (of viewing habits and of content) to reflect the complete pattern of television habits, and the complete universe of television content, specific to an individual. This sampling approach was the method adopted by TAS. Creating an indicator of sexual content exposure requires researchers to make multiple assumptions about television and how viewers perceive television. Fortunately, some of these assumptions are testable. Below, we describe how we went about constructing our measure and testing the implications of our measurement choices.

Measuring Viewing Habits

The TAS measure of viewing habits was based on a sample of television programs. A key issue in sampling is the size of the sample necessary to accurately represent the population from which it is drawn. Up to a certain point, larger sample sizes are better. The number of television programs studied by TAS was dictated by the need to reconcile this consideration with concerns regarding respondent burden. Through pre-testing, we learned that youth dislike responding to questions about television programs they are unfamiliar with, and tire after too many questions, even about shows they watch and like. We determined that the maximum number of programs we could ask about over the telephone was approximately 30 for the age group in our study, as long as the list included some popular programs (more might be possible using a paper-and-pencil survey or older youth, see Pardun, L'Engle, & Brown, 2005). Next, we set about determining which programs to incorporate in our measure.

One of our criteria was the program's Nielsen rating. In addition to the influence of program popularity on respondents' willingness to answer questions, the number of viewers a program typically attracts affects the likely distribution of a viewing-frequency measure. Even the most highly rated television programs generally attract only a modest proportion of all individuals in a given demographic group, and many of those who watch will miss a few or even most specific episodes that air. Because of this, if we included many shows in our survey with low ratings among teens, we would find that almost all of our respondents scored at the lowest point on our measure (i.e., "never" watched the shows). This would severely limit the variability of our indicator of exposure, variability from which we would hope to predict variations in sexual beliefs and behavior.

Using Nielsen ratings of the regularly scheduled prime-time programs, we selected those shows most watched (in the top 20) by any of four groups, male and female 12–14- and 15–17-year-olds, during the Fall season prior to our survey. We chose from four separate lists because some of the most popular programs within each of these demographic strata do not appear among the top programs for the more general group (12–17-year-olds of any gender), or for another stratum. Were we to omit programs popular with only a specific sub-group of teens (and the programs contained sexual content) we would underestimate exposure for this particular group, and thus bias tests of hypotheses toward null findings for that group but not for others. Because TAS wished to test whether findings differed for males versus females and for younger versus older teens, this was an important issue. We chose only prime-time programs because the majority of youth television viewing (other than sports) takes place during those hours. Eligible programs appeared on ABC, NBC, CBS, Fox, WB, UPN, or PAX networks.

Our second criterion was sexual content. It was critical, of course, to include all of the programs watched by teens that we knew (based on prior content analyses) or expected (based on reviews in the popular press) to contain high levels of sexual content. Thus, we selected any such programs appearing on the list of top-rated shows. We also included two additional sets of programs: (1) broadcast programs with high levels of sexual content that were highly rated by Nielsen overall, but not popular enough with teens to appear on the age-based list, and (2) highly rated cable programs with sexual content. We selected the cable shows separately because cable ratings are not directly comparable to ratings for broadcast shows. Cable programs have much smaller audiences than broadcast television, in part because fewer people are cable subscribers. By including these two additional sets of programs, we tapped into the viewing of adolescents whose habits were unusual for youth their age, and exposed them to sexual content to which others would not be exposed. This improved the validity of the measure, as well as its variability across participants.

We also created variability in our measure by choosing a few programs from the Nielsen list that we expected to include low levels of sexual content. Doing so also improved the acceptability of the survey to our participants, as noted earlier. Our final criteria were program characteristics and channel. Within the parameters described above, we sought to maximize our coverage of the television universe relevant to youth. Thus, we included programs appearing on broadcast networks and those on basic and premium cable channels. Our list also included both animated and live action shows, as well as reality shows, sitcoms, and dramas. Failure to include this full range of programs might have resulted in the underestimation of sexual content exposure for youth who consistently select one particular genre or channel, or have access to channels that other youth do not.

Applying these strategies resulted in a final list of 25 programs. Two of these programs were included in the survey but dropped from further consideration following initial analyses, because 5% or fewer of TAS participants had ever watched them. Although rated within the top 20 for one of our demographic sub-groups, both programs were cancelled during the television season. This is a hazard in selecting programs for use in surveys that will take place over a period of a few months, and should be allowed for in deciding how many programs to include in a survey. The characteristics of the 23 shows used in the TAS exposure measures are displayed in Table 10.2. As can be seen there, some shows were popular among all sub-groups of youth that we considered, while others drew their viewership from a specific demographic. The table also makes clear that Nielsen ratings were generally in line with the frequency of

Table 10.2 Characteristics of television series used to measure viewing habits in TAS

Television series	Top-rated younger boys	Top-rated older boys	Top-rated younger girls	Top-rated older girls	Average viewing frequency (1–4)	Average sex scenes per episode
One	*	*	*	*	2.53	0.0[a]
Two		*	*	*	2.06	2.1[a]
Three	*	*	*	*	1.92	0.0
Four	*		*	*	1.81	1.7
Five	Cable	Cable	Cable	Cable	1.80	12.0
Six	*	*		*	1.77	7.0
Seven		*	*	*	1.66	1.7
Eight	*	*	*		1.57	0.0[a]
Nine	*	*	*		1.57	1.4
Ten	*	*		*	1.55	4.4[a]
Eleven	Cable	Cable	Cable	Cable	1.51	13.0[a]
Twelve	*	*	*	*	1.49	2.6[a]
Thirteen	*	*	*	*	1.47	1.0
Fourteen				*	1.47	3.0[a]
Fifteen			*		1.42	5.0
Sixteen	*	*		*	1.42	8.3
Seventeen			*	*	1.41	3.7
Eighteen				*	1.38	4.0[a]
Nineteen			*		1.32	1.7
Twenty			*	*	1.26	1.5
Twenty-one		*		*	1.26	10.7
Twenty-two				*	1.21	8.3
Twenty-three	Cable	Cable	Cable	Cable	1.15	8.0

Note
a Indicates half-hour show; other shows are one hour in length.

self-reported viewing within our sample, increasing our faith in the validity of those reports. Shows with high ratings across multiple groups had the highest average viewing scores in our survey. In addition, the table bolsters a point made earlier, that even highly rated shows are viewed infrequently on average. Note that the highest mean score was 2.53 on a 1 to 4 scale. The percentage of our sample that watched each show at all in the prior season (not tabled) ranged from 69% (Show 1) to 12% (Show 23). Thus, a nontrivial minority of study participants "sometimes" watched even the shows that were viewed least frequently. Finally, the table indicates good variability and range in viewing frequency across the various programs. We discuss the basis for the last column in the table, the average amount of sexual content in each program, in the section below.

A final issue in choosing programs is the possibility that viewership of certain programs reflects some characteristic of the individual or the program unrelated to sexual content. For example, if the shows studied were mostly about romantic relationships, those who have a boyfriend or girlfriend might be more interested in them. These people might also be more likely to have sex, not because of the show's sexual content, but because of the relationship content. If nonsexual content drives the relationships we observed in our study, we should find that viewing the specific shows listed in our survey predicts sexual initiation as well as or better than a measure that weights viewing by amount of sexual content. To test this, we substituted participants' reports of how often they watched each of the 23 programs (i.e., 23 separate variables) for the sexual content exposure measure in the regression analysis reported by Collins et al. (2004). Only two of the 23 programs significantly predicted sexual initiation—and none did so when the p-value was adjusted to account for the 23 tests conducted. Nor did the set of programs predict intercourse initiation when their effects were tested jointly (Wald F (22, 1633) = 1.36, p = .12). This strongly supports the idea that it is exposure to the sexual content in television programs that predicts sexual initiation, rather than exposure to the relationships, characters, or other themes presented in the specific shows we studied.

Measuring Sexual Content

Sample Size

Sampling issues also influence measures of television content. Ideally, the best possible approach for TAS would have been to code all episodes of each of the 23 programs in the survey that appeared in the relevant season. However, it was not feasible to do so given the hundreds of hours of programming involved (20 or more episodes times 23 programs). Thus, TAS coded only a sample of episodes from each television series to determine the average amount of sexual content it portrayed. The number of episodes this involved was variable across television series. A minimum of three episodes were recorded and coded for each series, but for some programs more episodes (up to 14) were used. This variability in sample size stemmed from overlap between Kunkel's larger research agenda and that of TAS. When Kunkel had additional episodes of relevant series in his tape library, we coded all that were available. Our goal was to maximize the sample size for estimating the content of a given television series, and this resulted in averages based on variable numbers of episodes.

Three episodes constitute approximately 15% of the typical number of new episodes aired in a series each television season. This percentage was arrived at somewhat arbitrarily. We explored the reliability of our estimate of the total amount of sexual content for each television series by conducting a standard one-way ANOVA of the content data, predicting number of sex scenes. Episode was the unit of analysis, and the predictor variable was television series. Thus, the F-statistic is an estimate of the variability in amount of sexual content across different television series, divided by the variability in sexual content within the series, but across different episodes. The F-test was significant (F (22, 70) = 5.81, p < .0001) indicating that the sample of episodes coded was sufficient to distinguish one television series from another, in terms of its level of sexual content.

Unitizing Content

Other chapters in this volume have also raised the problem of properly unitizing content. Questions of how to unitize content in order to produce a valid and sensitive measure of sexual content exposure took multiple forms in TAS. Answering them required making some assumptions about how television content is perceived and processed. It was believed at the TAS project's outset that the unitizing approach employed in Kunkel et al.'s (2005) content study was appropriate to form the basis of an exposure measure. In Kunkel's work, content is described based on an analysis of discrete scenes.

Other methods of unitizing content could have been employed. For example, Pardun and colleagues (2005) unitized television sexual content according to "non-break sequences" or camera cuts. Other choices might be to unitize according to each interaction between characters or by time increments (e.g., 10-second segments). Pardun et al. chose their unit of analysis in part because they compared different media, ranging from television and film through the internet and song lyrics. Clearly a "scene" would be difficult to define for the latter two media. TAS was unconstrained by these considerations and indeed chose scenes as a content unit based on the specific medium under study. We postulated that experienced television viewers perceive and react to television by breaking it into scenes, following plot developments according to these scenes. Thus, we expected scenes to be the most meaningful unit to measure. That is, we assumed that each scene has an individual effect on viewers that does not vary significantly according to the scene's length or the number of interactions within the scene. Because this assumption may be false, we subjected the measure resulting from this approach to some preliminary tests.

As noted above, a reasonable alternative to counting scenes is to consider the time spent viewing sexual content. Table 10.2 displays the average number of sex scenes contained in each program in the TAS sample. As the table makes clear, the number of sex scenes in one-hour programs was typically *not* twice the number of scenes in a half-hour program. Indeed, the number of scenes containing sexual content in our set of 23 programs appears to be independent of program length. One might reasonably expect that watching a half-hour program with two scenes containing sexual content would have twice the impact of watching an hour-long program with two such scenes. That is, a scene every 15 minutes might be a stronger dose than a scene every 30 minutes.

We were able to test whether program length matters to the effects of a given number of sexual scenes with the TAS data. We did so by weighting viewing-frequency for each program by the program's length, so that our measure represented the number of sex scenes per hour of viewing, rather than the number of scenes per episode. We then entered this variable into the TAS regression equation shown in Table 10.1, in place of the measure of overall sexual content that did not account for show length. The coefficient for the new variable was positive and significant (beta = .38, p < .05), indicating that this approach can be used effectively to measure level of sexual content exposure. However, it did not appear to be superior to the measure that did not account for show length (beta = .32, p < .05; see Table 10.1). The two measures were equivalent in their association with sexual initiation, suggesting that accounting for show length does not improve the measurement of sexual content levels beyond that afforded by measuring number of scenes, alone.

Level of Specificity

A second issue related to content units in TAS was the level at which sexual behavior was best described. Although TAS employed only three exposure measures, Kunkel's coders actually described the episodes sampled in much greater detail. They indicated for each scene the presence of any of the following types of (1) sexual behavior: physical flirting, passionate kissing, intimate touch, intercourse implied, intercourse depicted; (2) sexual talk: about own/others' plans or desires, about sex that has occurred, talk toward sex, expert advice, and other; and (3) talk or behavior depicting sexual risk or responsibility issues: abstinence, waiting to have sex, portrayals mentioning or showing condoms or birth control, and portrayals related to AIDS, STDs, pregnancy, or abortion. Other codes not listed here were also employed.

It would have been possible, given this variety, to construct measures of exposure at a very specific level, for example, "exposure to intercourse depictions." We focused on only the broader categories of behavior, talk, and risk/responsibility for a variety of reasons. First, behavior and talk were frequent and variable enough to examine in statistical analyses. That is, the programs studied differed in their inclusion of such material more or less along a continuum. Choosing a smaller sub-category on which to focus might result in nearly uniform scores of "zero" across programs on a measure of intercourse or measure of some other specific (and relatively rare) depiction. If so, there would be little variability to examine for correspondence with variations in sexual behavior. Moreover, an important theoretical and policy-relevant question could be addressed with the broader measures: does exposure to talk about sex and to sexual behavior have an equivalent effect on sexual initiation? Since parents and policy-makers often object to depictions of behavior more strongly than to sexual references and innuendo, and because behavior is easier to regulate, this is a question of great practical significance.

Understanding the consequences of exposure to sexual risk or responsibility depictions is at least as significant as the talk versus behavior question. Exposure to portrayals highlighting the potential negative consequences of sexual activity (e.g., unintended pregnancy) should, according to social learning theory, inhibit sexual activity among viewers, rather than promote it. If this were the case, it would be possible for television producers to include sex in their programming without fear of promoting sexual activity, as long as they also include references to sexual risk. Parents could also rest easier, as long as they ensure that their teens are exposed to such programming in equal proportion to their exposure to less responsible fare. This hypothesis is difficult to test, however. Risk and responsibility content is not shown very frequently (Kunkel et al., 2005), rendering tests of its impact difficult to conduct reliably. The principal problem is that tests may suggest no effect of risk portrayals, when there is a true underlying association. It is less likely that a significant effect would be obtained where no association actually exists. Given the variable's import, TAS explored the effect of exposure to risk and responsibility information, but with the caveat that nonsignificant findings should not be strongly interpreted as a lack of effect for this variable. Others exploring effects of infrequent but theoretically important types of media content might wish to do the same in their research.

In general, choice of the level at which to code content, broad versus specific, depends on the breadth of the questions one wishes to address with the research and the theoretical importance of each potential category of content, as well as the practical limitations of statistical techniques that preclude examination of content characteristics that are close to uniformly present or absent.

TAS's main measure was of a program's sexual content in general. This variable was constructed very simply. It was the sum of the number of scenes with sexual behavior in an episode, plus the number of scenes with talk about sex in that same episode, averaged across episodes. This works because all sub-categories of sexual content coded by Kunkel reside exclusively within one or the other of these two broader classifications (i.e., all are either talk or behavior). However, the presence of one of these content categories does not preclude the presence of another—a given scene could contain sexual behavior, sexual talk, both kinds of content, or neither. Indeed, Kunkel's analysis for his larger study indicates that sexual behavior is almost uniformly accompanied by talk about sex within a television scene. This raised the issue as to whether TAS should weight a scene containing both talk and behavior twice as heavily as a scene with only one sub-type of content. Do two types of sexual content within a given scene affect viewers more than one type?

We decided to answer this question empirically. The results of applying the measure already described are displayed in Table 10.2. As the table indicates, the number of sex scenes calculated in this manner was broadly distributed across TAS programs. Estimates ranged from 0 to 13; the average across programs was 4.4. This score "double counts" exposure to scenes in which both talk and sex appear, relative to exposure to scenes with only talk or only behavior. When weighted by viewing frequency and summed across programs, the double-count measure produced the score entered in the regression equation by Collins et al. (2004) and displayed in Table 10.1. As noted previously, the effect was substantial in size and significant (beta = .32, p < .05).

To examine the role of double-counting in producing this effect, we created a second measure of sexual content. This index counted the number of scenes with *any* sexual content, thus giving equal weight to scenes that contain both talk and behavior and those that involve only one of these two sub-types of sexual content. Like the double-count measure, it was multiplied by viewing frequency and summed across programs. We then divided the double-count score obtained by each TAS participant by their score on this new measure. The resulting variable reflects the extra weight applied to watching scenes with multiple forms of content. When we added this measure to the basic TAS regression along with the double-count score, we found that it was a highly significant independent predictor of intercourse initiation ($p < .01$). In other words, accounting for multiple kinds of sexual content in a scene, rather than treating all scenes with any sexual content equally, adds to our ability to predict sexual behavior changes among teens.

Salience of Content

Kunkel's raters also coded the degree of focus (major or minor) on sexual behavior, talk, or risk/responsibility within each scene. Collins et al. (2004) based their measure of overall exposure to sexual content on counts of sexual talk and behavior that played a substantial part in a scene, i.e., those that were salient. We were uncertain whether references to sex that were not a substantial part of the scene would capture enough attention to be processed by viewers. If not, including them in our measure might have diluted any impact of portrayals in which the sexual content is more central to the scene (and thus more likely to be cognitively processed). To examine whether this was the case, TAS again tested an alternative model to that reported by Collins et al. (2004). In it, we substituted four indicators reflecting exposure to major- and minor-focus sexual talk and sexual behavior for the measure of overall exposure to sexual content. We found that, in this new equation, the effect of major-focus talk was positive and significant, but much smaller than the effect of overall exposure displayed in Table 10.1. All the other coefficients were nonsignificant or negative. (These values probably reflect collinearity between measures and should not be interpreted as indicating anything more than a weaker relationship between sex and these kinds of exposure relative to major-focus talk.) This suggests that had Collins et al. (2004) included minor-focus instances of sexual talk or behavior in their measure of television's sexual content, the effect of exposure would have been estimated to be smaller, probably as a result of diluting the effect of exposure to more prominent portrayals of sex.

Analytic Issues: Testing Media Effects Using Exposure Measures

As we have noted, and as shown in Table 10.1, Collins et al. (2004) employed three measures of sexual content exposure in their models. Total sexual content exposure was calculated by multiplying self-reported viewing frequency for each program by the average number of scenes in that program with a major focus on sexual behavior plus the average number of scenes with a major focus on sexual talk and summing across the 23 programs. Exposure to sexual behavior versus talk was calculated by first multiplying viewing frequency times the average number of scenes containing any major-focus sexual behavior and summing across programs, and subsequently dividing this measure by the measure of total sexual content exposure. The resulting score distinguished viewers of sexual content that mostly included behavior from those whose diet of sexual content was made up of something other than behavior. Given that the only alternative under our coding scheme was sexual talk, low scores on this proportion measure indicated more exposure to talk-only portrayals of sex. The measure of risk and responsibility exposure was based on viewing frequency times the average number of scenes containing *any* sexual risk or responsibility portrayals. The three measures had generally good distributional properties. All were standardized to a mean of 0 and standard deviation of 1. Scree plots indicated that exposure to sexual content and to risk and safety content was somewhat positively skewed (ranges were –1.43 to 4.49 and –.98 to 4.97, respectively), while the sexual behavior to total sex proportion measure was more normally distributed (range of –2.82 to 1.68).

In addition to these three measures of content exposure, TAS also created a measure of the average amount of time each participant spent viewing television each week. This measure was based on a set of five items tapping hours of viewing on various days of the week and at different times of day. Responses were averaged to create a continuous indicator of average viewing time. We included this measure in our study and in all analyses because we were concerned that the measures of sexual content exposure, if analyzed without controlling for total viewing, might "stand in" for it. That is, any associations between sexual content exposure and other variables might actually reflect associations with total viewing. This is possible because the sexual content exposure variable must necessarily reflect two underlying viewing tendencies, the frequency with which one watches television in general, and the frequency with which one watches programs with high levels of sexual content.

As indicated in Table 10.3, average time spent watching TV and overall exposure to sexual content were indeed correlated with one another. The table

Table 10.3 Correlations among television exposure variables in the TAS baseline

Television exposure variable	Sexual content	Behavior / total sexual content	Risk and responsibility	Average weekly viewing time
Sexual content	1.00	–.16	.63	.23
Behavior / total sexual content		1.00	.34	–.09
Risk and responsibility			1.00	.13
Average weekly viewing time				1.00

also displays correlations among the other exposure measures. The strongest association was between exposure to risk/responsibility portrayals and overall exposure to sexual content. It is important to emphasize that while this could indicate that programs with lots of sexual content have lots of risk and responsibility portrayals, there are also other factors that could produce such a correlation. For example, youth who are attracted to programs with high levels of sexual content may also be attracted to programs with smaller amounts of sex, but that contain risk and responsibility portrayals. Our measure does not allow examination of these distinctions. It does indicate what may be most important, however, which is that youth with high sexual content exposure are indeed those with the highest levels of risk and responsibility exposure. This is a promising pattern of results for promoting sexual safety, although risk and responsibility portrayals are so infrequent (Kunkel et al., 2005) that "high" levels of exposure relative to other youth may be insufficient to make a difference in behavior. Overall, Table 10.3 indicates that correlations among the TV exposure measures range from modest (–.09) to large (.63).

We had planned for such correlations in constructing our measures and designing our analyses. We expected from the outset of our study to include multiple complementary measures of television exposure in our multivariate models in order to account for overlap among the constructs and behaviors they tap. That is, we expected that the simple associations between each exposure measure and intercourse initiation would be different from the associations observed when each measure was tested in the context of the others, and that the latter set of correlations would be most readily interpretable. Results of preliminary TAS analyses were in line with expectations. The simple associations between intercourse initiation and sexual content exposure, exposure to sexual behavior versus talk, and exposure to sexual risk or responsibility portrayals produced coefficients of .35, –.18, and .10, respectively. In contrast, when we construct multivariate models in which we predict intercourse from all four exposure measures simultaneously (without including any of the other statistical controls displayed in Table 10.1) we find that the beta for overall exposure to sexual content is .47. The effect of exposure to sexual behavior (vs. talk) is close to zero, and the coefficient for risk and responsibility exposure becomes negative (–.19), although it is not statistically significant. The contrast between these estimates illustrates that assessments of exposure effects are highly sensitive to controls for other aspects of the content included in one's exposure measures.

Such results reinforce our caution to other researchers that it is critical to consider this kind of overlap in planning research. It is important to create exposure measures that allow one to control for any obvious confounds that might be inherent in one's key exposure variables. Had Collins et al. (2004) tested effects of exposure to sexual content without controlling for risk and responsibility portrayals in some of that content, results might have suggested that sexual content exposure *per se* had a smaller effect than seems to be the case. Importantly, Collins et al. also found that average number of viewing hours was unrelated to intercourse initiation, in both bivariate and multivariate models. This suggests that, had the study used only this measure to test for television effects, the results would have been nonsignificant—the apparent effects of exposure to sexual content on television would have been missed entirely without the use of content analytic methods to tap the specifics of exposure.

Conclusion

This chapter has described a number of issues that researchers should consider when testing effects of exposure to specific media content, and discussed in detail a case example of how they might be addressed. The methods described are by no means comprehensive—a variety of other techniques might be used to determine the manner in which to best derive exposure measures and test their effects. However, we hope that our in-depth description of the approach taken by TAS will familiarize readers with the landscape before they embark on research of this type, and perhaps provide a roadmap that guides them past some of the obstacles. While the methods undertaken by the TAS team were intensive and time-consuming, they bolstered our confidence that our final measurement approach was as good as or better than others we might have chosen. Thoroughly testing the effects of various methodological options not only resulted in greater scientific rigor, it also illuminated to some extent our understanding of how adolescents use, process, and react to television.

Interested researchers can extrapolate from our methods to test effects of other kinds of television content on other behaviors. For example, a number of studies link numbers of hours of television viewing among youth to overweight problems in this population (Marshall, Biddle, & Gorely, 2004), but most such studies have been unable to illuminate the processes responsible. As noted earlier in this chapter, one possibility is that television watching is substituted for physically active pursuits like playing sports or doing chores (Hancox et al., 2004). Another plausible explanation is that television advertising alters food preferences among viewers, leading them to make unhealthy choices like sugared cereals, potato chips, soda, or fast food (Horgen, Choate, & Brownell, 2001). These problematic diets may then contribute to weight gain.

Using hours spent viewing as a predictor makes it impossible to discriminate between these two processes. However, one could use survey techniques to measure individual children's viewing habits (which shows they watch and how often), identify the commercials aired during various television programs included in the survey, code the content of these commercials (e.g., number of ads per program promoting unhealthy food), and combine the two to create, for each child, an index of his or her relative amount of exposure to television ads for unhealthy food. If this measure is a predictor of overweight, independent of an association between hours spent viewing and weight problems (and remains so after controlling for factors that might affect both eating habits and viewing habits), it would provide evidence that television advertising contributes to weight problems among youth. Such a finding might lead to regulation of food advertising; such regulation would be an inappropriate remedy to the problem of child overweight if the source of overweight was inactivity. We have used this content-based approach to test for links between exposure to alcohol advertising on television and underage drinking (Collins, Ellickson, McCaffrey, & Hambarsoomians, 2007; Ellickson, Collins, Hambarsoomians, & McCaffrey, 2004).

The combination of content analysis and survey methods could also be used to explore the effects of exposure to content in media other than television. In a recent study using the TAS dataset (Martino et al., 2006), we coded for different types of sexual content in popular music lyrics, and linked these data to TAS reports of the frequency of listening to various artists. Results indicate that exposure to lyrics that portray sex as degrading is correlated with intercourse initiation, while exposure to other sexual references in music is not. Taking the survey/content analysis approach a step further, Pardun and colleagues (2005) have used these techniques to assess exposure to sexual content across a broad spectrum of media using a single measure. They find that such exposure is associated with teens' level of sexual experience. A similar approach could be used to examine exposure to portrayals of smoking, drinking, or violence across the variety of media that include them, and link these to substance use and aggressive behavior among youth.

We end this chapter by encouraging researchers to pursue these methods, while cautioning them to proceed carefully. As with any research, it is possible to obtain spurious associations between measures of exposure and hypothesized outcomes. Threats to validity include inadequate sampling of program content, inappropriate content unitization, and poor selection of programs to include in a survey, among others. Only a careful and detailed examination of the properties of an exposure measure, including the kinds of sensitivity, validity, and reliability analyses we describe here, will permit the investigator to rule out alternative explanations and confidently conclude that exposure to media content is truly related to health behavior.

References

American Psychological Association. (1993). *Violence and youth: Psychology's response.* Washington, DC: Author.

Andersen, R. E., Crespo, C. J., Bartlett, S. J., Cheskin, L. J., & Pratt, M. (1998). Relationship of physical activity and television watching with body weight and level of fatness among children. *The Journal of the American Medical Association, 279,* 938–942.

Bandura, A. (1986). *Social foundations of thought and action: A social cognitive theory.* Englewood Cliffs, NJ: Prentice Hall.

Bushman, B. J., & Huesmann, L. R. (2001). Effects of televised violence on aggression. In D. G. Singer and J. L. Singer (Eds.), *Handbook of children and the media* (pp. 223–254). Thousand Oaks, CA: Sage Publications.

CDC. (2006). Youth risk behavior surveillance—United States, 2005. *Morbidity and Mortality Weekly Report, 55*(SS-5), 1–108.

Collins, R. L., Ellickson, P. L., McCaffrey, D. F., & Hambarsoomians, K. (2007). Early adolescent exposure to alcohol advertising and its relationship to underage drinking. *Journal of Adolescent Health, 40*(6), 527–534.

Collins, R. L., Elliott, M. N., Berry, S. H., Kanouse, D. E., Kunkel, D., Hunter, S. M., & Mui, A. (2004). Watching sex on television predicts adolescent initiation of sexual behavior. *Pediatrics, 114*(3), e280–e289.

Ellickson, P. L., Collins, R. L., Hambarsoomians, K., & McCaffrey, D. F. (2004). Does alcohol advertising promote adolescent drinking? Results from a longitudinal assessment. *Addiction, 100,* 235–246.

Gerbner, G., Gross, L., Morgan, M., & Signorielli, N. (1994). Growing up with television: The cultivation perspective. In J. Bryant & D. Zillman (Eds.), *Media effects: Advances in theory and research.* Hillsdale, NJ: Lawrence Erlbaum.

Hancox, R. J., Milne, B. J., & Poulton, R. (2004). Association between child and adolescent television and adult health: A longitudinal birth cohort study. *Lancet, 364*(9430), 257–262.

Horgen, K. B., Choate, M., & Brownell, K. D. (2001). Television food advertising: Targeting children in a toxic environment. In D. G. Singer & J. L. Singer (Eds.), *Handbook of children and the media* (pp. 447–461). Thousand Oaks, CA: Sage Publications.

Kunkel, D., Eyal, K., Finnerty, K., Biely, E., & Donnerstein, E. (2005). *Sex on TV 4.* Menlo Park, CA: The Henry J. Kaiser Family Foundation.

Marshall, S. J., Biddle, S. J. H., Gorely, T., Cameron, N. & Murdey, I. (2004). Relationships between media use, body fatness and physical activity in children and youth: A meta-analysis. *International Journal of Obesity, 28*(10), 1238–1246.

Martino, S. C., Collins, R. L., Elliott, M. N., Strachman, A., Kanouse, D. E., & Berry, S. H. (2006). Exposure to degrading versus non-degrading music lyrics and sexual behavior among youth. *Pediatrics, 118*(2), e430–e441.

Nathanson, A. (2001). Parents versus peers: Exploring the significance of peer mediation of antisocial television. *Communication Research, 28*(3), 251–274.

Nielsen Media Research. Nielsen Analytics. (2007). *Benchmarking the digital household.* Retrieved June 14, 2007, from http://www.nielsenmedia.com/nc/portal/site/Public/menuitem.d7deb7344c5a8ffe818e6c1047a062a0/?vgnextoid=82387ccfd9 5d9010VgnVCM100000ac0a260aRCRD

Paik, H., & Comstock, G. (1994). The effects of television on antisocial behavior: A meta-analysis. *Communication Research, 21,* 516–546.

Pardun, C. J., L'Engle, K. L., & Brown, J. D. (2005). Linking exposure to outcomes: Early adolescents' consumption of sexual content in six media. *Mass Communication and Society, 8*(2), 75–91.

Peterson, J. L., Moore, K. A., & Furstenberg, F. F., Jr. (1991). Television and early initiation of sexual intercourse: Is there a link? *Journal of Homosexuality, 21,* 93–118.

Roberts, D. F., Foehr, U. G., Rideout, V. J., & Brodie, M. (2003). *Kids and media in America.* New York: Cambridge University Press.

11 Health Messages on Prime-time Television

A Longitudinal Content Analysis

Sheila T. Murphy, Holley A. Wilkin,
Michael J. Cody, and Grace C. Huang

For many Americans television provides an important, if not primary, source of health information (Beck, 2004; Kaiser Family Foundation, 2002; Murphy & Cody, 2003). According to a Porter Novelli HealthStyles survey, 26% of viewers list prime-time entertainment television shows among their top three sources of health information and over half, 52%, consider the health information contained in prime-time programs to be accurate (Beck, Huang, Pollard, & Johnson, 2003). But what health-related lessons, if any, are viewers learning from watching prime-time comedies or dramas? Although there have been several notable attempts to measure the impact of a single dramatic episode or series within the United States (Brodie et al., 2001; Sharf, Freimuth, Greenspon, & Plotnick, 1996; Whittier, Kennedy, Seeley, St. Lawrence, & Beck, 2005), there has been no systematic program of research to assess the impact of diverse media portrayals on the knowledge, beliefs, and actions of adult viewers.

The first step in assessing the impact of televised health information is to obtain an accurate assessment of what information is currently being conveyed. In January 2003, Vicki Beck, the director of Hollywood, Health & Society (HH&S) at the University of Southern California's Norman Lear Center, Sheila Murphy, and Michael Cody (faculty at the Annenberg School of Communication at USC) launched a pilot project to monitor the health-related content of popular prime-time television shows. Each spring season from 2003 to 2006 over two dozen of the most popular prime-time television shows among 18–49-year-old Hispanic, African American, and General (primarily Caucasian) audiences were content analyzed. In this chapter, we walk the reader through some of the key decisions made during the course of the Television Monitoring Project, as well as the rationale behind and consequences of each decision.

Why Prime-time Television?

At the height of its popularity, one out of every four television sets in the United States was tuned to NBC's *ER* on Thursday nights. It is because of this potential to reach millions of people instantaneously that the Kaiser Family Foundation and the CDC advocate that television programs be utilized to reach viewers who are difficult to reach through news releases and more traditional health campaigns (Beck, 2004; Brodie et al., 2001; Greenberg, Salmon, Patel, Beck & Cole, 2004). There are, in fact, compelling reasons for investigating television's potential to convey health-related information within the United States (Brown & Walsh-Childers, 2002). For example, the heaviest consumers of television—low socioeconomic status African American and Hispanic women—are also at disproportionate risk for life-threatening ailments such as cancer, diabetes, and heart disease (National Center for Chronic Disease Prevention and Health Promotion at the Centers for Disease Control and Prevention, 2008). Minority viewers also report being the most likely to act on information they learned on television (Beck, Huang, Pollard, & Johnson, 2003). Consequently, popular television programs have the potential to reach not only large audiences, but those most at risk for health problems.

Research also suggests that health information conveyed within an engaging narrative is more likely to be attended to than more traditional health campaigns (Singhal & Rogers, 1999; Singhal, Cody, Rogers & Sabido, 2004; Slater & Rouner, 2002). Television programs are designed to capture and hold an individual's attention. They do so by establishing a relationship between the viewer and the characters, involving liking, sympathy, identification, empathy, etc. (Brown & Fraser, 2004; Sood, 2002). The hour or half-hour television format allows for a combination of emotions to be experienced, the development of complex persuasive and informational messages, and observational learning to take place (Bandura, 2004; Sabido, 2004). Indeed, Bandura's concepts of observational learning, modeling, and perceived self-efficacy provide the theoretical underpinnings for virtually all entertainment education attempts.

Perhaps the most compelling argument, however, is that there is considerable evidence from developing countries that entertainment education programs have a significant impact on awareness, beliefs, attitudes and behaviors (Singhal et al., 2004). Yet Sherry (2002) and others have argued that unlike India or Africa, where the general population has few media options, developed countries such as the U.S. are "media saturated" commercial environments where it is virtually impossible to control the frequency and type of messages conveyed.

By focusing on popular prime-time programs, the Television Monitoring Project sought to provide an overview of health messages to which a large segment of Americans are exposed. The primary goal of the project was to gauge the frequency, content, and potential impact of health-related depictions in popular prime-time programming. For the remainder of this chapter, we focus on three distinct areas of concern to all content analyses—determining an appropriate sample, issues of measurement and data analysis, and, finally, a consideration of the potential impact of new technologies.

Determining an Appropriate Sample

A crucial first step in conducting a content analysis is to narrow down the scope of the project to a manageable, but meaningful, size. While a strong case could be made for analyzing the health content of newscasts, talk shows, or daytime programming, our selection of popular prime-time shows was guided largely by the number of individuals exposed to their content as reflected in their Nielsen ratings. It is important to recognize that an analysis involving a different selection of programs would likely produce a different set of results, thus limiting the generalizability of our findings. However, we felt that focusing on scripted comedies and dramas with the largest audiences made sense and had high face validity.

Thus, audience size was a key consideration in our selection of specific shows to content analyze. Each year of the project, our research team identified the scripted prime-time shows with the largest audience share using Nielsen ratings from the November sweeps (a week where the audience size and composition is used to set advertising fees). Notice that any new television shows starting in January would be excluded from this sample. Consequently, each year we also recorded promising new shows that we felt might break into the top tier during the spring season. The Nielsen ratings from the midseason February sweeps week determined our final sample.

It would have been relatively simple to identify, record, and analyze the shows with the largest overall audiences during the spring television season. But program preferences are far from random. For instance, an analysis of the five most popular shows in 2003 for Hispanic, African American, and General (primarily Caucasian) audiences as determined by Nielsen ratings reveals clear ethnic differences in viewing patterns. Only one show, *Friends*, was watched by both Hispanics and Caucasians in large numbers. There was no overlap in viewing preferences between African Americans and the other ethnic groups (Murphy et al., 2003). In short, African Americans and Hispanics—both groups at elevated risk for serious health problems—may be exposed to very different televised health messages than the largely Caucasian General audience.

As a result of these clear ethnic differences in program preferences (as reflected by Nielsen ratings) we made the decision to stratify shows on the basis of the ethnicity of viewers. However, this decision created another poten-tial confound. African Americans are heavy viewers of comedies that feature African American actors. In fact, in the first two years of the project, four of the five top-rated African American shows were UPN/CW comedies, with the fifth being an ABC comedy. If we compared the health content of these five comedies to the five top-rated shows for the largely Caucasian General audi-ence, which contained both comedies and dramas (including the medical show *ER*), the results of our content analysis would be preordained, showing that Caucasians are exposed to far more health-related content than African Ameri-cans. But we were uncomfortable comparing half-hour comedies to hour-long dramas. As a result we decided to stratify not only on ethnicity of viewers but also by genre, including the top five dramas and top five comedies for each of Nielsen's categories of African American, Hispanic, and General audiences. Because there was some overlap among the programs watched by each ethnic group, this resulted in content analyzing between 24 to 27 shows each spring season for a total of over 400 new episodes each year of the project. We felt this represented a manageable sample that could provide insight into how the health content in prime-time dramas and comedies might differ as a function of the ethnicity of viewers.

Our research team made several other key decisions regarding the selection of shows. For instance, it should be noted that we analyzed only English-language programs. One could certainly argue that many Hispanics living in the U.S. are also watching Spanish-language networks such as Univision or Telemundo. It is possible that audiences for certain Spanish-language prime-time shows could be larger than for some of the English-language shows in our sample. Nevertheless, we decided that content analyzing Spanish-language shows in addition to the English-language shows would be too overwhelming, particularly during the early stages of the project.

Moreover, we did not include "nonscripted" shows such as reality shows. The primary reason for this decision was that Hollywood, Health & Society often consults with various television shows to encourage writers and producers to include accurate health-related information in their storylines. Storyline consultation is not an option with nonscripted reality shows. Furthermore, reality shows typically do not follow the traditional television season schedule and often are used as midseason replacements for unsuccessful shows. Finally, unlike scripted programs, which tend to have a fairly loyal following, the ratings of most reality shows tend to be extremely variable from week to week and only rarely break into the top tier with respect to audience share. Some might legitimately argue that we should have included the 10 prime-time programs with the highest ratings each week, including reality shows. Although we feel comfortable with our decision it ultimately limits the generalizability of our results to prime-time scripted shows.

Measurement and Data Analysis

The sampling frame for the Television Monitoring Project includes all episodes of the 10 most popular prime-time comedies (five) and dramas (five) for Nielsen's General, African American and Hispanic audiences in the spring television seasons for 2004, 2005, and 2006. Our content analysis of these prime-time programs required two related but physically separate code sheets—a general content code sheet and a specific health content code sheet. The general code sheet was required for every episode of every show in our sample. Specific health code sheets were required for each separate health-related topic that rose to the level of at least a dialogue. Since the number of health topics in a given episode covered could range widely from 0, as was the case in almost half of all of the episodes coded, to 11, as happened in an episode of the medical drama *ER*, we decided to physically separate the two code sheets. This served two purposes. First, it reduced the overall number of pages required and saved paper. (Our coders still preferred to use paper code sheets for the initial coding despite having an electronic data entry system as described below.) Second, in the Television Monitoring Project we opted to analyze health-related content in two ways by maintaining two separate, but related, data files. In the first dataset, each case was a particular episode of a top-rated series. This "general" dataset of all episodes allows us to answer questions such as what percentage of episodes contained violence and whether this varied by genre, by series, or over time. In the second dataset, each case was a specific health-related issue. So if an episode of *Everybody Loves Raymond* contained absolutely no health-related content, it was included as a case in the general dataset but not in the specific health issue dataset. Other shows, like *ER* for example, also had a single entry in the general dataset but could have multiple entries for each episode in the second dataset—one for each separate health issue depicted. This second "specific health issue" dataset allows us to compare the relative prevalence and prominence of various health issues in popular prime-time programs. In other words, the unit of analysis in the general dataset was each individual episode, but the unit of analysis in the second dataset was each specific health issue. These two datasets allowed us to answer distinct, but related, questions.

As noted above, a general code sheet was required for every episode in our sample of prime-time shows. On the general code sheet each episode represented a case. Coders first entered the unique identifiers of a particular episode (e.g., show, episode name, time, date, length, new/repeat, genre, network, major character composition in terms of gender, ethnicity, etc.). As a result of ongoing concerns and controversies regarding medical coverage, the general sheet also asked coders to indicate whether any "access to care" issues were shown (e.g., inadequate health insurance, cutback of public health coverage programs or public medical facilities, immigration status concerns, confidentiality concerns, embarrassment/stigma concerns, lack of health/healthcare information, international concerns) and whether the healthcare received was adequate. In recognition of longstanding research on the impact of violence in the media, the general code sheet also recorded if violence occurred in a particular episode and, if so, what form it took, as well as the perpetrator's and victim's ethnicities.

One of the project's funders was responsible for the national "5 A Day" campaign to promote better nutrition. As a result coders were asked to identify what food or beverages were shown, discussed, and/or consumed, by whom and where (e.g., home, work, school, restaurant, etc.). Because Bandura's social learning theory holds a central role in entertainment education, it was crucial to distinguish between an apple sitting in a bowl on a counter versus an apple being consumed by a beloved character. If an item was consumed, then the coder filled out additional information about the gender, ethnicity, and body weight of the character. But perhaps the most important section of the general health code sheet was a grid which asked coders to identify which, if any, specific health issues appeared in the episode and how prominent the depiction was (e.g., a brief visual cue, a brief mention, a dialogue, a minor or major storyline). A specific health code sheet was completed for each health issue that rose to the level of a dialogue.

The specific health code sheet was designed to gauge what potential impact, if any, a particular health storyline might have on viewers. Each health-related storyline was coded on a number of dimensions, including whether the outcome was positive, negative, or neutral and whether the tone of the depiction was serious, comedic, etc. Since we were particularly interested in determining whether the health-related information conveyed in prime-time television was likely to help or hurt viewers, coders also indicated what type of health information—prevention, risk factors, symptoms, diagnosis, treatment, complications, prognosis—was included and whether they felt the information was misleading, neutral, or accurate. Similarly, our coders were asked to assess the educational content and the potential influence of the storyline on viewers' attitudes, values, and behaviors. Finally, coders provided basic demographic information on the primary characters involved in the specific health storyline, including their gender, age, ethnicity, SES, and the character's role (e.g., healthcare provider, ill or injured, etc.).

How did we determine what to include in our content analysis? As is often the case, our decisions were influenced by a number of factors. For instance, we were clearly influenced by prior research such as work by Gerbner and his colleagues on cultivation (e.g., Gerbner & Gross, 1976) as well as more recent research on violence on television and the potential effect on viewers (National Television Violence Study, 1998). These theories led us to use a more encompassing definition of health-related problems, including those caused by violence, as well as capturing the demographics of the characters involved in the violent acts. We were also persuaded by the previously mentioned potential of entertainment programs to change knowledge, attitudes, beliefs, and behaviors about a variety of health-related topics. Planned entertainment education programs are heavily driven by a particular set of attitude and behavioral change theories, including social learning theory (Bandura, 2004), self-efficacy (Bandura, 1997), the elaboration likelihood model and the processing of narrative dramas (Petty & Cacioppo, 1986; Slater & Rouner, 2002), the Sabido methodology (Sabido, 2004), theory of reasoned action (Fishbein & Ajzen, 1975), theory of planned action (Ajzen, 1991), the health belief model (Becker, 1974), hierarchy of effects and stages of change models (DiClemente & Prochaska, 1985; Singhal & Rogers, 1999; Sood, Menard, & Witte, 2004; Vaughan & Rogers, 2000). We were interested in the extent to which commercial entertainment programs, which are not developed with these theories in mind, nevertheless contained the same persuasive elements, such as modeling of behavior, peripheral and central cues, etc. Current controversies and campaigns also had an impact on our decisions, as can be seen by the inclusion of items measuring access to care, alternative medicine and the "5 A Day" campaign. However, the primary factor underlying many of our decisions was pragmatic. For each item coded we had to weigh our interest in examining that variable against the risk of making the coding too arduous or time-consuming for the coders.

For the purpose of this project, a health issue was defined as "something dealing with disease, injury or disability." This definition is broader than what may commonly be considered a "health issue" since it includes drug abuse, unintentional injury, violence, and mental health, in addition to topics more commonly considered "health problems" such as heart disease and cancer. Commonly occurring health conditions that were not seen as a "problem" were not coded. For instance, while a fertility problem or an unwanted pregnancy would be coded, a healthy, wanted pregnancy would not.

Episodes often contain overlapping, related health issues. For example, a person may have heart disease as a result of high cholesterol. In such cases, both "high cholesterol" and "heart disease" would be entered as separate health issues on the general form, with the relationship between the two indicated on the specific code sheet. In detective shows such as CBS's *CSI: Crime Scene Investigation*, multiple health issues may be associated with the death of a single character. Each possible cause of death put forth on the program would be coded as a separate health issue, along with its prominence in the overall storyline, ranging from a brief visual cue or mention to a major storyline.

In creating our list of health issues we had to strike a balance between being exhaustive, on the one hand, and ease of coding, on the other. While our list of health issues was fairly exhaustive, we nevertheless included several blank lines for "other" miscellaneous health issues. Our goal was to ensure that health issues that are listed as "other" are rare and appear on not more than one or two episodes during an entire season. Examples of health topics that have appeared in the "other" category include: shingles, gastric bypass surgery, frostbite, hemorrhoids, and macular degeneration. Medical shows depict a multitude of health issues and often include some that are relatively obscure. Therefore, we determined that there should be a limit to the number of "other" categories that could be added for a particular episode. There is one additional space on the coding sheet for "other cancer," "unintentional injury," "homicide/ attempted homicide," "other violence," as well as a maximum of five spaces for "other health issues." Coders were instructed that if the number of miscellaneous health issues exceeded the number of spaces provided, they were to record issues in the order of their prominence. Each year, we analyzed these miscellaneous health issues and if an issue appeared repeatedly it was added to the code sheet the following year. However, as discussed in more detail below, any additions or changes to an existing code sheet must be made with extreme care to avoid making the dataset incompatible from year to year.

In addition, we realized the need to limit our analysis of the food and beverages shown and consumed during shows. There are certain shows, such as NBC's *Will & Grace*, where eating and drinking occur almost continuously. If every morsel of food or drink shown or consumed on this show was coded, the amount of time for the coder to analyze an episode would have easily doubled or even tripled. In order to keep the coding manageable, coders recorded food consumption for the four most prominent characters shown eating and drinking for up to four foods or beverages per character. As a result, our dataset slightly under-reports the amount of food consumed on popular shows, but captures the type and frequency of foods that are consumed in popular prime-time shows.

Along similar lines, on the specific health sheet, coders were limited to identifying the four most prominent characters involved in each health storyline. On shows like *Law & Order* where there is generally a "victim," a "perpetrator," witnesses, cops, lawyers, judges, etc., the list of characters involved with the storyline could be endless. Clear guidelines that determine the order of importance among characters were essential to make the coding process manageable and comparable across coders. For example, our rule was that the person or persons experiencing the health problem—the ill, injured or deceased—should be listed first, followed by the perpetrator where appropriate, and then by the other characters involved in the health-related storyline in order of importance to the health issue. If multiple people are working with a patient or investigating a crime, the people taking the lead in the investigation or the primary caretaker are listed before others who may be more remotely involved. Again, we coded the four characters most involved with each health-related storyline and their respective roles. As a result of this decision, characters who were more tangential to the health storyline, such as a nurse who took a patient's temperature, are under-represented in our dataset. While we miss a level of detail that might be obtained by including everyone involved in the storyline, we capture those characters most centrally involved. According to the entertainment education literature (Singhal & Rogers, 1999; Singhal et al, 2004; Sood, 2002), it is these more prominent characters with whom viewers are most likely to identify, if they find themselves in a similar situation.

What Role Must a Health Issue Play Within the Show to "Count?"

In the first year of the project, any health issue appearing on the show—as a brief visual cue, brief mention, dialogue, minor storyline, and/or a major storyline—was identified and had a corresponding specific health coding sheet. But medical shows like *ER*, *Gray's Anatomy*, or *House* have doctors mentioning health topics in passing and background shots of patients coming into the hospital that are just part of a "typical hospital scene," and are not essential to a particular storyline. Filling out specific health sheets for every health-related image or brief mention quickly became cumbersome for the coders. Moreover, it raised questions about the impact these fleeting portrayals could actually have on viewers. Responding to these pragmatic and theoretical issues, we decided that in subsequent years brief visual and verbal cues of health issues would be noted, but not elaborated on using a specific health sheet.

Considerations Regarding Changes to Code Sheets

As indicated previously, from year to year we added health issues that occurred with some frequency in the "other" category to the general coding sheet. For analytic purposes, it was extremely important that all numeric codes used to identify specific health issues remain constant from year to year, otherwise merging the datasets and comparing data between years becomes problematic. For example, imagine that diabetes was assigned health issue number 15 in Year One's alphabetical list of 71 health issues. In Year Two, we wanted to add bioterrorism to the alphabetical list of health issues. While there might be a temptation to update the list alphabetically and renumber the health issues each year this would cause confusion and errors when looking across datasets. New items such as bioterrorism can easily be added to the code sheet in a way that is going to be easy for coders to find them, but the number and/or code assigned to it should be distinct from those used in the past and follow from whatever number and/ or code was assigned to the last option in the previous year's dataset. In other words, bioterrorism should appear alphabetically in the list but should be assigned the issue number 72. This compromise allows the datasets to remain consistent across years while presenting coders with an easy-to-use alphabetical list of health issues.

Coders will also occasionally generate new categories and ideas that were not included on the current code sheets. This often leads to pressure to make changes to a code sheet within a given year. However, we found that constantly modifying a code sheet to include additional categories or variables made it more difficult to begin the coding process in a timely manner. In Year One, training took place in mid-January, after the spring television season was already underway. Additional changes to the code sheet put the project even further behind schedule. This, in turn, put the data entry system creation behind schedule, making it unavailable to coders until they were already a month into the spring season.

The lesson learned? Unless they have uncovered a grievous oversight, coders' recommendations should be incorporated either before or after a particular coding period. In other words, training should either take place sufficiently in advance of actual coding to accommodate changes in the upcoming year's code sheet or suggested changes should wait until the next round of coding. In the meantime, the new data entry system could be created and coders can gain familiarity with it by entering their training data. This way, any glitches in the code sheets or entry system are caught in advance and everyone begins the season with finalized code sheets and a functional data entry system. Our experience suggests that changes to the code sheet and data entry system in the middle of a project may not only confuse coders, but may also undercut their confidence in the project. We resolved these issues in subsequent years by holding intensive training sessions in December, using 12 episodes with somewhat complicated health-related content from the previous spring season. As a consequence the very few changes that were made from year to year to the code sheets, coding manual, and the data entry system were finalized prior to the start of actual coding.

Reliability Issues

As a general rule, the highest inter-rater reliability occurs on simple dichotomous judgments such as present versus absent. Whenever a researcher attempts to measure greater levels of variation there will almost inevitably be an increase in disagreement between coders and a resultant decrease in inter-rater reliability. For instance, in Year One, the biggest disagreements between our coders occurred not over whether a health issue was depicted, but in distinguishing the prominence of the health issue (visual cue, brief mention, dialogue, minor storyline, major storyline). In Year Two, we tried to clarify problematic categories during training by generating specific decision rules like distinguishing the major and minor storylines by how many scenes they occurred in out of the entire show or whether they are alluded to in the episode title (always a clue to a major storyline).

Whenever possible, for more subjective judgments we also tried to give numerous examples during training until we were confident that the coders could successfully recognize the differences between categories. For example, to determine body weight we provided a picture chart of different weights along with characters from various television shows that fell into each of the five different weight categories. To ensure that coders would not forget these specific examples, we included them in a very detailed codebook that we used during training and continually referred to throughout the project.

It is important in any content analysis project to establish inter-rater reliability early on. During our training we had coders view and code a training reel of 12 shows from the prior season with increasingly complex health-related content. Note that we did not take a random selection of shows, because the majority of shows, particularly comedies, had relatively little health-related content. Each week three or four shows were coded at home using the code sheets and then subsequently discussed in a series of meetings led by the project manager. Differences in coding were discussed until coders understood the relevant decision rules. Even though roughly half of our coders had worked on the project the previous year, all coders attended training at the start of each spring season. In addition, we assessed inter-rater reliability throughout the season by having the project manager, who had been with the project several years and once been a coder herself, serve as a second coder on a sub-set of shows (at least 10%) for each current coder. This allowed us to identify and resolve any problems and to calculate inter-rater reliability between each coder and the project manager, who served as the gold standard.

The Potential Impact of New Technology

Identifying Health-related Content: Manual versus Automatic Content Monitoring

Advances in technology could revolutionize the way content analysis of television, newspapers, and even radio is conducted. One of the primary issues in the first year of the Television Monitoring Project was whether to rely exclusively on human coders or to take advantage of recent advances in computerized content monitoring. For instance, we spent time investigating the ShadowTV monitoring service, which automatically archives the major broadcast and cable television channels 24 hours a day, 7 days a week. This service provides researchers with the ability to search for shows using keywords and concepts either in the closed-captioning, speech-to-text transcription, or through speech recognition. In a pilot test designed to assess the feasibility of using ShadowTV for tracking health-related content, we found that ShadowTV's keyword search produced results virtually identical (96% agreement) to those of independent coders (who identified health-related content by viewing each of the shows). Errors using ShadowTV's closed-captioning search were rare and occurred mostly as a result of typographical errors. The 4% error rate of the closed-captioning search could be reduced to 2% by using the "soundex operator" function developed by ShadowTV that searches not only for certain keywords but also for words that are similar phonetically and in structure to the designated keywords.

ShadowTV and similar services have considerable appeal. The most obvious advantage is that the mechanical screening of content dramatically increases the number of channels and programs it is possible to content analyze. One could clearly argue that this larger universe of programs (we had contemplated monitoring 13 channels, 24 hours a day, 7 days a week) allows for a more complete picture of how health is depicted on television. However, these pros had to be weighed against the cons. This monitoring service did not eliminate the need for human coders. While the ShadowTV service would provide comprehensive coverage of verbal mentions of health topics, we would still need to rely on coders to manually code any visual components such as action/behaviors, foods shown/consumed, and certain demographic information on characters (e.g., ethnicity and age). Another consideration involved the quality of the images available from ShadowTV. When video images are streamed from their mainframe computer, they undergo a compression to save bandwidth and as a result, the clarity of the images is compromised. Given that one of the primary purposes of the Television Monitoring Project is to build an archive of health depictions, a higher degree of image clarity (comparable to that of videotaping from a home television set equipped with cable) was required. Finally, the cost, approximately $25,000 a year, for the monitoring service was not insignificant. A cost-benefit analysis revealed that the use of student coders to manually record and code the most popular prime-time shows was significantly more cost effective. Weighing these factors, we ultimately decided that until the technology improved, we would stay with the more traditional method of content analysis that relies primarily on human coders.

Recording: VCR versus DVR

In the pilot year of our project, student coders were responsible for taping and archiving each episode of the shows they were assigned using VHS recorders in their homes. At the conclusion of the spring 2003 television season, we had a list of 36 episodes that were not taped (a 9% error rate) as a result of last-minute programming changes, human error, equipment malfunctions, and other miscellaneous problems. This may have been a unique situation, because in spring 2003 many programs were cancelled or rescheduled because of the onset of the Iraq War. Regardless of the cause, significant time and effort was expended that summer trying to capture missing episodes, either as repeats or from the television networks, and data analysis was significantly delayed.

As a direct result of this experience, in the second year of the study we decided to use digital video recorders in order to increase the reliability of our archiving. DVR (Digital Video Recording) units such as TiVo or Replay had become vastly popular and could be purchased at a reasonable cost. Once a "season pass" is programmed for a designated show, a DVR automatically records all episodes of that particular show to its hard drive. Importantly for our purposes, updated *TV Guide* information is automatically uploaded to the hard drive via phone or internet connections, allowing the unit to capture programs of interest even when they are shown in different time slots. Broadcast image quality is also guaranteed when the DVR is connected through cable television. And unlike most VHS tapes, which can accommodate a maximum of 6 hours of material at low resolution, the DVRs available at that time could hold up to 42 hours of programming (and now can accommodate 140 hours). This enhanced technology and increased capacity to record shows meant that we decided to equip each student coder with a DVR unit to track the shows to which they were assigned. Given the DVR's larger storage capacity we were also able to assign each show to be recorded by two coders, with one of them serving as a back-up in case of power outage or some other problem. In 2004, using these "smart" DVRs that directly tracked programs using *TV Guide*, our percentage of missed programs fell to approximately 1%.

It is important to note, however, that DVRs still have limitations with respect to recording and archiving programs. For instance, once the internal drive is full the DVR will begin to either erase stored programs or stop recording additional programs. Consequently, to save a permanent copy of programs for coders it is critical to download and delete shows from the internal drive on a regular basis. Moreover, while the system we used automatically updated the television schedule periodically, it did not adjust itself for situations where a program exceeded its time slot by more than two minutes. In fact, during the 2004 and 2005 spring television seasons some of the broadcast networks were threatened by the widespread popularity of DVR recording (which allows users to fast forward through commercials) and fought back by making programs of irregular length. This typically involved "supersizing" a program to run between 5 and 15 minutes into the next time slot. As a result, viewers who recorded these programs were left hanging as to how a particular episode ended. Our method of circumventing this problem was to use a feature that allowed manual setting of the start and end recording time.

Archiving: VHS versus DVD

Another technological consideration was whether to use VHS tapes or DVDs when archiving the television shows. Because in 2002 the technology for burning television shows to DVDs was still expensive and somewhat unreliable, VHS tapes were used to archive shows for the first two years of the Television Monitoring Project. By the spring of 2004, however, we decided to switch to a DVD archival system for a number of reasons. Storage space became a key consideration, because of the large number of shows we were archiving (more than 400 per season). After we switched to DVDs we were able to store an entire season's worth of episodes in one tenth the amount of space taken up by the previous year's VHS tapes. Although we decided to record only a single episode on a disc, it should be noted that one disc could accommodate several episodes (up to two hours of programming at SP (slow play) quality). If several episodes were recorded onto one disc, a navigation menu would allow viewers to easily select the desired episode, without having to fast forward or rewind, as would be the case on a VHS tape. In addition to taking up less storage space DVDs are more resistant to deterioration (breakage, warping, and degradation of viewing quality) over time. Digital archiving also allows for more rapid duplication without compromising image quality.

The decision to switch to DVRs and DVDs was not made lightly. Academic researchers, many of whom are operating on a tight budget, cannot risk jumping on the bandwagon of the latest, greatest technology. Technology is constantly evolving and early adoption of new technology can prove both expensive (costs inevitably come down over time) and risky (as anyone stuck with a Beta recording system can testify).

Data Entry

Advances in technology have also influenced the data entry and analysis end of content analyses. A decade ago, it was common for researchers to enter data from paper code sheets by hand into some sort of data spreadsheet. Given the large number of variables often involved in content analysis, this manual data entry could easily result in data entry errors. One way to reduce the number of data entry errors is to utilize a data entry system that checks the range of values and responses permissible for each variable as the data are entered. For example, in the Television Monitoring Project, while our coders still preferred to initially code television programs using paper code sheets, the data was then entered into an electronic database using a data entry program. We compared a few existing data entry options, specifically, a web-based data entry system called SurveyMonkey, Microsoft Access, and SPSS Data Entry Builder/Station. Below, we describe the benefits and drawbacks of these software programs that guided our decision.

Web-based Data Entry systems

Web-based data entry software such as SurveyMonkey is typically very user-friendly and includes simple skip-logic features for data entry. Moreover, because they are web-based, these services generally allow for simultaneous data entry and instantaneous compilation into a single database. Thus, multiple users can simply log in with a username and password from any terminal with internet connection and enter data. They are also relatively inexpensive, requiring a monthly service fee of approximately US$20 a month as opposed to software programs that can run into hundreds or even thousands of dollars. On the negative side, these services tend to offer limited options for layout design and may place restrictions on open-ended responses. Moreover, had we chosen to use SurveyMonkey or any of its web-based competitors, the data entry interface would have looked vastly different from the layout of our paper code sheet. Maintaining a similar layout to the paper code sheets was crucial in order to minimize confusion among coders during data entry, and therefore was a major factor in our decision. A second strike against using SurveyMonkey or similar web-based survey services for data entry is that while the final data can be exported to a Microsoft Excel file, this may not be seamless. For example, the limited rule functions in SurveyMonkey that restrict open-ended questions make data cleaning a laborious task. After cleaning, data must be exported a second time to SPSS for labeling and data analysis. As a result of these drawbacks we decided not to go with SurveyMonkey or any of its web-based competitors.

Microsoft Access

One clear benefit of using Microsoft Access is that it is ubiquitous. Most computers with Microsoft operating systems, including those at the Annenberg School, already had the program installed. Consequently, individual coders would conveniently be able to enter data through almost any computer and then send their data files electronically to the project manager, who would then compile a master dataset. In the pilot year of the Television Monitoring Project, we hired a computer programmer to build an Access data entry database from scratch. Our consultant was able to make the data entry interface look identical to the paper code sheets, thus reducing confusion among the coders.

Unfortunately, the programming fees ran to several thousand dollars and once the data entry system was constructed, we were severely limited in our ability to make changes. Moreover, data had to be transported from Access to Excel, and then to SPSS for analysis. Programming errors and incompatibility between the data entry and data analysis programs meant that transfers were not always completely successful, and occasionally some data and labels were lost in the process.

Statistical Program for the Social Sciences (SPSS) Data Entry Builder

Most researchers in the social sciences are familiar with SPSS, a widely used statistical software program. For those who plan to use SPSS for subsequent data analysis, using this companion program for data entry would seem an obvious choice. Not surprisingly, of all the data entry programs we considered the SPSS Data Entry Builder provided the most seamless transition into a final SPSS dataset. Indeed, the main benefit of this software is the integration between the SPSS data entry and analysis programs. As data is entered through the entry interface, the Data Entry program automatically creates a parallel data file along with variable names and data labels. Individual datasets from different coders can also be easily merged into a master dataset. For example, we had each coder enter and send us their data files electronically roughly once a month. This served several purposes: it permitted us to run periodic checks on inter-coder reliability where the project manager compared a coder's interpretation of an episode against their own; it reassured us that the coders were not falling behind in their coding; and it allowed us to look for trends prior to the end of the spring television season. Because the data was entered directly through SPSS, it avoided the potentially arduous process of exporting, cleaning, and labeling the data. Moreover, SPSS Data Entry Station is available as a supplemental program allowing only data entry, which prevents tampering with the database structure while entering data.

On the downside, although this SPSS-based data collection software program requires only minimal knowledge of programming, it is only somewhat user-friendly, with an intermediate learning curve. It does, however, come with more options for layout design, allowing in-house creation and management of the database, without relying on outside consultants. Consequently, the data entry can be customized at a higher level with graphics, annotations, rules, and various other features, allowing researchers to design the interface to mirror the paper code sheets if they so desire. The major drawback to the SPSS Data Entry system was the size of the software. This requires a computer with at least 256 MB of RAM and a 2.4 GHz processor for the program to run at a reasonable speed. Moreover, the immense size of our database slowed data entry by the lag time between interface changes, which resulted in occasional computer malfunctions. In the final analysis, however, when we weighed relevant factors such as ease of programming, the ability to make modifications, the ability to design the data entry system to physically resemble the paper coding sheets, and the ease of transferring data into a statistical software program, we decided in Year Two to switch to the SPSS Data Builder and Station system.

The lesson we learned is that while technological advances can make content analysis significantly less labor-intensive and error prone, one should proceed with caution. As with any product, it is not wise to immediately adopt the first or even the second version of a new technology or software. Within a relatively short period of time the price will almost inevitably decrease and the reliability will increase. And, if one can afford it, it often makes sense to give preference to established companies that specialize in data entry or analysis who have a vested interest in improving both their product and their customer relations over time.

We predict that the wealth of new technologies such as voice, text, and image recognition already available and on the horizon will spark a renaissance in content analysis. These tools will allow researchers to analyze vast amounts of source material with exponential efficiency. For example, one can now search 6 months' worth of television programming on 13 channels, 7 days a week, 24 hours a day for all occurrences of the word "cancer"—a task that 10 years ago would have taken multiple coders the better part of a year—within hours. But while new technology is particularly useful at finding the "needle in the haystack" it will never completely eliminate the need for human coders to interpret the more subjective elements of a text. It is our hope that this chapter will prove helpful in navigating the theoretical, practical, and technological tradeoffs one must make when embarking on a content analysis.

Conclusion

In closing, this chapter has attempted to give readers a clearer understanding of the numerous issues involved in conducting a content analysis. To do so, we have essentially walked the reader through the key decisions made during the course of the Television Monitoring Project, as well as the rationale behind and consequences of each decision. We would be remiss, however, if we did not underscore that other scholars could legitimately disagree with any or all of our decisions. A divergent decision at any point could have yielded vastly different results. For example, our decision to focus on scripted prime-time dramas and comedies limits the generalizability of our findings to those types of shows.

These caveats aside, findings from this project have already provided public health professionals at the Centers for Disease Control and Prevention, National Cancer Institute, and others with valuable insights into how various ailments are being depicted to the American public (Murphy, Hether & Rideout, 2008). Hollywood, Health and Society also presents data from this ongoing content analysis to television writers and producers on a regular basis, emphasizing the need for more accurate and educational health storylines. Each year exemplary health storylines are identified by our coders and nominated for the "Sentinel for Health" award, providing both recognition and incentive for television writers to incorporate material that motivates viewers to lead healthier lives. Moreover, when used in combination with other methodologies such as pre-test/post-test surveys of specific storylines, the Television Monitoring Project illuminates how factors such as the age, gender, or ethnicity of a character can influence what information viewers retain from a storyline. Our hope is that this chapter may inspire other content analyses that will provide additional insights into one of America's primary sources of health information.

Acknowledgments

We would like to thank Heather J. Hether, Mandy Shaivitz Berkowitz, and Vicki Beck for their contribution to both the Television Monitoring Project and this chapter. We also would like to acknowledge the hard work of all coders past and present, as well as our funding agencies, the Centers for Disease Control and Prevention, the NCI, and the Annenberg School for Communication at the University of Southern California.

References

Ajzen, I. (1991). The theory of planned behavior. *Organizational Behavior and Human Decision Practices, 50*, 179–211.

Bandura, A. (1997). *Self-efficacy: The exercise of control.* New York: Freeman Press.

Bandura, A. (2004). Social cognitive theory for personal and social change by enabling media. In A. Singhal, M. J. Cody, E. M. Rogers, & M. Sabido (Eds.), *Entertainment-education and social change: History, research, and practice* (pp. 75–96). Mahwah, NJ: Lawrence Erlbaum Associates.

Beck, V. (2004). Working with daytime and prime time TV shows in the United States to promote health. In A. Singhal, M. J. Cody, M. Sabido, & E. M. Rogers (Eds.), *Entertainment-education and social change: History, research, and practice* (pp. 207–224). Mahwah, NJ: Lawrence Erlbaum Associates.

Beck, V., Huang, G. C., Pollard, W. E., & Johnson, T. J. (2003). TV drama viewers and health information. Paper presented at the American Public Health Association 131st Annual Meeting and Exposition, San Francisco, CA.

Becker, M. (1974). The health belief model and personal health behavior. *Health Education Monographs, 2*, 241–251.

Brodie, M., Foehr, U., Rideout, V., Baer, N., Miller, C., Flournoy, R., & Altman, D. (2001). Communicating health information through the electronic media. *Health Affairs, 20*, 192–199.

Brown, J. D., & Walsh-Childers, K. (2002). Effects of media on personal and public health. In J. Bryant and D. Zillman (Eds.), *Media effects: Advanced in theory and research* (pp. 453–488). Mahwah, NJ: Lawrence Erlbaum Associates.

Brown, W. J., & Fraser, B. P. (2004). Celebrity identification in entertainment-education. In A. Singhal, M. J. Cody, M. Sabido, & E. M. Rogers (Eds.), *Entertainment-*

education and social change: History, research, and practice (pp. 97–106). Mahwah, NJ: Lawrence Erlbaum Associates.

DiClemente, C. C., & Prochaska, J. O. (1985). Processes and stages of change: Coping and competence in smoking behavior change. In S. Shiffman & T. A. Wills (Eds.), *Coping and substance abuse* (pp. 319–342) New York: Academic Press.

Fishbein, M. & Ajzen, I. (1975). *Belief, attitude, intention and behavior: An introduction to theory and research*. Boston: Addison-Wesley.

Gerbner, G., & Gross, L. (1976). Living with television: The violence profile. *Journal of Communication, 26*, 172–199.

Greenberg, B., Salmon, C. T., Patel, D., Beck, V. & Cole, G. (2004). Evolution of an E-E research agenda. In A. Singhal, M. J. Cody, M. Sabido, & E. M. Rogers (Eds.), *Entertainment-education and social change: History, research, and practice* (pp. 191–204). Mahwah, NJ: Lawrence Erlbaum Associates.

Kaiser Family Foundation, *Health Poll Report*, February 2001 to February 2002. Menlo Park, CA: The Kaiser Family Foundation. Available at: www.kff.org.

Murphy, S. T., & Cody, M. J. (2003). *Summary report: Developing a research agenda for entertainment education and multicultural audiences*. Atlanta, GA: Centers of Disease Control and Prevention. Available at: http://www.learcenter.org.

Murphy, S. T., Cody, M. J., Beck, V., Burkett, H., Shavitz, M., & Huang, G. (2003). An analysis of health content in popular television shows. Paper presented at the 131st Annual Meeting of the American Public Health Association, November 17, San Diego.

Murphy, S. T., Hether, H. J., & Rideout, V. (2008). How healthy is prime time? An analysis of health content in popular prime time television programs. A report to The Kaiser Family Foundation. Available online at: http://www.kaisernetwork.org.

National Center for Chronic Disease Prevention and Health Promotion at the Centers for Disease Control and Prevention. (2008). *Overweight and obesity*. Retrieved May 30, 2008, from www.cdc.gov/nccdphp/dnpa/obesity.

National Television Violence Study. (1998). *Report of the University of California, Santa Barbara, Center for Communication and Social Policy. Executive summary* (J. Federman, Ed.). Available online: http://www.ccsp.ucsb.edu/execsum.pdf

Petty, R. E., & Cacioppo, J. T. (1986). *Communication and persuasion: Central and peripheral routes to attitude change*. New York: Springer-Verlag.

Sabido, M. (2004). The origins of entertainment-education. In A. Singhal, M. J. Cody, M. Sabido, & E. M. Rogers (Eds.), *Entertainment-education and social change: History, research, and practice* (pp. 61–74). Mahwah, NJ: Lawrence Erlbaum Associates.

Sharf, B. F., Freimuth, V. S., Greenspon, P., & Plotnick, C. (1996). Confronting cancer on *thirtysomething*: Audience response to health content on entertainment television. *Journal of Health Communication, 1*, 157–172.

Sherry, J. (2002). Media saturation and entertainment education. *Communication Theory, 12*, 206–224.

Singhal, A., Cody, M. J., Rogers, E. M., & Sabido, M. (Eds.). (2004). *Entertainment-education and social change: History, research, and practice*. Mahwah, NJ: Lawrence Erlbaum Associates.

Singhal, A., & Rogers, E. M. (1999). *Entertainment-education: A communication strategy for social change*. Mahwah, NJ: Lawrence Erlbaum Associates.

Slater, M. D., & Rouner, D. (2002). Entertainment-education and elaboration likelihood: Understanding the processing of narrative persuasion. *Communication Theory, 12*, 173–191.

Sood, S. (2002). Audience involvement and entertainment-education. *Communication Theory, 12,* 153–172.

Sood, S., Menard, T., & Witte, K. (2004). The theory behind entertainment-education. In A. Singhal, M. J. Cody, E. M. Rogers, & M. Sabido (Eds.), *Entertainment-education and social change: History, research, and practice.* Mahwah, NJ: Lawrence Erlbaum Associates.

Vaughan, P. W., & Rogers, E. M. (2000). A staged model of communication effects: Evidence from an entertainment-education radio soap opera in Tanzania. *Journal of Health Communication, 5,* 203–227.

Whittier, D. K., Kennedy, M. G., Seeley, S., St. Lawrence, J. S., & Beck, V. (2005). Embedding health messages into entertainment television: Effect on gay men's response to a syphilis outbreak. *Journal of Health Communication, 10*(2), 251–259.

12 Receiver-oriented Message Analysis

Lessons from Alcohol Advertising

Erica Weintraub Austin

Message meaning interests most of us because we presume that message content reflects the motives of media producers and has effects on receivers (Shoemaker & Reese, 1990; Stroman & Jones, 1998). For example, beer commercials frequently attract criticism because they contain elements such as humor, extreme sports, and sexual themes, which appeal to adolescent boys (Atkin, Hocking, & Block, 1984; Aitken, Leathar, & Scott, 1988; Grube, 1993; Grube & Wallack, 1994; Jones & Donovan, 2001). Critics of the media often infer motives and effects from the presence of content elements, such as that (1) the alcohol industry intends to target adolescent boys, and (2) the advertisements make adolescent boys more likely to want to drink beer and engage in risky, promiscuous activities. But how can we verify whether the alcohol industry actually uses these elements to target underage males—when they say they don't (Beer Institute, 1999; Beer Institute, 2003)? And how do we know that boys will agree with trained coders on what is funny, appealing, and sexy, as opposed to stupid, ridiculous, and degrading? How do we know the ads do not contain additional elements that appeal to boys but that carefully trained coders may miss?

Because content analysis research cannot address these questions on its own, my colleagues and I have been exploring a way to do so, which we call "receiver-oriented message analysis" (ROMA). Using this method, we have confirmed that underage males believe they often are the intended targets for certain alcohol ads. They find many of the ads appealing, but they also see things in the ads that offend them. Perhaps most importantly, we have verified that young adults notice content elements in the ads that trained coders do not see (Austin et al., 2003; Austin, Pinkleton, Hust, & Miller, 2007).

Scholars typically use content analysis to reliably establish "common" meaning; that is, meaning on which most people can agree (Berelson, 1952). Some hold the view that the purpose of content analysis is to separate the actual meaning of content from its intended or received meanings (Kassarijn, 1977; Kepplinger, 1989). Communication, however, is "a social process, within a context, in which signs are produced and transmitted, perceived, and treated as messages from which meaning can be inferred" (Worth & Gross, 1974, p. 30). This means that receivers have to figure out, or infer, what the signs in messages are supposed to symbolize. As a result, researchers—particularly in a public health context—want to establish how informational signs are perceived by receivers, in whom meaning resides and resonates.

Because the assignment of meaning requires inference, researchers need to understand how inferences made by content analysts relate to those made by typical message receivers. Trained coders typically make few inferences, depending instead on explicitly defined categories described in a coding protocol. The typical message receiver, however, may assign meaning based on a variety of available information. This makes message meaning a variable, not a constant. Shared meaning can fracture along lines created by expectations (Darley & Smith, 1995), developmental level (Collins, 1983; Kunkel et al., 2004), and processing strategy (Chaiken, Liberman and Eagly, 1989; MacDonald & MacDonald, 1999; Meyers-Levy & Tybout, 1997; Petty & Cacioppo, 1986; Vakratsas & Ambler, 1999).

Kiecker, Palan, and Areni (2000) have noted that the interpretations even of well-trained content coders may differ as a result of characteristics such as gender roles and influenceability. As a result, content analysts who intend to theorize about effects need to understand how and why receiver interpretations might vary from a presumed common meaning. As Krippendorff (2004) has cautioned, "the popular and simplistic notion of 'content' has outlived its explanatory capabilities ... this development calls for a redefinition of content analysis, one that aligns content—the target of the research—with how contemporary society operates and understands itself" (pp. xix–xx). In other words, content analysis must be a dynamic process that is sensitive to the meanings likely to be received by different types of relevant audiences. ROMA helps to accomplish this goal.

Developmental Considerations

Age-related developmental differences in information processing are especially important to consider when examining potential media effects on children and adolescents. For example, studies have shown that children are exposed to a substantial amount of alcohol advertising (Center on Alcohol Marketing and Youth, 2002a,b, 2004), but also that children often interpret advertising messages differently than adults (Kunkel et al., 2004). This raises questions about the extent to which traditional content analysis provides accurate information about the meanings children take away from alcohol advertising messages.

As this chapter will explain, we have found evidence that young adults may come away with different impressions of content than trained coders. It seems even more likely that the same is true for children and adolescents. During middle childhood and adolescence, children gradually develop a mature understanding of most message content and production techniques. Some scholars have indicated that fifth grade represents a critical turning point in children's understanding of communication, in that at this age they become better able to understand messages but more susceptible to social influence

(Austin & Knaus, 2000; Miller, Smith, & Goldman, 1990). Children prior to and shortly after reaching this critical juncture therefore may notice somewhat different things in messages, and they also may interpret them differently. These differences are likely to affect the impact of the messages.

Children prior to fourth and fifth grade still are developing their understanding of the difference between television programming and advertising. They tend to be less confident about identifying public service announcements (Dorr, 1986), an atypical message category that appears only infrequently on television. Children in this age range also have difficulty understanding persuasive intent (Austin, 1995), sometimes treating persuasive messages as informational messages instead (Blosser & Roberts, 1985). Being more literal and less flexible in their thinking abilities, they alternatively may consider all ads as entirely untrue instead of understanding that a middle ground exists (Dorr, 1986).

By adolescence, children tend to understand that advertising may have some truth but is not entirely truthful. A mature understanding of explicit and implicit information, perspective and intentions, and production techniques does not develop until approximately the eighth grade (Dorr, 1980; Austin, 1995). Even then, adolescents appear to learn more and interpret messages differently if they receive media literacy education programs (Austin, Chen, Pinkleton, & Quintero-Johnson, 2006; Hobbs & Frost, 2003). Indeed, one of the purposes of media literacy education is to teach students to "read" messages more reflectively, recognizing elements they may not have noticed before (Center for Media Literacy, 2005).

The Role of Reflection

Even adults can vary in what they notice about a media message based on how reflectively they approach it. Individuals use cognitive shortcuts when they need or want efficiency, or when they do not have the time or desire to devote to careful message processing. Individuals also may use cognitive shortcuts when they do not have the ability to analyze a message in depth, leading again to the probability of developmental differences in message evaluations. For example, children often miss implicit messages or do not consider the intentions of programmers and characters, and they also can misunderstand the meaning behind techniques such as slow motion and flashbacks (Collins, 1983; Dorr, 1980). This limits their understanding of latent (i.e., implied) content.

In addition, it is likely that some of the decision-making shortcuts available to adults have yet to be learned by children. Conversely, some shortcuts rejected by adults as too simplistic may be embraced by children. This too could lead to different conclusions about the meaning present in various messages.

The Role of Affect

Affect also is likely to influence observations and interpretations of content. Although trained adults doing traditional content analysis will be analyzing messages logically against carefully constructed definitions, typical receivers are more likely to incorporate affect into their evaluations, particularly given that this type of message is designed carefully to produce positive emotional response (Dorr, 1986; McNeal, 1992). According to Clore and colleagues (Clore et al., 2001), positive affect can shut down processing by signaling success, or it can motivate more creative processing. Bless (2001) notes that "happy" participants in a problem-solving task may outperform emotionally neutral participants. Negative affect, on the other hand, tends to motivate more analytical processing. Erber and Erber (2001) similarly caution that individuals may choose to process messages in a way that maintains a mood or, alternatively, in a way that changes their mood. According to theorists studying heuristic and systematic approaches to processing, individuals' defense motivations may bias their systematic interpretations of content (Chen & Chaiken, 1999). As a result, people using media for enjoyment may be motivated to maintain that enjoyment, and therefore may not process messages in an analytical fashion.

The Value of Receiver-oriented Message Analysis

If inferences can vary for such a variety of reasons, traditional content analysis can obtain a reliable assessment of *potential* message elements. Researchers then need to consult receivers to obtain realistic assessments of content as it is actually perceived by particular types of audiences. The application of receiver-oriented message analysis makes it possible to verify assumptions about common meaning and investigate the potential role of developmental differences, cultural differences, and processing styles on observations and interpretations of message content. This chapter attempts to illustrate the usefulness of the ROMA method by reviewing some of our findings to date, with a particular focus on one study that examined how young-adult men and women perceive and respond to alcohol advertising (Austin et al., 2003).

For that study, we chose to consult young-adult men and women about alcohol advertising because recent content analysis research has indicated that alcohol advertising appears to target males more than females, and other research has suggested that males and females drink alcohol for somewhat different reasons. If the ads target men, this implies that gender differences should exist in perceptions of alcohol advertisements. Even if men and women observe the same content elements in alcohol ads, which has not been previously verified, the research on their respective motivations for drinking suggests that they may respond to these persuasive appeals different ways. Applying the ROMA method can help to build a clearer link between reliably obtained content analysis findings and clearly varying audience interpretations and effects.

Receiver-oriented message analysis examines content from the perspective of particular audiences, using quantitative measures that take into account the unique characteristics that help to shape message meaning for that specific group. This approach differs from interpretative analysis (also called reception analysis), in which scholars analyze content for latent meanings by employing qualitative methods such as interviews, focus groups, and ethnographies (Ahuvia, 2001; Jensen, 1991). As Ahuvia has explained, these studies typically focus on a small number of messages in order to analyze them in depth for their received meaning, whereas quantitative content analyses focus on a larger number of messages but cannot analyze them in as much depth. Nor can quantitative content analysis verify that message receivers draw the same conclusions about messages that carefully trained coders do. The tradeoff between these two approaches, notes Ahuvia, is between emic (subjective) interpretations that provide depth but limited applicability, or less rich, etic (researcher-defined) analyses that provide generalizability but less depth.

The value of ROMA is its ability to tap message meaning as it resides in the inferences audience members make, which traditional content analysis cannot verify on its own and interpretive analysis cannot investigate reliably. In particular, the ROMA approach can address three specific issues: (1) the extent to which content analysis results coincide with meanings common to a particular audience; (2) the correlates of differences in perceived meaning within an audience; and (3) the extent to which exposure to objectively identified content, as well as perceived content, can be connected validly to beliefs and behaviors. This chapter reviews the basic process of conducting a ROMA study, offering examples of how it addresses each of these three issues.

How Receiver-oriented Content Analysis Works

In receiver-oriented message analysis, respondents who are members of a particular message audience code content quantitatively—just like trained coders do in traditional content analysis—but without relying on predetermined definitions. This enables researchers to draw valid and reliable conclusions about content elements as identified by a message's receivers. Gathering a large, diverse sample of "coders" makes it possible to explore cultural, individual, and situational differences in observations. ROMA results can be compared with traditional content analysis to see what factors predict that receivers will come close to (or stray far from) the common meaning identified by trained coders.

A receiver-oriented message analysis systematically assigns a sample of messages to a large subject pool so that a sub-sample of respondents codes each message. The sample of respondents can be selected purposively to represent any socio-cultural groups of interest. In one study, for example, we compared young-adult males and young-adult females. One also might compare age groups or ethnic groups. The sample of messages is selected to be generalizable to the relevant population of messages. For our study of young-adult men and women, we selected advertisements from a population of magazines popular among young adults. Each message in the sample gets coded by a group of "receiver-coders" (i.e., individuals in the target population), paralleling the methodology of a repeated-measures experimental design.

Because ROMA is controlled less tightly than traditional content analysis, but more naturalistic, it acts as a counterpart to traditional content analysis in much the same way as a field test serves as a naturalistic counterpart to a lab experiment. The receiver-coders are not trained as are traditional coders, much as scholars do not control the environment for a field experiment the way they would for an experimental manipulation in a lab. This is because the purpose of ROMA is not to compare what naive receivers can find versus what trained coders can find. Instead, just as a field experiment tests what *does* happen in a realistic situation versus what *can* happen in a laboratory situation, a ROMA study examines what naive receivers *do* find versus what trained coders *can* find.

Planning a ROMA Study

The goal for ROMA analysis is to provide generalizable findings about message meaning from the perspective of a message's focal interpreters. Ideally, the sample of content elements *and* the sample of receiver-coders will be generalizable. At minimum, studies must avoid the limitations of message-specific findings so that results can speak more broadly to message types and content variables, rather than only to specific examples.

To accomplish this, each message needs to be coded by a group of typical message receivers to establish reliability or, alternatively, to provide an opportunity for varied perceptions to emerge. To develop a realistic design for a particular study, researchers need to consider how much time receivers will require to code each message, along with how much time is available. For example, researchers are not likely to get 400 participants to code 80 messages apiece. Fortunately, the principles of repeated-measures designs make this unnecessary anyway. We have found that we can get responses to 4–8 messages from each receiver during a typical 45–50-minute session, depending on the type of message and level of analytical detail desired.

For example, in the primary study described in this chapter (Austin et al., 2003), we used receiver-oriented message analysis to examine the perceptions of males and females regarding advertisements for alcohol contained in the most popular men's and women's magazines. We thought this was important to do because scholars have found empirically derived links between exposure to alcohol advertisements and alcohol consumption among young people inconsistently (Saffer, 2002). This raises questions about the implications of content analyses and econometric analyses that have indicated that alcohol advertising appears to target young people in terms of advertising placements and in the content of advertising appeals (Austin & Hust, 2005; Center on Alcohol Marketing and Youth, 2002a, 2004; Strickland, Finn, & Lambert, 1982). Most important to our study, even though content analysis consistently has shown that alcohol advertising targets males more often than females (Austin & Hust, 2005; Garfield, Chung, & Rathouz, 2003; Pfau, 1995) adolescent girls have caught up to boys in the rates at which they use alcohol

(Martin et al., 2002) and, in comparison to adults, girls see more alcohol advertising in magazines than boys do (Jernigan, Ostroff, Ross, & O'Hara, 2004). To illuminate how they might internalize these messages differently, we thought it would be useful to begin by investigating the extent to which men and women would differ or concur in the content elements they perceive in print-based alcohol advertisements.

Assessing a Content Population's Relationship to the Receivers of Interest

One of the challenges in any content analysis is to select a sample with potential audiences in mind. A researcher, for example, might want to distinguish the content in G- or PG-rated movies from the content in R-rated movies. This challenge is a little different in a ROMA study because the targeting of the message also can be a variable of interest. In our study of young-adult men and women, for example, we wanted to be able to test whether receivers perceived the content differently in ads ostensibly aimed at men rather than women. To select an appropriate message sample, we therefore decided it was important first to verify assumptions we held regarding the use of "men's" and "women's" magazines by men and women. Accordingly, we distributed a questionnaire to 160 undergraduate students and asked them to list magazines they had read during the previous two months. To confirm our assumptions about targeting, we also had them indicate whether each magazine was geared toward women, men, or both.

This gave us the information we needed to be able to compare viewers' perceptions across male- and female-targeted ads. The respondents listed a total of 106 magazines, and we selected the six most frequently read magazines for use as the content population for our study. Respondents consistently identified three of these magazines as targeted toward men and three magazines as targeted toward women. Then, to verify receivers' perceptions of messages that content analysis has established as heavily gender-stereotyped, we kept the respondents in our main study blind to whether the particular ads they were viewing came from a men's magazine or a women's magazine.

Avoiding Message-specific and Order Effects

To draw conclusions about magazine types instead of about particular ads, we decided to employ a repeated-measures design. We had each respondent code at least two ads from each type of magazine. To prevent findings from being skewed by primacy or recency effects, we presented the ads in a variety of balanced orders, much as one would approach a repeated-measures experimental design. To maximize the opportunity provided by data collection taking place in a multiple-classroom setting, we settled on a design that randomly assigned groups to a set of stimuli consisting of four alcohol advertisements, selected from the six magazines (*Playboy, Maxim, Sports Illustrated, Glamour,*

Vogue, and *Cosmopolitan*) identified as the most frequently read magazines among the sample population (Center on Alcohol Marketing and Youth, 2002). We selected ads that appeared in either a men's or women's magazine but not in both.

We assigned ads randomly to stimulus groups that included four advertisements per group (two men's and two women's). To control for order effects and ensure that each ad would appear an equal number of times, we presented the ads in six different arrangements based on the type of magazine the ad was selected from (i.e., MFMF, FMFM, MMFF, FFMM, MFFM, FMMF). We then repeated two of these patterns to accommodate a total of 32 ads (16 men's and 16 women's), presented in eight different groups. By reversing the order of presentation of the advertisements, we created an additional eight groups. This arrangement ensured that each participant would code two ads from men's magazines and two ads from women's magazines and also ensured that each individual message would be coded by at least two groups of individuals.

Similarly, in another study intended to compare young-adult receiver interpretations with a traditional content analysis performed by trained coders (Austin, Pinkleton, & Hust, 2007), we used a sample of 40 previously coded alcohol ads and randomly assigned each ad to one of ten orders, always presenting the ads in groups of four. This procedure ensured that each respondent would view a random sample of four alcoholic beverage ads, and that the group of student participants as a whole would view the entire set of 40 ads in a randomly assigned manner.

In a study comparing televised beer ads and public service announcements (Pinkleton, Austin, & Fujioka, 2001), adolescent participants viewed a total of eight clips selected to represent a variety of message strategies. In this case our content sample was purposive rather than randomly selected. We presented the clips in eight balanced orders. Each order included four beer ads and four public service announcements. We did not embed the clips in programming because we saw no need to conceal the purpose of the study. Instead, we asked the respondents to pay careful attention so they could answer questions about the clips after viewing. We had them provide their responses to each particular clip immediately after that segment was shown, but before the next one was presented. This tactic helped ensure that they would not miss any of the content in order to complete the instruments.

Planning Tactics for Data Collection

Researchers can collect receiver-oriented data from individuals in a laboratory or home-based setting, but real-world constraints often require data collection in group settings such as classrooms. To run studies such as our print-based alcohol advertising studies in a classroom setting (Austin et al., 2002; Austin et al., 2007), we display each ad on a color transparency for approximately four minutes while participants complete the receiver-oriented message analysis measures. Respondents are free to move if they need to examine the ad more closely. As already noted, for responses to video-based ads we typically show one message at a time and then ask for their responses to each message before going on to the next.

After participants finish viewing the content sample, they can complete a series of measures representing a relevant theoretical model, provide demographic information and answer other questions of interest to researchers. For example, we have asked respondents to answer questions about their media use, liking of and trust toward the messages, perceived norms and expectancies for alcohol use, and other variables with theoretical relevance (Austin et al., 2002; Austin et al., 2007). We have found that collecting the measures prior to message exposure can alter the processing strategy they apply to the messages, making them more reflective than they normally might be (Austin et al., 2002). If the point of ROMA is to obtain realistic assessments of messages from typical message recipients, it seems best to avoid making an already manufactured situation even more unrealistic.

To obtain the receiver-oriented message analysis of each message, we give respondents a survey-like questionnaire that prompts them to identify things they see in the messages. For example, the questionnaire for the alcohol advertising studies has included lists of demographic variables such as "men," "women," "people under 21," and so on. The questionnaire also has included lists of themes such as "friendship," "instant gratification," and other variables of interest, such as the existence of moderation messages. We make the lists as similar as possible to coding protocols used by trained coders. In some cases we modify measures a bit—for example, we don't ask receivers to delineate whether women appear in the foreground or in the background. Also, we can ask respondents whether they think they themselves are targets for the messages.

Comparing Traditional Content Analysis Results with Received Meanings

In the primary study for which data collection procedures are described here in depth, and in which we assessed young adults' responses to magazine ads, we found that men and women agreed both with each other and with traditional coders that men more often were the targets of alcohol advertisements in both men's and women's magazines. More specifically, they agreed that the ads targeted men more often than women—by about 90% to 63%. These estimates far outstripped those of trained coders, who found that 52% of alcohol ads featuring human models from these magazines targeted men, while 25% targeted women (Austin & Hust, 2005). In addition, although respondents agreed with traditional coders that men more often are the targets of alcohol advertising overall, they disagreed with the trained coders' conclusion that ads in men's magazines tended to target men and ads in women's magazines tended to target women. Both sexes thought that men were targeted more often than women even in women's magazines.

Our respondents' perceptions regarding targeting also differed from traditional coders in other respects. The receivers' estimates of underage targeting were far higher than those of traditional coders, perceiving that college students were targeted 86% of the time in men's magazines and 72% of the time in women's magazines. Trained coders had concluded that only one of every six ads (17%) had targeted underage readers. Respondents further indicated that the ads in men's magazines targeted underage drinkers 65% of the time versus 54% of the time in women's magazines. Respondents also reported that college students were targeted more often in men's magazines than in women's magazines. In other words, our ROMA studies showed that these receivers of alcoholic beverage ads perceived they were the targets of the ads far more often than the estimates generated by traditional coders.

These results were similar to those obtained from another ROMA study of college students in which our focus was on how their perceptions corresponded to the findings of trained coders (Austin, Pinkleton, Hust, & Miller, 2007). In that study we found that message receivers and trained coders disagreed on virtually all types of content. In general, they noticed many specific message features more often than coders trained to search for these features did, suggesting that these characteristics were more salient to the message receivers, just as an advertiser would intend. Of most concern, message receivers tended to perceive more frequent portrayals of underage individuals, more appeal to underage drinkers, more frequent sexual connotations, more frequent messages that encouraged drinking a lot of alcohol, and fewer moderation messages. We concluded that the untrained receiver-coders noticed things that may have gone under the radar of the trained coders. In other words, message attributes that are not typically measured by traditional content analysis may be contributing meaning to audience members, and that meaning is then reflected in the judgments of receiver-coders.

Understanding How and Why Perceived Meaning May Differ Among Audience Sub-groups

Within a general demographic such as a college-student audience, sub-groups' observations of message content may vary in ways that have implications for message effects. For example, studies frequently show that women tend to process messages at deeper levels of elaboration than men (Andsager, Austin, & Pinkleton, 2002; Meyers-Levy & Sternthal, 1991) and that men tend to rely on schemas or overall message themes when processing ads (Meyers-Levy & Maheswaran, 1991). Given that alcohol ads employ a variety of themes designed to appeal to men's sex-role stereotypes (Austin & Hust, 2005; Finn & Strickland, 1982), this presumably would make these characteristics especially salient and memorable to male observers. In addition, because of women's tendency to process in a more relational and contextual way (Putrevu, 2001), men and women might differ in their perceptions of how males and females are portrayed in ads featured in men's and women's magazines.

When we tested these possibilities in the primary data collection described here, we found that men and women concurred in their reports of the themes used in men's and women's magazine advertisements for alcohol. This study was analyzed by trained coders for this target public, although the results cannot be generalized to other groups such as younger adolescents or children. Differences arose, however, in men's and women's analyses of content elements related to portrayals of women, particularly regarding those in women's magazines. Male observers reported that women in the ads seemed happier and had more fun than did female observers. Male observers also reported that women in the women's magazines were more seductive and sexually aroused than female observers indicated. Finally, male observers indicated that men seemed more desirable in the women's magazines than female observers reported. We surmised that men and women evaluated the latent (i.e., implied) content according to different cues or different scripts regarding indicators of women's happiness and sexuality.

For content analysts, this result suggests that we can have more confidence in objectively obtained measurements of manifest content than of latent content susceptible to perceptual bias. Latent content embodies context, personal experience, and symbolism (Graber, 1989) and holds the most significance for individuals' responses to messages and their uses of message meanings in decision-making (Austin, Pinkleton, & Fujioka, 2000; Bandura, 1994; Fischhoff, 1992; Worth & Gross, 1974). This underscores the importance of validating observed content with different audiences and, where differences exist, of developing and testing explanations for variations in "common" meanings.

Ensuring the Validity of Connections Between Objectively Identified Content and Effects

The data show that we have established that observed content elements can vary, and interpretations of those observed content elements can also vary. These variations can provide important information about latent meaning to researchers trying to understand uses and effects. To the extent perceived content varies across groups of receivers, these variations obviously can affect the links between exposure and outcomes such as attitudes, beliefs, and behaviors. Accounting for these variations should reduce error variance in estimations of potential relationships.

In our study of young-adult men and women, for example, we realized we did not have to assume that content identified as male-targeted actually would be especially appealing to men. In addition, the fact that our respondents had perceived that ads in women's magazines nevertheless seemed male-targeted raised questions about how appealing ads identified by trained coders as targeted to women actually would be to women. Finally, because research has indicated that women tend to counter-argue more than men with television ads (Rouner, Slater, & Domenech-Rodriguez, 2003) and elaborate more than men do on negative information (MacDonald & MacDonald, 1999), male-targeted and sexually stereotyped content in alcohol ads could make the ads less persuasive to women.

When we investigated these possibilities, we found that our expectations held mainly for the ads published in men's magazines. Men judged those ads as more appealing than women did. Nevertheless, even though they thought women's ads often were targeted to them, they did not find women's ads more appealing than women did. This perhaps reflected successful gender targeting of those messages despite the receivers' beliefs that most of the ads targeted men. Similarly, women found men's ads more offensive than men did, but they did not find women's ads more offensive than men did. This also seemed to reflect successful gender targeting.

If both genders were targeted successfully, the advertising should have demonstrated equal effectiveness across genders, perhaps varying according to frequency of exposure. In fact, this could indicate that trained coders' observations regarding targeting actually were more valid than the receivers' observations from an effects point of view. In other words, regardless of what they thought they saw, men and women could have responded to what trained coders observed in the messages.

Even if that were not the case, we could test whether exposure to consistently observed/perceived content predicted expectancies. Whether or not they agreed with the conclusions of traditional coders, men and women had converged on their identification of content elements in advertising. Differences between genders in apparent message effects thus could relate mainly to levels of message exposure. Content analysis, however, has shown that exposure to magazines does not equate to exposure to alcohol advertising. Men and women tend to read magazines that are targeted more toward their own gender (Jernigan et al., 2004; Taveras et al., 2004), and alcohol advertisements are concentrated in men's magazines (Austin & Hust, 2005). Even though adolescent girls see almost twice as much print-based alcohol advertising as adult women do (Jernigan et al., 2004), the concentration of alcohol advertising in women's magazines is much lower than in men's magazines (Austin & Hust, 2005; Center on Alcohol Marketing and Youth, 2002b).

Separating exposure by type of magazine could account for this disparity. If men or women tend to see a magazine type more frequently, and frequency of exposure to consistent content explains effects, then both men and women should be more affected by the ads in same-gender-oriented magazines. That is, both sexes should be affected similarly. We found, however, that the frequency of men's magazine use positively predicted expectancies only for men. More frequent use of women's magazines did not predict perceptions for either sex. Of course, given that our study was cross-sectional in design, it should be noted that expectancies could have predicted magazine use rather than the other way around.

Nevertheless, this result suggested to us that the higher concentration of alcohol ads in men's magazines made them more salient to heavier users, who tended to be male. This also suggested that a certain threshold of content saturation must exist before repeated exposure to content elements with common meaning has an effect independent from more individualistic inter- pretations of those elements. Further research combining message interpreta- tion process measures with traditional and receiver-oriented message analysis could establish whether threshold levels of content elements of interest exist in certain types of messages, such as popular television programs.

Although frequency of exposure did not predict alcohol expectancies for women, research suggests that women are also affected by alcohol adver- tising. As Greenberg pointed out some time ago (1988), exposure need not be frequent for content to have a significant impact. We therefore used ROMA to examine links between identified content elements and resonant interpretations. We expected that men and women would respond differently to similar content elements. Indeed, we found that men and women largely converged on the meaning of the ads but that the meanings associated with the ad content resonated with them in somewhat different ways, primarily in terms of emotional responses.

Theorists have shown that emotion can provide important information (Clore et al., 2001). We saw this most plainly by investigating a finding that had initially surprised us: women reported higher desirability scores for the ads than men did despite finding them more offensive. We had reasoned that men would respond positively to the gender-stereotyped content because, even though men also have been shown to criticize the portrayals of women in alcohol ads (Rouner et al., 2003), they nonetheless would respond to gender schemas primed by the ads. This should have led them to higher desirability ratings. Indeed, men's desirability scores were positively predicted by overall appeal of men's magazines. Women's desirability scores, however, were nega- tively predicted by overall offensiveness of men's magazines. Overall appeal or offensiveness of women's magazines did not predict desirability for either sex.

This indicated to us that, for men, the degree to which individuals portrayed in ads seemed likeable, successful, or attractive—the operationalizations of desirability—straightforwardly reflected how appealing the ad seemed to receivers. Potential offensiveness did not detract from apparent desirability. For women, however, the opposite occurred, in that perceived offensiveness drove their perceptions of desirability more than apparent appeal did. This shows that content analysts should find it useful to verify how message receivers respond to message elements on an emotional level. We have seen in other studies that what observed content means on a latent level can change depending on how receivers process the information (Austin, Chen, & Grube, 2006; Austin, Pinkleton, & Funabiki, 2005; Pinkleton, Austin, Cohen, Miller, & Fitzgerald, 2007).

Summary and Implications of Using Receiver-oriented Message Analysis

This chapter has explored the usefulness of employing receiver-oriented message analysis (ROMA) to increase the true-to-life context of content evaluations. A unique feature of the ROMA design is that it systematically assigns a sample of messages across a large subject pool. The sample of respondents who evaluate the content may be purposively selected to represent particular socio-cultural groups of interest. The goal is to give the results reliability in terms of their reflection of the population of relevant messages. The content sample can be employed with a variety of respondent groups to verify commonalities and explore differences in message analysis and response.

In general, our ROMA studies to date have found that a good deal of common meaning exists between young-adult receivers and trained coders on measures of manifest content. Where differences arise, they tend to be relatively modest. Some findings regarding latent content, however, differ considerably. In some cases, such as the apparent targeting of the ads, the ROMA studies found reliability across the sexes but considerable differences from the conclusions drawn by trained coders. Male and female receivers' conclusions about targeting, for example, were consistent but far outstripped the estimates from traditional content analysis. Given that these respondents were members of the target readership for the magazines, and two-thirds still were underage for drinking alcohol, it seems likely that their judgments about whether the ads target these groups would be valid. This demonstrates the potential for receiver-oriented message analysis to provide important information about latent content beyond that which is measured by traditional content analysis research. In this case traditional content analysis appeared to underestimate latent meaning evident to the target public. With an audience of children or younger adolescents, the disparities might be reversed.

The ROMA analyses also have shown that audiences can see similar techniques employed in a message but draw different meanings from those elements and then respond to them differently. For example, in our study of young-adult men and women, the sexes reacted similarly to the content in the women's magazines but differed in striking ways with regard to the men's magazines. Men reported that the ads overall were more "cool," interesting, entertaining, persuasive, appealing, and funny than women who viewed the same ads. Men then incorporated the appeal of the ads into their conclusions about the desirability of the characters portrayed in the ads, in terms of whether they were having fun and looked popular, powerful, and cool. Meanwhile, women judged the ads as more annoying, stupid, and offensive than men did. Women then incorporated the offensiveness of the ads into their conclusions about the desirability of characters in the ads.

These results show that men and women held shared meaning at some level but divergent meaning at a deeper level. That women generally reported higher levels of desirability appeared to indicate that their reports reflected an observation of the content rather than an endorsement of the content, a result that has been found among more skeptical or media-literacy-trained individuals in other studies of message interpretation (Austin, Chen, & Grube, 2006; Austin, Pinkleton, Cohen, & Hust, 2005; Austin, Pinkleton, & Funabiki, 2005; Pinkleton et al., 2007).

Because men and women coded much of the content similarly, differences found in men's and women's evaluative reactions seem especially significant because they illustrate potential drawbacks in predicting effects from a combination of content analysis and exposure measures. Receiver-oriented message analysis data as a complement to traditional content analysis data can help to bridge the gap between content and effects by accounting for the relationships between observed content and received meaning. The results illustrate the need to interpret data with an understanding of the differing reactions that the same content can produce in different audiences.

From a methodological perspective, ROMA studies demonstrate a way to tap message meaning as it resides in the inferences audience members make, which traditional content analysis cannot verify on its own and interpretive analysis cannot investigate with reliability.

The ROMA method makes it possible to explore: (1) the extent to which content analysis results coincide with meanings common to a particular audience; (2) the correlates of differences in perceived meaning within an audience; and (3) the extent to which objectively identified perceptions of content can validly be connected to exposure, beliefs and behaviors. The method responds to the need expressed by Ahuvia to consider that the variance in perceptions among typical audience members is "not a problem, it's a finding" (Ahuvia, 2001, p. 155).

Quantitatively based content analysis provides a valuable starting-point from which to examine naturally occurring variations in meaning where it resides and resonates in the message receiver. The additional use of receiver-oriented message analysis makes it possible to examine reliably the existence and implications of cultural, developmental, and situational differences from empirically determined common meanings. As shown in this study, the ROMA method can reveal latent meanings common to a particular audience that would not be identified by traditional "objective" content analysis. This methodology can strengthen researchers' ability to test relationships between message content and audience effects.

Acknowledgments

This study was funded in part by National Institute on Alcohol Abuse and Alcoholism Grant R01-AA12136.

References

Ahuvia, A. (2001). Traditional, interpretive, and reception based content analyses: Improving the ability of content analysis to address issues of pragmatic and theoretical concern. *Social Indicators Research, 54,* 139–172.

Aitken, P., Leathar, D., & Scott, A. (1988). Ten- to sixteen-year-olds' perceptions of advertising for alcoholic drinks. *Alcohol and Alcoholism, 23,* 491–500.

Andsager, J. L., Austin, E., & Pinkleton, B. E. (2002). Gender as a variable in interpretation of alcohol-related messages. *Communication Research, 29*(3), 246–269.

Atkin, C. K., Hocking, J., & Block, M. (1984). Teenage drinking: Does advertising make a difference? *Journal of Communication, 34*(2), 157–167.

Atkin, C. K., Neuendorf, K., & McDermott, S. (1983). The role of alcohol advertising in excessive and hazardous drinking. *Journal of Drug Education, 13*, 313–325.

Austin, E. W. (1995). Developmental considerations in health promotion campaigns. In R. Parrott & E. Maibach (Eds.), *Designing health messages: Approaches from communication theory and public health practice* (pp.114–144). Newbury Park, CA: Sage.

Austin, E. W., Chen, M., & Grube, J. W. (2006). How does alcohol advertising influence underage drinking? The role of desirability, identification and skepticism. *Journal of Adolescent Health, 38*, 376–384.

Austin, E. W., Chen, Y., Pinkleton, B. E, & Quintero-Johnson, J. (2006). The benefits and costs of Channel One in a middle school setting and the role of media literacy training. *Pediatrics, 117*, e423–e433.

Austin, E. W., & Hust, S. J. T. (2005). Targeting adolescents? The content and frequency of alcoholic and nonalcoholic beverage ads in magazine and video formats, November 1999–April 2000. *Journal of Health Communication, 10*, 769–785.

Austin, E. W., & Knaus, C. S. (2000). Predicting the potential for risky behaviors among those "too young" to drink, as the result of appealing advertising. *Journal of Health Communication, 5*, 13–27.

Austin, E. W., Miller, A., Sain, R., Andersen, K., Ryabovolova, A., Barber, L., Johnson, A., Severance, K., Beal, T., & Clinkenbeard, C. (2003). Similarities and differences in college-age men's and women's responses to alcohol advertisements in men's and women's magazines. Paper presented to the Communication Theory and Methodology Division of the Association for Education in Journalism and Mass Communication, Kansas City, August.

Austin, E. W., Miller, A. C., Silva, J., Guerra, P., Geisler, N., Gamboa, L., Phakakayai, O., & Kuechle, B. (2002). The effects of increased cognitive involvement on college students' interpretations of magazine advertisements for alcohol. *Communication Research, 29*(2) 155–179.

Austin, E. W., Pinkleton, B. P., Cohen, M., & Hust, S. (2005). Evaluation of American Legacy Foundation/Washington State Department of Health media literacy pilot study. *Health Communication, 18*(1), 75–95.

Austin, E. W., Pinkleton, B. E., & Fujioka, Y. (2000). The role of interpretation processes and parental discussion in the media's effects on adolescents' use of alcohol. *Pediatrics, 105*, 343–349.

Austin, E. W., Pinkleton, B. P., & Funabiki, R. (2005). The desirability paradox in the effects of media literacy training. Paper presented to the Health Communication Division of the International Communication Association, New York City, May.

Austin, E. W., Pinkleton, B. E., & Hust, S. J. T. (2007). The locus of message meaning: Differences between trained coders and untrained message recipients in the analysis of alcoholic beverage advertising. *Communication Methods & Measures, 1*, 91–111.

Austin, E. W., Pinkleton, B. E., Hust, S. J. T., & Miller, A. (2007). The locus of message meaning: Differences between trained coders and untrained message recipients in the analysis of alcoholic beverage advertising. *Communication Methods and Measures, 1*(2), 91–111.

Bandura, A. (1994). Social cognitive theory of mass communication. In J. Bryant & D. Zillmann (Eds.), *Media effects* (pp. 61–90). Hillsdale, NJ: Lawrence Erlbaum Associates.

Beer Institute (1999, September). *Issue backgrounder: Beer Institute facts.* Washington, DC: Beer Institute.

Beer Institute (2003, December). *Beer Institute Bulletin, 1–2.* Washington, DC: Beer Institute.

Berelson, B. (1952). *Content analysis in communication research.* New York: Hafner.

Bless, H. (2001). Mood and the use of general knowledge structures. In L. L. Martin & G. L. Clore (Eds.), *Theories of mood and cognition: A user's guide* (pp. 9–26). Mahwah, NJ: Lawrence Erlbaum Associates.

Blosser, B. J., & Roberts, D. F. (1985). Age differences in children's perceptions of message intent: Responses to TV news, commercials, educational spots, and public service announcements. *Communication Research, 12,* 455–484.

Center for Media Literacy. (2005). Media kit: Five key questions of media literacy. Retrieved April 1, 2005, from http://www.medialit.org/reading_room/article661.html

Center on Alcohol Marketing and Youth (2002a). *Out of control: Alcohol advertising taking aim at America's youth.* Washington, DC: Center on Alcohol Marketing and Youth.

Center on Alcohol Marketing and Youth (2002b, September 24). Overexposed: Youth a target of alcohol advertising in magazines. Washington, DC: Center on Alcohol Marketing and Youth. Available at www.camy.org.

Center on Alcohol Marketing and Youth (2004, April 21). Youth exposure to alcohol ads on television, 2002: From 2001 to 2002, alcohol's adland grew vaster. Washington, DC: Center on Alcohol Marketing and Youth. Available at www.camy.org.

Chaiken, S., Liberman, A., & Eagly, A. H. (1989). Heuristic and systematic processing within and beyond the persuasion context. In J. S. Uleman & J. A. Bargh (Eds.), *Unintended thought* (pp. 212–252). New York: Guilford Press.

Chen, S., & Chaiken, S. (1999). The heuristic-systematic model in its broader context. In S. Chaiken & Y. Trope (Eds.), *Dual-process theories in social psychology* (pp. 73–96). New York: Guilford Press.

Clore, G. L., Wyer, R. S., Jr., Dienes, B., Gasper, K., Gohm, C., & Isbell, L. (2001). Affective feelings as feedback: Some cognitive consequences. In L. L. Martin & G. L. Clore (Eds.), *Theories of mood and cognition: A user's guide* (pp. 27–62). Mahwah, NJ: Lawrence Erlbaum Associates.

Collins, W. A. (1983). Social antecedents, cognitive processing, and comprehension of social portrayals on television. In E. T. Higgins, D. N. Ruble, & W. W. Hartup (Eds.), *Social cognition and social development* (pp. 110–133). New York: Cambridge University Press.

Darley, W. K., & Smith, R. E. (1995). Gender differences in information processing strategies: An empirical test of the selectivity model in advertising response. *Journal of Advertising, 24,* 41–56.

Dorr, A. (1980). When I was a child, I thought as a child. In S. Withey & R. Abeles (Eds.), *Television and social behavior: Beyond violence and children* (pp. 199–220). New York: Academic Press.

Dorr, A. (1986). *Television and children: A special medium for a special audience.* Beverly Hills, CA: Sage.

Erber, R., & Erber, M. W. (2001). Mood and processing: A view from a self-regulation perspective. In L. L. Martin & G. L. Clore (Eds.), *Theories of mood and cognition: A user's guide.* Mahwah, NJ: Lawrence Erlbaum Associates.

Finn, T. A., & Strickland, D. E. (1982). A content analysis of beverage alcohol advertising: II. Television advertising. *Journal of Studies on Alcohol, 43*(9) 964–89.

Fischhoff, B. (1992). Decisions about alcohol: Prevention, intervention and policy. *Alcohol Health & Research World, 16,* 257–266.

Garfield, C. F., Chung, P. J., & Rathouz, P. J. (2003). Alcohol advertising in magazines and adolescent readership. *Journal of the American Medical Association, 289,* 2424–2429.

Graber, D. A. (1989). Content and meaning: What's it all about? *American Behavioral Scientist, 33,* 144–152.

Greenberg, B. S. (1988). Some uncommon television images and the drench hypothesis. In S. Oskamp (Ed.), *Applied social psychology annual* (Vol. 8): *Television as a social issue.* Newbury Park, CA: Sage.

Grube, J. W. (1993). Alcohol portrayals and alcohol advertising on television: Content and effects on children and adolescents. *Alcohol Health & Research World, 17,* 61–66.

Grube, J. W., & Wallack, L. (1994). Television beer advertising and drinking knowledge, beliefs and intentions among schoolchildren. *American Journal of Public Health, 84,* 254–259.

Hobbs, R. & Frost, R. (2003). Measuring the acquisition of media-literacy skills. *Reading Research Quarterly, 38*(3), 330–355.

Jensen, K. B. (1991): Reception analysis: Mass communication as the social production of meaning. In K. B. Jensen & N. Jankowski (Eds.), *A handbook of qualitative methodologies for mass communication research* (pp. 135–148). London: Routledge.

Jernigan, D. H., Ostroff, J., Ross, C., & O'Hara, J. A. (2004). Sex differences in adolescent exposure to alcohol advertising in magazines. *Archives of Pediatrics & Adolescent Medicine, 158,* 629–634.

Jones, S. C., & Donovan, R. J. (2001). Messages in alcohol advertising targeted to youth. *Australian and New Zealand Journal of Public Health, 25*(2), 126–131.

Kassarjian, H. H. (1977). Content analysis in consumer research. *Journal of Consumer Research, 4,* 8–18.

Kepplinger, H. M. (1989). Content analysis and reception analysis. *American Behavioral Scientist, 33,* 175–182.

Kiecker, P., Palan, K. M., & Areni, C. S. (2000). Different ways of "seeing": How gender differences in information processing influence the content analysis of narrative texts. *Marketing Letters, 11,* 49–65.

Krippendorff, K. (2004). *Content analysis: An introduction to its methodology.* Thousand Oaks, CA: Sage.

Kunkel, D., Wilcox, B. L., Cantor, J., Palmer, E., Linn, S., & Dowrick, P. (2004). Report of the APA task force on advertising and children. Section: Psychological issues in the increasing commercialization of childhood. Washington, DC: American Psychological Association.

MacDonald, J. B., & MacDonald, E. N. (1999). Gender differences in information processing: Retesting the selectivity hypothesis. *American Marketing Association Conference Proceedings, 10,* 23–30.

Martin, S. E., Snyder, L., Hamilton, M., Fleming-Milici, F., Slater, M. D., Chen, S. A., & Grube, J. W. (2002). Alcohol advertising and youth. *Alcoholism: Clinical and Experimental Research, 26,* 900–906.

McNeal, J. U. (1992). *Kids as customers: A handbook of marketing to children.* New York: Lexington Books.

Meyers-Levy, J., & Maheswaran, D. (1991). Exploring differences in males' and females' processing strategies. *Journal of Consumer Research, 18,* 63–70.

Meyers-Levy, J., & Sternthal, B. (1991). Gender differences in the use of message cues and judgments. *Journal of Marketing Research, 28,* 84–96.

Meyers-Levy, J., & Tybout, A. M. (1997). Context effects at encoding and judgment in consumption settings: The role of cognitive resources. *Journal of Consumer Research, 24,* 1–14.

Miller, P. M., Smith, G. T., & Goldman, M. S. (1990). Emergence of alcohol expectancies in childhood: A possible critical period. *Journal of Studies on Alcohol, 51*(4), 343–349.

Petty, R. E., & Cacioppo, J. T. (1986). *Communication and persuasion: Central and peripheral routes to attitude change.* New York: Springer-Verlag.

Pfau, M. (1995). Designing messages for behavioral inoculation. In E. Maibach & R. Parrott (Eds.), *Designing health messages: Approaches from communication theory and public health practice.* Thousand Oaks, CA: Sage.

Pinkleton, B. E., Austin, E. W., Cohen, M., Miller, A., & Fitzgerald, E. (2007). Effects of media literacy training among adolescents and the role of previous experience. *Health Communication, 21,* 23–34.

Pinkleton, B., Austin, E. W., & Fujioka, Y. (2001). The relationship of perceived beer ad and PSA quality to high school students' alcohol-related beliefs and behaviors. *Journal of Broadcasting & Electronic Media, 45*(4), 575–597.

Putrevu, S. (2001). Exploring the origins and information processing differences between men and women: Implications for advertisers. *Academy of Marketing Science Review, 2001,* 1–14.

Rouner, D., Slater, M. D., & Domenech-Rodriguez, M. (2003). Adolescent evaluation of gender role and sexual imagery in television advertisements. *Journal of Broadcasting & Electronic Media, 47,* 435–454.

Saffer, H. (2002). Alcohol advertising and youth. *Journal of Studies on Alcohol, 14,* 173–181.

Shoemaker, P. J., & Reese, S. D. (1990). Exposure to what? Integrating media content and effects studies. *Journalism Quarterly, 67,* 649–652.

Strickland, D. E., Finn, T. A., & Lambert, M.D. (1982). A content analysis of beverage alcohol advertising: Magazine advertising. *Journal of Studies on Alcohol, 43*(7), 655–682.

Stroman, C. A., & Jones, K. E. (1998). The analysis of TV content. In J. K. Asamen & G. L. Berry (Eds.), *Research paradigms, television, and social behavior* (pp. 271–285). Thousand Oaks, CA: Sage.

Taveras, E. M., Rifas-Shiman, S. L., Field, A. E., Frazier, A. L., Colditz, G. A., & Gillman, M. W. (2004). The influence of wanting to look like media figures on adolescent physical activity. *Journal of Adolescent Health, 35,* 41–50.

Vakratsas, D., & Ambler, T. (1999). How advertising works: What do we really know? *Journal of Marketing, 63,* 26–43.

Worth, S., & Gross, L. (1974). Symbolic strategies. *Journal of Communication, Autumn,* 27–39.

13 Violent Video Games
Challenges to Assessing Content Patterns

Katherine M. Pieper, Elaine Chan, and Stacy L. Smith

In 2006, the video game *25 to Life* came under fire from police groups across the country for its depiction of violence toward law enforcement officers (House Democrats, 2006). This is not the first instance of public outcry or legislative action focused on interactive games. Pereira (2003, p. B1) indicates that "16 anti-videogame bills have been introduced in states and cities from New York state to Fairbanks, Alaska." More recently, the debate continues between California State Assembly and U.S. District Courts as to whether to allow minors to access games that "depict serious injury to human beings in a manner that is especially heinous, atrocious or cruel" (Editorial, 2007, p. 3).

Such legislation should be built upon reliable and valid scientific evidence regarding the harmful effects associated with specific content patterns in violent video games. Researchers must conduct methodologically sound analyses of this medium in order to inform public policy, experimental studies, child advocates, and parents on the nature of games. However, the nature of video game technology and play (e.g., interactivity, unscripted patterns of play) poses unique challenges to content analytic research. Our research team has conducted multiple content studies in this domain (Downs & Smith, 2005; Lachlan, Smith, & Tamborini, 2005; Smith, Lachlan, & Tamborini, 2003; Smith & Pieper, 2004). Thus, we feel particularly well suited to comment on the obstacles faced with this type of empirical work, and to provide insights for scholars to consider when designing their own content-based investigations. To that end, this chapter focuses on several challenges in measuring video game content.

To date, there have been over a dozen content analyses of console- or arcade-based video games. Although violent messages are found in other gaming environments (e.g., online multi-player games such as *Asheron's Call*, *EverQuest*), they will not be reviewed in this chapter. First, most of the pending legislation in the United States, as well as existing law in other countries (e.g., Germany, Australia), mainly stems from concern regarding violence in platform-based games, such as the *Grand Theft Auto* series. Additionally, console-based games are most popular with youth (Roberts, Foehr, Rideout, & Brodie, 1999), especially boys in the tween and adolescent years. Finally, the complexities of multi-player environments have already been considered (for a complete review of topic, see Vorderer & Byrant, 2006) and, more importantly, are beyond the scope of our collective expertise in this content domain.

Before we address the challenges associated with examining the content of video games, we urge the reader to consider another, more fundamental question regarding this method of study: Is content analysis an appropriate method for the study of video games? Put differently, can we be certain that the results of such studies provide scientifically reliable and valid evidence, given the nature of the medium itself and the limitations of the methodology? Certain elements of content analysis (sampling, units of analysis, etc.) make sense when used with more stable, traditional media like newspapers and television. However, the content of video games is inherently unpredictable, as newer games depart from conventions of linearity and provide more variable and open-ended experiences to players. Our goal, therefore, is not only to provide a means for educating researchers on interpreting and conducting content analyses of this medium, but also to explore the underlying tension of attempting to quantify variable messages in continuously evolving environments.

Given this situation, we may therefore raise more questions than provide answers about measuring messages in video games. This chapter addresses five major challenges associated with this type of work. Each challenge will be tackled by introducing the problem; illuminating how previous researchers have dealt with the issue; addressing the potential consequences of these methodological choices in terms of research findings; and offering recommendations for future research.

Challenge #1: Choosing a Sample

Regardless of the type of study, a sample represents the link to the population of interest, and can heavily influence the type of results found by researchers. Four different approaches to sampling video game content have been employed in the literature. When evaluating the strengths and weaknesses of an approach, researchers should consider how samples may focus results on a particular effect, and in some cases may resemble sampling strategies from other methodological domains. Table 13.1 provides a list of video game content analyses to date, including sampling and other methodological information.

The first approach has been to sample "popular" games (Braun & Giroux, 1989; Dietz, 1998; Shibuya & Sakamoto, 2004). Several different criteria have established which games to include in samples, such as observing players in coin-operated arcades (Braun & Giroux, 1989), using rental data and magazine rankings (Dietz, 1998), and soliciting nominations from children (Shibuya & Sakamoto, 2004).

As with surveys using volunteers, this approach depends completely on the sample of individuals studied, and not the universe of games. In other words, using "popular" games prioritizes nominations by gamers sampled in a particular study over the preferences of the general public. The resulting non-representative

Table 13.1 Methods of video game content analyses

Author and year	N	Sample	ESRB rating	Type of sample	Console	Unit of analysis	Duration of game play	# of game players	Skill of game players	% of violence
Provenzo (1991)	47	Console games	n/a	Top-rated games	Nintendo	Game covers, game theme	n/a	n/a	n/a	85%
Braun & Giroux (1989)	21 games	Arcade games	n/a	Popular games	n/a	Game	n/a	n/a	n/a	71%
Dietz (1998)	33 games	Console games	not in article	Most popular games	Sega Genesis, Nintendo	Game	not in article	not in article	Not in article	79%
Children Now (2000)	24 games	Console games	E, T, M	Top-selling games	Sony PS, Sega DC, Nintendo 64	Game cover, character, game	1st level	not in article	Not in article	46%
Children Now (2001)	70 games, 1,716 characters	Console games, handhelds, PC games	E, T, M	Top-selling games	Sega DC, Sony PS & PS2, Nintendo 64	Character, game	1st level	2	Not in article	89%
Thompson & Haninger (2001)	55 games	Console games	E	Convenience sample	Sega DC, Sony PS & PS2, Nintendo 64	Violent incident, game	90 min/ end of game	1	Expert	64%
Schierbeck & Carstens (2000)	338 games	Console games, PC games	n/a	All games available 1998	Playstation, Nintendo 64	Game	not in article	not in article	Not in article	53%

Continued

Table 13.1 Continues

Author and year	N	Sample	ESRB rating	Type of sample	Console	Unit of analysis	Duration of game play	# of game players	Skill of game players	% of violence
Brand & Knight (2002)	130 games	Console games, handhelds, PC games	n/a	Top-selling games	Sony PS2, Xbox, Game Cube	Game covers, two lead characters, game	10 min	4	Had played games or became familiar	
Smith et al. (2003)	60 games 1,389 interactions	Console games	E, K-A, T, M	Top-selling games	Sony PS, Sega DC, Nintendo 64	Violent interaction, game	10 min	3	3–5 yrs gaming experience	68%
Smith & Pieper (2004)		Console games	E, K-A, T, M	Top-selling games		Violent interaction, game	10 min	3		
Shibuya & Sakamoto (2004)	41 games	Not specified	n/a	Most popular by 5th grade children	Not in article	Game	Up to 2 hours	11	Not in article	85%
Haninger & Thompson (2004b)	81 games	Console games	T	Random sample of T games	Sega DC, Sony PS & PS2, Nintendo 64	1 sec. epoch, game	1 hour	1	Expert	98%
Haninger et al. (2004)	9 new games (81 games from H & T 04)	Console games	T	Not in article	Xbox, Game Cube	1 sec. epoch, game	1 hour	2	Played games several hours	89%

Note
Adapted from Smith (2006).

samples fail to account for individual differences in liking, and may feature a disproportionate amount of one type of game (e.g., first-person shooter games). Therefore, findings may be difficult to generalize, and such studies may artificially inflate or suppress the amount of violence identified. An additional risk is the potential to place unfair blame on the gaming industry by overestimating harmful effects on players because a small number of individuals like violent games.

A second method for sampling game content is convenience sampling. Thompson and Haninger (2001) selected 55 games out of a total of 672 E-rated games released before April 1, 2001. The advantage here involves including some games which may not have been on top-selling lists at the time of data collection (e.g., *Q*bert, Paperboy*; cf. Thompson & Haninger, 2001) while allowing researchers to hold out unavailable games. The major problem with convenience sampling in all domains is that it includes only those games available to researchers. Findings are restricted to games in the sample; characteristics or general trends for all games remain a mystery. Moreover, this method sheds little light on potential effects—convenience sampling does not consider enjoyment or purchase, leaving researchers in the dark regarding the degree of impact of such games.

Third, researchers sample video game content by randomly selecting games from the population, or those distinguished by a particular commonality, such as sharing the same product rating category. For example, Haninger and Thompson (2004) sampled 81 games out of 396 T-rated games released before April 1, 2001. Sampling games at random provides information about the universe of games, thus supplying a description of the content patterns generalizable to all games. Random sampling is not without disadvantages, however. This method does not focus on games receiving the most attention at the time of the study and may include games many people have not heard of or do not play. Researchers must balance the utility of understanding the universe of games (including games that have long been out of vogue) with the practicality of taking a snapshot of current content patterns.

The most utilized sample is that of top-selling games (Children Now, 2000, 2001; Brand & Knight, 2002; Smith et al., 2003, Smith & Pieper, 2004). When using this tactic researchers rely upon sales data compiled over a particular time period to determine which games to include. Sampling top-selling games provides researchers with the ability to determine content patterns—and estimate the degree of harm therein—in what are often the most cutting-edge or technologically advanced games. Additionally, researchers can note the most problematic areas in games to determine if particular elements (e.g., violence) are actually more likely to sell games.

This is a double-edged sword, however, since by definition, what is top-selling will change over time. We have three particular concerns related to this method. First, there seems to be no standard length of time used to determine how long a game must be "best selling" to be sampled. The role of release dates, revenue calculation and accumulation has been largely unconsidered when assigning the moniker of "top selling." If game sales decline or increase sharply, should games sold during this time period be compared to those sold in another time period? Game release dates make comparisons more complicated, as sales figures are totaled from the first date a game became available, which is frequently inconsistent across titles. The relationship between violent content and higher sales remains unknown, but the complexity surrounding this issue must be considered when constructing a sample.

Second, newer games may contain more (or less) violence and might be briefly popular, threatening the generalizability of findings. The length of time between data collection, analysis, write-up, and publication can be extensive, making games in the sample even less likely to be popular. Delaying the release of findings may result in outdated research, or an under- (or over-) estimation of harmful content. One remedy is to regularly update findings via longitudinal studies. Researchers can draw comparisons over time. However, we know of only one such study to undertake this type of analysis (Smith & Pieper, 2004).

Finally, rental data is not included in sales data. Game players may rent a game rather than purchase it, and popular rental games may be overlooked if researchers rely on sales data. Unlike sales data, "rental activity also reveals interesting patterns of lingering interest in titles that don't show up in retail reports or show up too late for marketers to act upon" ("Home video essentials," 2004, p. 6). Similarly, purchasing a game does not necessarily predict exposure to its content. By selecting games based on units sold, studies may overlook games played most often, and thus wrongly estimate problematic or beneficial content within those games.

Minimizing the problem of sampling bias may require a multi-method approach to sampling. Researchers could make initial choices using sales data, and then include those games played most often, utilizing gamer self-reports. The best solution to the issue of sampling choice, though, is to select a method to answer particular research questions. For instance, Children Now (2001) and Smith et al. (2003) specifically selected top-selling games to update the literature on violent content in games children play. Operating with the assumption that newer games are played more than older games, the researchers realized that using a random sample would not have allowed them to determine if new games on new platforms were more violent. Their choice to sample top-selling content allowed for conclusions that reflected the popular gaming environment at the time of their studies.

A second important consideration is the potential effects of playing games. Investigations of violent games often attempt to quantify violence to make claims about possible harm, especially to vulnerable segments of the population. Thus, considering the potential effects of games (i.e., aggression, desensitization) may lead researchers to sample titles which have been demonstrated to have an effect on players.

In sum, researchers should remain mindful of the costs and benefits that exist when choosing a particular sample, particularly the issues of representation, generalizability, and selection. Additionally, multi-method approaches should be considered to minimize inherent sampling bias. Finally, content analysts should keep in mind that, while each sampling method has weaknesses, the best sample is the one most suited to answer the research question of interest.

Challenge #2: Choosing Gamers

Alongside sampling questions, one of the first challenges facing a content analyst is to decide "who will play the games" in the study's sample. Because the individual player directly impacts how the game is played and, thus, what appears on the screen, who is chosen to play a sample of video games can seriously influence the amount and context of violence to be coded later. Demographic (e.g., age, gender) and personality (e.g., levels of aggression, empathy, sensation-seeking) factors may affect individual attraction to and enjoyment of television violence (see Cantor, 1998). Similarly, individual differences may dictate how a person plays a video game, the character the gamer chooses to be, and the overall level of aggressiveness in fending off virtual rivals. In our own work, we have witnessed several instances in which a different player can alter the course and outcome of a game, in the process influencing the amount of violence that occurs.

We are not aware of any content study that has grappled with these issues systematically. Indeed, most scholars have dealt with issues of expertise or skill with video games inconsistently. For instance, Thompson and Haninger (2001) and Haninger and Thompson (2004) used a single expert video game player, although the researchers did not specify the criteria used to determine expertise. Without rationale, Smith et al. (2003) employed three video game players with 3–5 years of gaming experience. Individuals in Brand and Knight's (2002) study had either played the games before or played to familiarize themselves with the content. Other content analyses do not articulate information about the skill of the individuals who played in their studies (Children Now, 2000, 2001; Dietz, 1998; Schierbeck & Carstens, 2000; Shibuya & Sakamoto, 2004).

Despite the lack of attention to this important selection criterion, we believe that player skill may account for some of the variability in findings. Imagine playing a video game for the first time: the logic is unknown and the overall mission or purpose is often not readily ascertainable. With repeat play and practice (Newman, 2004), the novice may transform into an expert with a well-defined schema for different types of games, the commonality in missions played across games, and the often used codes or "cheats" for scoring more points.

Researchers may need to confront this problem by thinking about video games like sports, and gamers like athletes (Bainbridge, 2002; Scanlon, 2003). The Cyberathlete Professional League (http://www.thecpl.com/), for example, was created with the purpose of turning computer gaming into a professional sport. We believe the nature of expertise in these domains is analogous, as both are knowledge- and skill-based activities. Thomas and Thomas (1994) argue that expertise in sport includes both knowledge and performance aspects. Interestingly, knowledge about how to perform and performance are not necessarily related, as "[it] is possible to know when and how to do a movement, yet not be able to actually execute the movement" (Thomas & Thomas, 1994, p. 296). This distinction between knowledge and performance applies to game playing, which requires declarative and procedural knowledge, and also fine motor skills, timing, and hand–eye coordination.

With regard to effects of violent games, Sherry (2001) has argued that "the amount of exposure to violence in a given amount of time varies by individual player depending on his or her skill level. Highly skilled players may engage in more violence more frequently than players learning the game" (p. 412). Smith (2006) has also claimed that individual player differences may be important for video game content analysis, and suggested that gender, playing style, and expertise may all significantly influence content patterns found in interactive media. Several studies examining expert–novice differences in video games have considered the potential positive effects of video games, for example, for visual attention and perceptual learning (Green & Bavelier, 2003; Greenfield, DeWinstanley, Kilpatrick, & Kaye, 1994) or manipulation of three-dimensional spatial representations of objects (Greenfield, Brannon, & Lohr, 1994). Keeping these effects, as well as more negative effects (e.g., desensitization), in mind when selecting players will allow researchers to control for individual differences in game play and draw more precise conclusions about data trends.

VanDeventer and White (2002) observed expert game-playing 10- and 11-year-old children as they taught non-expert adults how to play either *Super Mario World* or *Super Mario Kart*. They demonstrated that outstanding video game-playing children frequently exhibited the characteristics found in experts in other domains, with the more highly skilled players displaying these characteristics more frequently than less highly skilled players. Using Chi and Glaser's (1988) itemization of expert characteristics, they found that the greater the players' skill, the more they showed evidence of pattern perception, superior memory, and representation of problems at principled levels. Hong and Liu (2002) also found significant differences between expert and novice computer game player thinking strategies, in particular, that expert players showed a greater variety of problem-solving types than did non-experts.

Insofar as pattern perception, problem solving, and strategizing by the player influences game playing, player expertise may also lead to variation in content patterns. As Smith (2006) has cautioned, results may vary widely across studies because of the content-producing players' differing levels of skill. Such skill may vary either for video game playing generally, or with regard to a particular game. Knowledge and performance expertise may even lead to asymmetric or contrasting outcomes for particular content observations. For example, expertise manifested as manual dexterity may allow the player to shoot more accurately, engage in efficient killing, and experience an increased rate of violence per unit of time. On the other hand, expertise in the form of tactics or knowledge of secret routes in a game may lead to less onscreen violence, allowing players to more easily elude their foes. Clearly, the decision of how much or how little game-specific experience the content-producing player should have before the investigators record game play will influence the nature of the content produced.

The interdependent relationship between player skill and violent content patterns needs further exploration. Researchers first need to establish criteria for expertise in the gaming arena, particularly if expertise is related to a general knowledge of games or specifically to an ability to play a single game well. Scholars must then turn to the delicate task of trying to understand exactly how player skill impacts game content, and use these results to inform future content studies.

To address the issue of player skill variance, we believe investigators should assess how differences in expertise contribute to differences in content via experiments. These studies would manipulate as the independent variable a number of factors hypothesized to impact manifest content, using content analysis to analyze the dependent variable of violence. In addition, researchers could determine the impact of variables other than play experience that may be responsible for variance in content patterns, such as trait aggressiveness or sensation-seeking. These can be assessed alongside content patterns to determine, for example, if more aggressive individuals actually play games differently, on average, than non-aggressive individuals.

To illustrate, our data demonstrate that individual differences may alter the amount of violence experienced. Smith and Pieper (2004) sampled 60 games across three platforms, and used three different "expert" players to investigate the amount of violence. As part of this investigation, two game titles were sampled over all three platforms, with a single expert assigned to each. Thus, we can compare differences in violence for each player on what should be, if not identical, at least very similar games. Using *The Hulk* and *Enter the Matrix,* two T-rated games in which the main goal is to dispense with enemies (usually via force) to accomplish some task, chi-square analyses were executed to assess several aspects of violence. Investigations that employ a larger sample may find more significant and meaningful differences between players. However, these numbers at least demonstrate that a somewhat different picture of violence results from allowing a different individual to take the controls.

Table 13.2 reveals that a few significant differences were noted across the players. In terms of sheer amount, in *The Hulk* player 1 produced a greater proportion of overall violence, and relied on firearms significantly more often to commit acts of violence, while players 2 and 3 relied on other means to accomplish the task. This difference may also explain why players 2 and 3 witnessed a higher degree of harm or pain than player 1; using different means may impact the consequences of violence.

The game *Enter the Matrix* provided other interesting differences. Here, player 2 executed more blows to deal with opponents than player 1, and player

Table 13.2 Player skill variance

Player	The Hulk			Enter the Matrix		
	1	2	3	1	2	3
Acts of violence	79	37	54	52	63	84
Type of violence						
Credible threat	14% (n=11)	11% (n=4)	9% (n=5)	19% (n=10)	22% (n=14)	30% (n=25)
Behavioral act	86% (n=68)	89% (n=33)	91% (n=49)	81% (n=42)	78% (n=49)	70% (n=59)
Weapon						
Firearm	47%[a] (n=37)	14%[b] (n=5)	20%[b] (n=11)	27% (n=14)	13% (n=8)	24% (n=20)
Harm/pain depicted						
None	88%[a] (n=60)	48%[b] (n=16)	54%[b] (n=25)	48% (n=20)	6% (n=3)	41% (n=24)
Mild	6%[c] (n=4)	45%[a] (n=15)	24%[b] (n=11)	50% (n=21)	84% (n=41)	56% (n=33)
Extent of violence						
Single act	25% (n=17)	18% (n=6)	21% (n=10)	21%[a] (n=9)	12%[b] (n=6)	15%[b] (n=9)
2–9 acts	68% (n=46)	58% (n=19)	66% (n=31)	48%[c] (n=20)	84%[a] (n=41)	67%[b] (n=41)
10–20 acts	2% (n=1)	12% (n=4)	11% (n=5)	17% (n=7)	4% (n=2)	16% (n=10)
21+ acts	6% (n=4)	12% (n=4)	2% (n=1)	14% (n=6)	0% (n=0)	2% (n=1)

Note
Items with different superscripts are statistically significant at least at the $p < .05$ level.

3 demonstrated the highest amount of violence. Whether extent reflects unfamiliarity with the game or more aggressive tendencies on the part of the player is unknown. However, extent of violence in this case indicates that player 3 might have seen more acts of aggression than the others, despite playing the same game. Overall, these findings illustrate that even among experts play differs in important ways.

The practical task of determining who should play can be boiled down to a few guidelines: (1) consider whether an "expert" or "novice" should be used; (2) determine whether more than one individual will play; (3) match players on skill level, experience, and applicable personality traits; and (4) justify these methods in the report. Interactivity affords games a great degree of unpredictability, but researchers can control some error caused by differences in player skill with careful thought and planning. Ultimately, however, we need more research on exactly how player skill affects content patterns.

Challenge #3: Time Frames

Another major challenge associated with content analyses of video games regards time frames. Two issues arise here (a) the length of time play should be assessed; and (b) the level of game play at which analysis should begin. We examine each concern below.

Researchers have employed varying approaches to how much play to capture for study. Some scholars did not specify the amount of time played in their studies (Dietz, 1998; Schierbeck & Carstens, 2002). Brand and Knight (2002), Smith et al. (2003), and Smith and Pieper (2004) used 10-minute time frames of recorded play. Haninger, Ryan, & Thompson (2004) and Haninger and Thompson (2004) sampled one hour. Thompson and Haninger (2001) sampled either 90 minutes or until the end of the game. Shibuya and Sakamoto (2004) used up to two hours of video game play in their investigation. Studies by Children Now (2000, 2001) used the first level of play rather than a designated amount of time.

It is possible that different amounts or types of violent content would appear, given differing approaches to sampling. Longer samples may lead to more explicit and graphic content (Smith, 2006). Smith (2006) has suggested that researchers may want to sample longer time frames to assess "whether and how violence or any other objectionable content escalates with time" (p. 69). Additionally, different samples (i.e., a segment of similar time length but from a different point of progress in the game) may also change the amount of objectionable content. To illustrate, a game in which the main character scores points by scouring a jungle, stalking and sniping hidden enemies, may begin with a high frequency of violent gun acts. However, once most immediate threats are disposed of, the frequency of violence may diminish. Similarly, as the supply of ammunition dwindles, instead of shooting to kill, the player may be forced to dispense with opponents *mano a mano*, leading to their violent but less graphic deaths. Thus, researchers should not assume that more offensive content necessarily appears later, rather than earlier, in a game, particularly those with linear play.

Some games violate the assumption of linearity because they allow the player many more choices. The *Grand Theft Auto* series of games, for example, is known for its nonlinearity and open-ended game play (Colayco, 2004). A major feature highlighted in the marketing of *GTA: Vice City* was that the game would allow players to "go where you want, when you want" (*Grand Theft Auto: Vice City*—Pre-played, 2005, p. 7). In this case, it is unlikely that recording game play in its entirety would show natural patterns of violence progression.

Players' ability to "save" their games (i.e., store game progress in order to continue in subsequent episodes of play) makes it even more important for researchers to consider the time frames they sample. Saving a game allows players to experience initial game play once and move on, potentially encountering more or different violent content than they would by playing from the beginning of a game each time. Without knowledge about how frequently gamers save play for subsequent resumption, it is hard for researchers to design study strategies that best mirror actual playing conditions.

This underscores the fact that scholars have insufficient depth of knowledge regarding actual household video game play. If content analyses are to be representative of the range of actual video game-playing experience, they should be comparable to actual video game playing. Consider the amount of time played as a variable of interest. Roberts, Foehr, & Rideout (2005) found that 8–18-year-olds play close to 49 minutes a day on average. However, it is not clear how long the typical session actually lasts. A child might play 50 minutes every day, or for nearly 3 hours each on Saturday and Sunday but not at all the rest of the week. Either scenario yields the same overall average. In addition, these data include children who spend no time playing video games, further obscuring the norm. Thus, content analyses that sample only 20 minutes (or less) of play may not actually estimate the amount of violence children will see in a typical session of game play, and may be using imprecise information to make judgments about how much time to sample. As Sherry (2001) has noted, differences in time frame have led to different findings in studies on video games and aggression.

Our own data allow us to examine the relationship between play time and amount of violence (Smith & Pieper, 2004). When examining the amount of violence in 60 top-selling games, we sampled the initial 20 minutes of play time, separating this into two distinct 10-minute segments. We then compared the percentage of games featuring violence in the first 10 minutes to the percentage featuring violence in the second 10-minute segment. We found that violence did not increase significantly between 10 and 20 minutes of game play. Seventy-seven percent of games in our sample featured violence in the first 10 minutes, while 82% of these games featured violence in the second 10 minutes. Additionally, violence in the second 10 minutes was not more graphic or explicit than in the first 10 minutes of play. One major flaw in this example is that we did not consider the level at which play took place, and focused only on time of play. Though the players were allowed to familiarize themselves with the game, it may be that they were still in the initial stages of play during the whole of their 20-minute session. Our data may only be indicative of the need to sample beyond 20 minutes of play or to sample by level of play, not length of time.

Beyond the question of just how much time to capture, fatigue or desensitization in the player providing the game content may also affect variance in content patterns. If players used for a content analysis play differently at the beginning of the investigation than at the end, the results of the analysis will be biased. Additionally, the relationship between exposure to violence and desensitization to game content is unknown. From the effects literature, it is clear that a relationship between exposure to violent games and aggressive behaviors, cognitions, and affect exists (Anderson, 2004; Anderson & Bushman, 2001; Sherry, 2001). If researchers continue to use expert players in their analyses, they must consider levels of desensitization the player has before play and what will occur as the individual is systematically exposed to further violent content. To control for this variability, researchers undertaking content analysis must balance how much time is sampled with demands on players, contemplating what they believe the potential effects of playing violent games may be.

We believe that future investigations should systematically assess differences in content as a function of time of play. Again, we recommend that experimental studies be utilized to clarify the relationship between time frame and the amount of violence in manifest content. Some researchers have applied such a method; one study of video game violence and brain-mapping paired content observed to brain wave activity in order to determine how neurological responses changed as a result of violent actions during play (Weber, Ritterfeld, & Mathiak, 2005). Researchers must control for other factors, namely player expertise, fatigue, desensitization, and individual differences (e.g., aggressiveness) while attempting to determine thresholds for play length. Subjects might be asked to play for anywhere between 10 minutes and 2 hours, and content should be analyzed for significant increases in the amount of violence as the duration of play lengthens.

Overall, little empirical data has been collected on game play in natural settings. The average number of hours spent playing a particular game, or an estimate of the percentage of people who play a game to its conclusion, are unknown. Such information would help to better define how much and what content to analyze, and is imperative to consider in future investigations. Researchers must decide at the outset of a content analysis what limits to set on play time, considering the issues mentioned above. These choices should be based on such factors as concern about particular audiences, particular types of effects, or the effects of particular types of content.

Challenge #4: Units of Analysis

Content analysts must clearly articulate what constitutes the unit of analysis for their particular study. Essentially, content analysis represents the "counting" of a particular type of subject matter. Thus, the unit of analysis typically represents the smallest piece of subject matter that can be described or explained by researchers. Findings must then be interpreted in relation to the unit of analysis employed. Four main units of analysis have been used in content analyses of violence in video games: the entire game (Braun & Giroux, 1989; Beasley & Standley, 2002; Brand & Knight, 2002; Dietz, 1998; Children Now, 2000, 2001; Haninger et al., 2004; Haninger & Thompson, 2004; Shibuya & Sakamoto, 2004; Smith et al., 2003; Thompson & Haninger, 2001); the character (Beasley & Standley, 2002; Brand & Knight, 2002; Children Now, 2000, 2001); the violent incident (Smith et al., 2003; Thompson & Haninger, 2001); and the one-second epoch (Haninger & Thompson, 2004; Haninger et al., 2004).

The selection of an appropriate unit of analysis for an investigation must be justified. In our studies (Smith et al., 2003, Smith & Pieper, 2004), the violent interaction was chosen as the unit of analysis to correspond to the definition of violence and several related contextual variables set out in the National Television Violence Study (NTVS) (Smith et al., 1998). Other researchers may employ different theories or rely on their own proclivities to determine a unit of analysis.

Considering the unit of analysis in relation to the questions of interest is crucial to any content study. Overall trends for violence can be examined across games, characters, acts, or seconds, but the interpretation and conclusions drawn from all those results will differ. Determining the percentage of games rated T or M that feature violence (e.g., 90%, Smith et al., 2003; 98%, Haninger et al., 2004) is related to the unit of analysis. Smith et al. (2003) measured violent interactions, and found that violence occurred 4.59 times per minute in T- and M-rated games, while Haninger et al. (2004) used one-second epochs, and found that 39% of game play time (or about 24 minutes of an hour) in T-rated games involves violence. Extrapolating from these figures, Smith et al. (2003) would expect to find approximately 275 acts of violence in an hour of game play, while Haninger et al. (2004) would estimate approximately 1,404 seconds of violence in an hour of game play. These numbers look very different because of their metric (i.e., acts vs. seconds). We cannot know the length of each act Smith et al. (2003) measured, nor can we know if the number of seconds Haninger et al. (2004) counted is consecutive. Each finding has different implications for what the average hour of game play would contain, and outlines a different picture of violence. Clearly, when discussing video game content, it is crucial to determine the unit of analysis at the outset.

Focusing on the characters involved in the action is one way to answer questions regarding representation (i.e., minorities, women) of the roles that individuals play in a story-based game (e.g., *Enter the Matrix*) or other related questions about individuals on screen. Relying on characters as the unit of analysis in video games can be advantageous because games often rely on a single character to drive the action through multiple levels of play. Examples of such games include *Lara Croft: Tomb Raider*, in which the female lead moves through different levels of a particular quest, and *Luigi's Mansion*, in which the main character moves through different rooms of a house to fulfill his task.

On the surface, this type of play seems deceptively suitable for capturing character traits or patterns; a character is static throughout the game and should thus serve as an appropriate unit of analysis. When one looks just below the surface, however, it becomes apparent that choosing a different character at the start of play can impact the content that is analyzed. Each character in a game is outfitted with particular strengths and weaknesses that must be taken into account. One example is *Dynasty Warriors 4*. Choosing one player over another can impact the type of violence that occurs, not to mention the overall outcome of the game. In this game, players select a warrior equipped with a unique weapon. If, the character Huang Gai is chosen, the player would be outfitted with a club. The choice of Sun Shang Xiang, however bestows large sword-like rings as a weapon. It is possible, given these differences in characters, that the amount, or more likely the contextual elements, of violence would be altered significantly. One solution is to capture all unique characters and content. Children Now (2001) sampled every character encountered in non-sports play.

Further complicating this problem is the fact that not all characters are immediately available. Some characters serve as "rewards" for successful game play. That is, only after a player has completed a particular level or challenge is a new character "unlocked" and available for play. New characters may feature different weapons or skills that make play easier or more challenging. Moreover, they may unlock even more characters later in the game. For instance, in *Brute Force* the player must complete the first level—rescuing an ally—to make another character available for play. This continues until, as the ad copy claims, players can "instantly switch between 4 elite super-commandos, each with unique skills and special abilities" (Microsoft, n.d.).

Additional characters may be announced in the instruction manual, the primary means of learning about the game, and may be overlooked or never encountered if the players in a content study are not well trained, or if the time frame for sampling is not long enough. As noted above, it is important to complete all the levels of the game—a process that can be very time-consuming—in order to discover secret characters or weapons. Systematically excluding elements may result in findings unrepresentative of the most problematic, beneficial, or interesting aspects of video games. In the example above from *Brute Force* (Smith & Pieper, 2004), only two main characters, both male, were seen during 20 minutes of game play. Two additional female characters are also included in the game but were never observed during the 20-minute sample that was content coded. In content analyses focused on hypersexuality or gender differences in game play, the addition of these two characters would provide two important data points. Achieving bonus or hidden characters may be what motivates longer play sessions. By overlooking these aspects of game play, researchers may miss the full picture of game content.

In sum, units of analysis serve as both a counting and explanatory mechanism for researchers. We know how much of something occurs in video games by how many units of analysis we find. Researchers must therefore consider what unit of analysis will most clearly explicate their questions of interest and what will be most parsimonious.

Challenge #5: Definitional Discrepancies

Closely related to units of analysis are the definitions researchers use to identify key content categories. Definitions make it possible for coders to know when to "stop the tape" because they have found an example of violence. Thompson and Haninger (2001) and Haninger et al. (2004) defined violence as "acts in which the aggressor causes or attempts to cause physical injury or death to another character" (Thompson & Haninger, 2001, p. 593). The researchers eliminated accidental violence or sports violence, but included every kick or punch in a boxing match. Smith et al. (2003) adapted the definition of violence from the NTVS for their research. NTVS defined violence as:

> any overt depiction of a credible threat of physical force or the actual use of such force intended to harm an animate being or group of beings. Violence also includes certain depictions of physically harmful consequences against an animate being/s that results from unseen violent means (Smith et al., 1998, p. 30).

Children Now (2001) defined violence on three levels: incidental, significant, and major, and each was distinguished on the basis of the use of violence related to the outcome of the game (i.e., incidental violence had "no effect on the outcome of the game," p. 8).

While each definition of violence is concise and accurate, the use of multiple definitions reduces the chance of drawing precise comparisons over time or across samples or studies. The variation in at least two of these definitions restricts such analyses. Moreover, variation in content pattern findings could also be explained by confounding the application of those disparate definitions across different time frames. As noted previously, Thompson's research team looks for violence in every one second of content, while Smith et al. (2003) look for a violent act, harmful consequences, or credible threats of violence. Although these two research teams espouse similar definitions of violence, subtle differences may produce inconsistent findings by changing the application criteria.

Definitional variety is not unique to the content analysis literature. Experimental studies also assign terms like "violence" and "aggression" different meanings. In their meta-analysis, Anderson and Bushman (2001) describe violent media, aggression, and violence as three separate entities, yet do not apply these definitions to effects. Sherry (2001) borrows from Funk's (1993) typology to separate game violence into human, fantasy and sports violence, with other categories for non-violent games. While these studies clarify what overall effect video games have on aggressive behavior, the underlying assumptions made by the authors with respect to the definitions employed reflect the same disparity that plagues content analytic research. Investigators must clearly and consistently define "aggression" and "violence" and their relation to harm. Content analysts can then apply these elements to investigations to discover how often truly "harmful" content appears.

Definitional differences are only part of the problem contributing to inconsistent findings across content studies of video game violence. In addition, discrepancies in definitions may be magnified by other problems (e.g., time frame differences, sampling divides) which are to blame for large variations in the amount of violence identified in video games. Researchers must carefully create sound, precise definitions of violence. Definitions of violence—whether for content analytic work or in the experimental literature—must be based on sound empirical evidence and practical consideration. Researchers must rely on previous work to inform projects and craft meticulous definitions which reflect knowledge of why violent content may be harmful.

Conclusion

In this chapter, we have considered five major issues that accompany content analysis of video games: sampling, player skill, time frame, units of analysis, and definitional discrepancies. These topics are uniquely impacted by the interactive nature of games and demand special methodological consideration, especially in the realm of content analysis.

Expertise, time frames, and units of analysis are especially new realms for investigators to conquer. To be sure that content analysis research will provide a truly valid estimate of violence in video games, it is important to know exactly how different time frames impact violent content, how expert players stack up against novices, and whether bonus characters or advanced levels of play feature significantly more or less violent behavior. Besides contributing to variation in content findings, we suspect that differences in player expertise and time frame studied are related to variability in the results of experiments regarding the effects of game play. Such factors might explain, for example, Sherry's (2001) finding that length of play is negatively related to aggressive outcomes. Thus, each of these areas presents an important and promising new venue for research, and we encourage scholars to investigate how such factors may alter research outcomes.

The continuous evolution of games poses another challenge to content analysis. The "solutions" offered in this chapter may represent answers to questions posed by the current gaming environment. With the introduction of the Xbox 360 and other new consoles or game types, the approaches used by content analysts may become outdated. How should scholars seek to overcome these challenges? One important step is for researchers to engage with the medium by experimenting. While it is likely that most researchers studying games already play, they may not be "experts" or play as the general public does. It is crucial to incorporate those more familiar with games into the process in order to provide an informed perspective on naturalistic game play. Our research team has benefited from the creation of a group of faculty, graduate, and undergraduate students (Annenberg Studies on Computer Games Group) that provide discussions and opportunities for criticism and suggestion as researchers consider new studies.

Investigations should also be guided by specific research questions, with the methodology selected matched to those questions. Research design decisions involving sampling, player expertise, time frame, and units of analysis must be closely linked to the purpose of the study and the outcomes of interest. At the outset of a content study, scholars should specify what knowledge they hope to gain from their analysis and formulate a plan for data collection that will best provide answers, even if it means that the study takes longer or is more burdensome to complete. Researchers must prize methodology over efficiency in order to produce the most valuable results.

References

Anderson, C. A. (2004). An update on the effects of playing violent video games. *Journal of Adolescence, 27*, 113–122.

Anderson, C. A., & Bushman, B. (2001). Effects of violent video games on aggressive behavior, aggressive cognition, aggressive affect, physiological arousal, and prosocial behavior: A meta-analytic review of the scientific literature. *Psychological Science, 12*, 353–359.

Bainbridge, R. (2002). Why gamers are athletes. *Wired.* Retrieved June 12, 2004, from http://www.wired.com/wired/archive/10.04/mustread.html?pg=2

Beasley, B., & Standley, T. C. (2002). Shirts vs. skins: Clothing as an indicator of gender role stereotyping in video games. *Mass Communication & Society, 5*, 279–293.

Brand, J., & Knight, S. J. (2002). *Diverse worlds project.* Retrieved June 12, 2004, from http://www.diverseworlds.bond.edu.au/Default.htm

Braun, C. M. J., & Giroux, J. (1989). Arcade video games: Proxemic, cognitive, and content analyses. *Journal of Leisure Research, 21*, 92–105.

Cantor, J. (1998). Children's attraction to violent television programming. In J. Goldstein (Ed.), *Why we watch: The attraction of violent entertainment* (pp. 88–115). New York: Oxford University Press.

Chi, M., & Glaser, R. (1988). Introduction. In M. Chi, R. Glaser, & M. Farr (Eds.), *The nature of expertise* (pp. xv–xxviii). Hillsdale, NJ: Erlbaum.

Children Now. (2000). *Girls and gaming: A console video game content analysis.* Oakland, CA: Author. Retrieved May 17, 2004, from http://www.childrennow.org/media/video-games-girls.pdf

Children Now. (2001). *Fair play? Violence, gender, and race in video games.* Oakland, CA: Author.

Colayco, B. (2004). The history of *Grand Theft Auto. Gamespot.* Retrieved June 12, 2004, from http://www.gamespot.com/features/6111834/

Dietz, T. L. (1998). An examination of violence and gender role portrayals in video games: Implications for gender socialization and aggressive behavior. *Sex Roles, 38*, 425–442.

Downs, E. P., & Smith, S. L. (2005, May). Keeping abreast of hypersexuality: A video game content analysis. Paper presented at the annual conference of the International Communication Association, New York, NY.

Editorial: Battle against violent video games continues. (2007, September 7). *San Jose Mercury News.* Retrieved September 18, 2007, from http://www.mercurynews.com/portlet/article/html/fragments/print_article.jsp?articleId=6824970&siteId=568

Funk, J. (1993). Reevaluating the impact of video games. *Clinical Pediatrics, 32*, 86–90.

Grand Theft Auto: Vice City—Pre-played. (n.d.) Retrieved August 8, 2005, from http://www.ebgames.com/ebx/product/223735.asp

Green, C. S., & Bavelier, D. (2003). Action video game modifies visual selective attention. *Nature, 423,* 534–537.

Greenfield, P. M., Brannon, C., & Lohr, D. (1994). Two-dimensional representation of movement through three-dimensional space: The role of video game expertise. *Journal of Applied Developmental Psychology, 15,* 87–103.

Greenfield, P. M., DeWinstanley, P., Kilpatrick, H., & Kaye, D. (1994). Action video games and informal education: Effects on strategies for dividing visual attention. *Journal of Applied Developmental Psychology, 15,* 105–123.

Haninger, K., Ryan, S. M., & Thompson, K. M. (2004). Violence in teen rated video games. *Medscape General Medicine.* Retrieved May 14, 2004, from http://www.medscape.com/viewarticle

Haninger, K., & Thompson, K. M. (2004). Content and ratings of teen-rated videogames. *Journal of the American Medical Association, 291*(7), 856–865.

Home video essentials takes the pulse of game rentals. (2004, November 17). *Electronic Gaming Business.* Retrieved August 7, 2005, from http://www.findarticles.com/p/articles/mi_m0PJQ/is_22_2/ai_n6364562

Hong, J., & Liu, M. (2002). A study on thinking strategy between experts and novices of computer games. *Computers in Human Behavior, 19,* 245–258.

House Democrats support boycott of *25 to Life* video game. (2006, March 6). *The Associated Press State & Local Wire.* Retrieved September 18, 2007, from http://www.lexisnexis.com.

Lachlan, K., Smith, S. L., & Tamborini, R. (2005). Models for aggressive behavior: The attributes of violent characters in popular video games. *Communication Studies, 56*(4), 313–329.

Microsoft (n.d.) *Brute Force.* [Video game packaging]. Redmond, WA: Microsoft Corporation.

Newman, J. (2004). *Videogames.* New York: Routledge.

Pereira, J. (2003, January 10). Just how far does First Amendment protection go? Videogame makers use free speech to thwart proposals to keep violent, adult fare from kids. *Wall Street Journal,* p. B1.

Roberts, D., Foehr, U.G., & Rideout, V.J. (2005). *Generation M: Media in the lives of 8–18-year-olds.* Menlo Park, CA: Kaiser Family Foundation.

Roberts, D., Foehr, U. G., Rideout, V. J., & Brodie, M. (1999). *Kids & media @ the new millennium.* Menlo Park, CA: Kaiser Family Foundation.

Scanlon, C. (2003). South Korea's professional gamers. *BBC News.* Retrieved August 7, 2005, from http://news.bbc.co.uk/2/hi/asia-pacific/3321537.stm

Schierbeck, L., & Carstens, B. (2000). Violent elements in computer games: An analysis of games published in Denmark. In C. von Feilitzen & U. Carlsson (Eds.), *Children in the new media landscape: Games, pornography, perceptions* (pp. 127–131). Gothenburg, Sweden: Nordicom, for UNESCO International Clearinghouse on Children and Violence on the Screen.

Sherry, J. (2001). The effects of violent video games on aggression: A meta-analysis. *Human Communication Research, 27,* 409–431.

Shibuya, A., & Sakamoto, A. (2004). The quantity and context of video game violence in Japan: Toward creating an ethical standard. In R. Shiratori (Ed.), *Gaming, simulations, and society.* Tokyo: Springer-Verlag.

Smith, S. L. (2006). Perps, pimps, & provocative clothing: Examining negative content patterns in video games. In P. Vorderer & J. Bryant (Eds.), *Playing computer games: Motives, responses, and consequences* (pp. 57–76). Mahwah, NJ: Erlbaum.

Smith, S. L., Lachlan, K., & Tamborini, R. (2003). Popular video games: Quantifying the presentation of violence and its context. *Journal of Broadcasting and Electronic Media, 47,* 58–76.

Smith, S. L. & Pieper, K. M. (2004, November). Video game violence: Examining the amount and context over time. Paper presented at the annual meeting of the National Communication Association, Chicago, IL.

Smith, S. L., Wilson, B. J., Kunkel, D., Linz, D., Potter, W. J., Colvin, C., & Donnerstein, E. (1998). Violence in television programming overall: University of California, Santa Barbara. *National television violence study* (Vol. 3, pp. 5–220). Newbury Park, CA: Sage Publications.

Thomas, K. T., & Thomas, J. R. (1994). Developing expertise in sport: The relation of knowledge and performance. *International Journal of Sport Psychology, 25,* 295–312.

Thompson, K. M., & Haninger, K. (2001). Violence in E-rated video games. *Journal of the American Medical Association, 286*(5), 591–598, 920.

VanDeventer, S. S. & White, J. A. (2002). Expert behavior in children's video game play. *Simulation & Gaming, 33,* 28–48.

Vorderer, P. & Bryant, J. (Eds.). (2006). *Playing computer games: Motives, responses, and consequences.* Mahwah, NJ: Erlbaum.

Weber, R., Ritterfeld, U., & Mathiak, K. (2005, May). Neuroscience in video games research: Functional magnetic resonance imaging of virtual violence. Paper presented at the International Communication Association, New York, NY.

Wright, B. (2004). Sounding the alarm on video game ratings. Retrieved June 13, 2004, from http://www.cnn.com/2002/TECH/fun.games/12/19/games.ratings/

Part 4
The Big Picture

14 Non-academic Audiences for Content Analysis Research

D. Charles Whitney, Ellen Wartella, and Dale Kunkel

Two decades ago, Wartella and Reeves (1985) observed that throughout the history of mass media, the introduction of each new media technology prompts a patterned social response. The first phase emphasizes initial euphoria about a medium's potential to improve society. Historical examples include Edison's grandiose claim that the advent of motion pictures might lead to schools being replaced, and wildly optimistic suggestions that the emergence of interactive cable television might lead to instantaneous national referenda on important political issues. The second phase that typically follows in societal reaction to new media is the growth of concern for how that medium impacts its audiences, particularly the most vulnerable segments such as children. It is only then, Wartella and Reeves (1985) argue, that a research community develops and begins to gauge the content of the new medium as well as its effects on audiences. Their view is that scholars who study communication in society have been largely reactive to the social concerns about media voiced by the larger population. From this perspective, the stimulus for media and social effects research typically originates from politically active groups and organizations in the wider society, rather than emanating directly from any scholarly theory or evidence.

Wartella and Reeves' historical analysis concludes with the advent of television. In the media-saturated twenty-first century, this pattern may well have shifted. That is, the field of communication research and related social sciences has at this point established a compelling body of media effects research which establishes that many types of content pose potential concerns for society. These include messages related to sexuality, violence and aggression, alcohol, smoking, and illicit drugs, among others. It seems quite feasible to suggest that communication scholars may now be leading the charge to investigate the influence of the internet and other new technologies, rather than merely pursuing the agenda of concerns raised by other segments of society. But regardless of whether this pattern has changed, Wartella and Reeves' (1985) analysis underscores the important relationship that exists between academic research and those who seek to apply it in real-world contexts such as public policy debates about media influence or controversies involving questions about media industry social responsibility. Participants in these exchanges are among the most important of the non-academic audiences for content analysis research.

There are a variety of aims for this chapter. The first is a discussion of the uses of content analysis by those outside of the community of scholars who seek to apply such research to further goals in their organizations, institutions, or efforts to improve society. The second is an elaboration of our title—the non-academic audiences for content analyses—with more specific attention to the utility of the technique for them. Finally come two recommendations for the applied use of content analysis research: first, that truly useful content analyses must forefront the consideration of content in context; and second, that applied audiences for content analysis must be more sensitive to rigor in such reports.

The Uses of Content Analysis

Content analytic data, like all social scientific evidence, serve three types of purposes for traditional academic audiences: description, explanation, and prediction. Such applications, of course, depend upon the broader frame of investigation to which they are linked, and the case studies in this volume demonstrate a range of potential applications. For example, scholars who seek to understand the implications of adolescents' exposure to sexually explicit online material study the content patterns of such sites visited most frequently by their sample of subjects, as Salazar et al. (Chapter 8) report in this volume. Similarly, researchers such as Austin (Chapter 12) who want to understand the role of alcohol advertising as a factor in underage drinking explore the predominant messages presented by beer commercials. Regardless of the specific focus, the primary goal in most media content analysis research conducted by academics is to gain a more precise understanding of the patterns of message content. When that evidence is linked with studies of audience effects, content-based research may afford the opportunity to draw conclusions that hold important implications for explaining and predicting the role of media as a social force.

For those outside academe, however, content analysis research can fulfill many corporate, political, or social advocacy goals. Business interests may track how individual companies or entire industries are covered by the news media in order to best anticipate how public perceptions may shape their future opportunities. The research firm Media Tenor (www.mediatenor. com) specializes in news media analyses using exactly this type of technique, which incorporates agenda-setting theory in its investigations. Other organizations seek to apply the knowledge produced by empirical research to alter media industry practices, or to promote regulation of media behavior. For example, the advocacy group Children Now (2004) has marshaled content analysis research that examines the ethnic diversity of characters in prime-time television programming in an effort to encourage television networks to diversify their portrayals. Existing audience effects research demonstrates that children's self-esteem benefits when they can view positive "role-model" characters of their own race or ethnic background (Berry & Asamen, 1993). In a different example, the Parents Television Council (2003a, 2003b) has employed content analysis research to demonstrate that material it defines as inappropriate on television (i.e., containing excessive sex, violence, or offensive language) is so widespread that indecency regulation by the Federal Communications Commission should be strengthened.

For those who employ content analysis research in applied issue contexts, it is important to think of the findings that are produced in terms of their *location in an argument*—often practical or political—about the process of communication and its likely outcomes. Riffe, Lacy, & Fico (1998) identify two distinct frames for content analysis research: the first engages arguments about content as the outcome of processes of production, including industry self-regulation or public policy mandates, while the second treats the content evidence as an antecedent or agent of communication effects. In other words, researchers study content either to understand aspects of its production, or to infer social effects as a consequence of media messages, drawing upon previously existing evidence that documents the outcomes of exposure.

In the first of these two areas, tracking industry practices as an outcome variable, content studies have examined whether a law such as the Children's Television Act actually led to an increase in educational programming for youth as it was intended to do (Jordan, 2000; Kunkel & Goette, 1997). Similarly, researchers have examined alcohol advertising on television to evaluate the degree of compliance with industry self-regulatory policies (Pinsky & Silva, 1999; Zwarun & Farrar, 2005). Besides providing evidence evaluating the efficacy of self-regulation, the findings produced from such research also reveal information about the willingness of media companies to accept alcohol advertising placements. The examples in both of these areas provide valuable evidence about media message patterns, even though the content analysis data are not used to draw any obvious implications for viewer effects.

In contrast, the second of the two orientations identified by Riffe et al. (1998) involves using content analysis research to draw implications for audience influence. Like many mass media textbooks, Sparks (2006) reminds us that "it is important to understand that *the results of a content analysis do not permit one to make inferences about the effects of that content*" (p. 21; emphasis in original). This is of course true for a variety of reasons: an audience cannot be assumed to have attended to, or to have understood the analyzed content; and individual differences among audience members may lead to varying interpretations and impacts. Nonetheless, we argue that there are cases in which effects can, with due caution, be imputed to content. Indeed, that theme is prevalent throughout this volume. Numerous chapters report study designs in which the message categories that are measured in content analysis research are specifically designed to facilitate optimal linkage with existing effects research.

Both of these two types of studies are of interest to those who seek to apply content analysis research in real-world contexts, such as to shape media industry regulatory policy or practice. It is quite apparent that both the public and policymakers find it useful to track and debate media content patterns, and hence the press always seems ready to highlight the latest twist or turn in the available evidence.

The Key Audiences for Content Analysis

Virtually anyone who cares about the role of media in society can be considered a potential audience for content analysis research. It goes without saying that this includes media scholars in the field of communication, as well as academics in related fields such as public health who are interested in media influence. But beyond the traditional academic audience, content analysis resonates with several key types of audience members—*government policymakers* who seek to promote and protect the public interest; *media industry leaders* who seek to achieve an optimal balance between social responsibility and corporate profitability; *issue advocates* who seek to influence policy agendas; and lay members of *the public*, particularly parents, who seek advice and perspective to help guide them in their efforts to safely navigate the media environment. In addition, it is important to consider *the press* as an important audience for content analysis research. News media journalists play a central role in informing all of the other audiences about any research evidence produced regarding media content. In the examples discussed below, we illustrate how content analysis research can and often does speak in important ways to all of these key audiences.

The National Television Violence Study (NTVS) (1998) is one of the largest content analysis studies yet produced by the scientific community. Conducted over a three-year period in the mid-1990s, it examined roughly 10,000 programs on a broad range of content attributes surrounding the presentation of televised violence. NTVS grew out of a mandate from the U.S. Senate Commerce Committee, spearheaded by the late Sen. Paul Simon (D-Illinois), in an effort to hold the broadcasting and cable industries accountable for public commitments they had made to reduce and/or to more responsibly portray violence on television. The study was widely referred to as a "report card" assessing how well the industry was making good on its commitments in this regard.

In developing the design of the study, the researchers met with television writers and producers and consulted frequently with an advisory board that included representatives from a variety of academic, professional, and public interest organizations in areas of education, health, and child welfare. The goal was to consider the perspectives and interests represented by all of these potential audiences for the research. In the end, NTVS framed its reporting of the data in a manner that offered specific recommendations for several of the key audiences for content analysis research. For the television industry, the study provided recommendations about programming content, ratings and advisories, and anti-violence media campaigns, including, for example, more frequent portrayal of remorse, criticism, or penalty associated with violent acts as well as depiction of more of the serious negative consequences of violence. For policymakers, it counseled that any regulatory initiative must recognize the critical importance of the context of televised violence, and emphasized the need for ongoing monitoring of televised violence. For parents, the study offered a range of suggestions about appropriate television viewing for their children, such as recommending that parents be aware that younger children are developmentally unable to distinguish fantasy from reality or to connect punishments for violence to the acts if the two are presented in distant scenes. Both of these factors make violent cartoons more "risky" for younger children, though not for older children or adults (Federman, 1998).

Another example involves the role of food marketing to children as a possible contributor to the growing epidemic of childhood obesity. A recent report from the National Academy of Sciences' Institute of Medicine (McGinnis, Gootman, & Kraak, 2006) reviewed all existing research on the topic. From an effects perspective, the review established that children's exposure to food advertising on television exerts significant influence on child viewers' product preferences, purchase requests, and food consumption. But the press coverage surrounding the report, along with the subsequent policy debate that is still unfolding, has centered largely on content analysis evidence. Content-based studies demonstrate that roughly half of all advertising in children's television programs has long comprised commercials for food products, and of that base, the large majority are for foods that are unhealthy when consumed in abundance, or so-called "junk food."

Policymakers reacted to the report with serious concern. Congressman Edward Markey, chair of the House Subcommittee on Telecommunications and the Internet, conducted hearings on the topic and wrote to the chief executives of many major food corporations, calling on them to limit their advertising of unhealthy foods to children (Eggerton, 2007b). Two U.S. Senators, Samuel Brownback and Tom Harkin, partnered with two FCC members to form a task force to examine the issue (Eggerton, 2007c). The food marketing industry responded with an initiative whereby many large corporations agreed to improve the nutritional quality of the foods marketed to children, and/or to restrict the advertising to children of foods that do not meet healthy nutritional criteria (Council of Better Business Bureaus, 2007).

Public interest advocates continue to spar with the industry to achieve stronger concessions, while food industry officials maintain that they are already well on the path to solving the problem (Eggerton, 2007a). It is almost certain that the future landscape of this debate will be shaped importantly by content analysis research that tracks the nutritional quality of the foods advertised to children, comparing and contrasting the current practices with those of the past. Such evidence will likely shape public concern about the issue over time. If that concern were to grow sufficiently, it might well prove a catalyst to more formal governmental regulation restricting the advertising of so-called junk foods targeted at children. That outcome recently occurred in the United

Kingdom, where that country's Food Standards Agency partnered with the telecommunications regulator OFCOM (Office of Communications) to ban television commercials for unhealthy food products during any programming viewed by significant audiences of children (BBC News, 2006).

Both of these examples demonstrate the ways in which media content research plays an important role in the debate about media social policy concerns regarding critical public health issues such as violence and obesity. Content analysis research in these areas tends to receive prominent attention in the news media, which often heightens public awareness and concern, triggering both policymakers' interest as well as media industry efforts to address the issue. Although concerns regarding televised violence or junk-food marketing to children are based upon a broad range of diverse types of evidence, including audience effects research, once such issues become well established it is often the ongoing content analysis studies in the area that drive the policy agenda.

The Importance of Context

Violence on U.S. television has been one of the most consistently controversial issues surrounding the medium, waxing and waning, but never receding far from view. Each public eruption of the issue has pitted largely an academic and advocacy community against largely an industry-oriented defense. In the past, that defense challenged the critics on many points meant to deter public concern with the issue, arguing that the effects research showed only trivial or inconsistent negative impacts, and that the impact of television violence on real-world violence was far less than that of other agents such as poverty, presence of guns, and peer or family influence. These criticisms have been countered successfully elsewhere (Anderson et al., 2003; Bushman & Anderson, 2001; Wilson et al., 2002). Of particular concern for this chapter, the industry has also argued that content studies, which constitute a large segment of TV violence research, could be dismissed for two reasons: that measuring content patterns is not the same as measuring effects, and that most content analysis of TV violence suffers from fatal conceptual and methodological flaws. These latter two criticisms merit further discussion.

The pioneering content analyses that were part of George Gerbner's cultural indicators project in the 1970s and beyond (e.g., Gerbner & Gross, 1976; Gerbner, Gross, Morgan, & Signorielli, 1980) were benchmarks that were widely reported in the press. These reports contributed significantly to the policy debate about whether there was "too much" violence on television. Television industry executives countered that Gerbner's research oversimplified the issue of violence by decontextualizing the assessment of violent portrayals, reporting data at gross levels such as rates of violence per hour. Implicit in such analysis is the assumption that all acts of violence portrayed on television are equivalent; otherwise, how could they be tallied equally in such reductionistic fashion? However, they are not equivalent, at least not in terms of implications for audience effects. Moreover, the unit of analysis for reporting is a pivotal question: Should reports focus on any "acts of violence" or should they more carefully parse out the frequency of violent portrayals that are known to pose a risk of harmful effects on viewers?

We earlier noted that logically, effects cannot be "read off" of content; however, plausible inferences can be made. Of critical importance is the degree to which consideration is given to the *context* in which a given behavior is depicted. To draw inferences about effects, there must be strong correspondence between the content characteristics observed and demonstrable impacts of that content-in-context, usually derived from previously existing experimental research. The three-year NTVS content analysis project began by exhaustively reviewing the research literature on media-violence effects on both young people and adults to find evidence of *what sorts* of violent portrayals were linked to which effects. For example, because prior research had indicated that the learning of aggression was associated with attractive perpetrators of violence, coding categories were established to judge violent characters on this element. Similarly, because effects studies show that violence that is rewarded and/or presented as justifiable increases the likelihood of subsequent aggressive behavior, coding categories were constructed for each of these variables, among many others that were grounded in the existing effects research. In all, NTVS gleaned from the literature several dozen context characteristics that, with varying degrees of confidence in the experimental literature, had been shown to contribute to three key types of effects from exposure to televised violence: learning of aggressive attitudes and behaviors, desensitization (i.e., increased callousness to victims of violence), and exaggerated fear of being victimized by violence (NTVS, 1997, 1998).

Of paramount importance in maintaining the integrity of content analytic research is the way data are reported and framed. When the time came for NTVS researchers to report data, extensive discussions led to a considered strategy for reporting. Integral to this was a consideration of the likely audiences for the research and the uses to which each audience might put the data. Two dimensions underlay this strategy: first was a press release to a general public, coupled with a release of a technical report of interest primarily to specialized, academic audiences. Second was identification, early in the formulation of the project, of specialized publics with specific interests in the topic, namely policymakers, the broadcast and cable television industries, and parents/childcare providers.

The general public would be reached by a press conference with an executive summary of the data. It was early agreed that there would be no news release featuring a rate of violence in programs, but the researchers also realized that a complex report with *no* summary measures would attract little mass media attention. The strategy was to issue a final report that included summary measures, but these were presented only after an articulation of the reasons why a complex and nuanced approach was necessary: that not all forms of TV violence are equal in their impacts; that child audiences are different in their comprehension of television than adult audiences; and that differing contextual features affect the risks associated with exposure to televised violence. Only then were summary measures reported, including such findings as the percentage of programs with violence, as well as the frequency of violent scenes within programs across genres of programming, across outlet types (network, independent stations, basic cable, premium cable, public TV), and across time periods of the programming broadcast.

While the analysis comprised more than 10,000 hours of programming on 23 channels over 3 television seasons, data were never reported for individual series programs because the relatively small numbers of any individual program did not allow for stable findings at this level. Indeed, the sampling strategy reflected the finding that most media violence effects stem from cumulative exposure to large numbers of violent depictions over time, rather than to viewing particularly influential episodes of specific programs. Hence, the content analysis sampling strategy sought to accurately represent the overall television environment as a whole, but not necessarily to capture multiple episodes of individual violent series. Because coding categories had been specifically designed to reflect content characteristics (e.g., presence of humor, presence of rewards/absence of punishment for commission of acts of violence) that the experimental literature linked to the learning of aggression or other harmful effects, the researchers' sensitivity to context afforded confident conclusions about the risks posed by viewing of the violent content, and hence led to recommendations for parents, media producers, and public policymakers.

In conclusion, the lessons derived from the study of televised violence underscore that it is essential to consider context when measuring content attributes in entertainment media when that context is likely to be critical in shaping audience interpretation and effects. Categorizing content without sensitivity to context can lead to unintended and problematic outcomes, such as when internet filtering software designed to screen out sexually explicit material inadvertently blocks access to sites with breast cancer information. Whether intended for academic or applied audiences, it is important for content analysis research to be sensitive to the context of all messages examined.

Content Analysis: a Consumer's Guide

In part because doing a content analysis seems on the surface a fairly simple task, content analyses have joined polls and surveys among the most frequently published types of social science research. However, just like opinion surveys, the rigor of the research is often disproportionate to the degree of attention some findings receive from the press and the public. That is because most non-scientific observers are ill-equipped to scrutinize the quality of the research process involved with either polls or content analysis studies.

For polls and surveys, there are two widely available, published standards for reporting data and evaluating its quality, and they are both reasonably well diffused among professional journalists. The National Council on Public Polls (NCPP) offers a document called "20 Questions a Journalist Should Ask about Poll Results," which includes explanations for why each element is important for assessing poll reliability and validity (Gawiser & Witt, n.d.). Similarly, the American Association for Public Opinion Research (2005a) includes in its code of ethics and practices an eight-item disclosure-standards list.

In contrast, there are no comparable guidelines upon which consumers of content analysis research may rely. Drawing upon the examples noted above as a template, we offer the following as a checklist for evaluating the adequacy of a content analytic study.

1 Where, and in what form, does the research appear?

Studies appearing in refereed scholarly journals generally can be assumed to have undergone peer review, as can analyses appearing in books from scholarly publishers. Likewise, studies published by scientific organizations and institutions with reputations for quality and credibility (e.g., the National Academies of Science, the Institute of Medicine) have undergone rigorous review. In contrast, studies produced by independent parties, such as advocacy organizations which are likely to prefer one outcome over another in promoting their policy agenda, warrant much more careful scrutiny.

2 Who sponsored the study, and who conducted it?

As in survey research, sponsorship is not necessarily an indicator of bias, but by the same token, survey sponsors rarely release results that conflict with their own interests. There are wide variations in the quality and reputation of research organizations and firms conducting content analysis. Those who sponsor and conduct research can be investigated to gain information about their motives and reputations.

3 Are a codebook and coding instructions available for inspection?

Examination of a codebook allows evaluation of the adequacy and specificity of directions and definitions used in the study. Where studies employ computerized analysis rather than human coders for text-scanning, full dictionaries of terms searched are important to consider in weighing the comprehensiveness of the study.

4 Is the population of interest for the study clearly specified?

By "population" we mean the entire range of content to which a study is meant to be generalized. For example, some studies of television content are conducted with a narrow focus on broadcast network prime-time programming, or children's programming, rather than "all of television." If a study implies it is applicable to all aspects of a broad population such as all "news media" or "video games," it is important to consider whether the sampling strategy is sufficient to warrant such generalization, as indicated in the question below.

5   Is the sampling strategy representative of the population of interest?

Because most media populations of interest are huge, sampling is an aspect of virtually all content analyses. Random selection of units within the overall population is the optimal tactic to employ to enhance generalizability. Yet many studies employ a sampling strategy that privileges "popularity" of content. For example, a retrospective study of smoking in motion pictures over time might sample films once every five years in the past, selecting the top 20 films with the highest box office sales in the target years, or selecting the films nominated for Academy Award Best Picture. The findings of studies with such samples might look very different than a study that randomly sampled all films produced in each year examined. The latter study would provide the more accurate estimate of what all films are likely to include in terms of smoking behavior, whereas the former would be more reflective of films that people were more likely to have seen.

6   Is information provided about sample size?

Sample size is important for two central reasons. For all samples, larger sample sizes assure more stability and relatively less measurement error. However, for nonprobability samples (e.g., convenience samples or purposive samples), even large sample sizes may be misleading unless there is a strong argument for the representativeness of the content selected. For random or probability samples, sample size is inversely related to sampling error. All other things being equal, larger samples produce more accurate, reliable, valid results.

7   Which results are based on parts of the sample, rather than on the total sample?

Where sub-sample results are employed for specific analyses, the sampling error of the sub-sample is calculated from the sub-sample size rather than the full sample size. Thus, for example, any discussion of a content analysis of cartoons drawn from several children's channels would, in reporting data from each channel individually (e.g., Nickelodeon, Cartoon Network), need to interpret results with more caution than for the full sample. Sub-sample sizes with small Ns should be interpreted with great caution.

8   How is data on coder reliability reported?

Reliability of coding is essential for validity of findings. Hence, data on coder reliability must be reported, and should be indicated separately for individual variables, not as overall averages. Many commercial and interest-group studies either fail to report reliability coefficients, or report overall or average reliability data that may disguise low reliability on key indicators. For example, some obvious coding judgments (e.g., channel, program genre, gender of lead characters) are easy to code reliably, at virtually 100% coder agreement. In contrast, critical content attributes (e.g., presence of sexual talk, degree of justification for violent behavior) are much more difficult to classify consistently. Reporting reliability coefficients that are summed across all measures in a study would inevitably inflate the actual level of inter-coder agreement obtained on the critical content variables in any study. Moreover, it is important for researchers to employ statistics that correct for chance agreement in assessing reliability, rather than to merely assess the raw percentage of agreement.

Like all research, content analysis studies vary in quality. While the list provided above is hardly exhaustive of all possible criteria that may be used to evaluate content analysis projects, it nonetheless provides a model for assessing the key attributes that are critical to consider in most studies. These evaluative standards should be carefully considered by all audiences for content analysis research, and most particularly journalists, who play a pivotal role in disseminating research information to the public.

Conclusion

Content analyses serve a wide variety of purposes for those in the public health communities as well as in other policy arenas served by communication research more generally. Content data can suggest prophylactic interventions to health professionals, can direct media professionals to ways of producing content that would either minimize harm or even improve health outcomes for their audiences, can suggest to parents and educators ways to direct young people's attentions and modify unhealthy behaviors, and can inform policy-makers' deliberations. The likelihood that any such beneficial outcomes will occur is increased to the extent that content analysis research is conducted with sophisticated rigor by the scholars who practice the technique. It is similarly important that when content analysis research is applied by non-academic audiences, such as the press or public policymakers, the quality of the evidence receives careful consideration. By identifying criteria to help scrutinize the strength of content analysis investigations, it is hoped that this chapter will benefit the more active and effective use of content-based research in applied, non-academic settings.

References

American Association for Public Opinion Research (2005a). Code of professional ethics and practices. Retrieved December 7, 2007, from http://aapor.org/standardsethics?s=Code%20of%20professional%20Ethics%20and%20Practices

American Association for Public Opinion Research (2005b). Standards and best practices. Retrieved 9 October, 2006, from http://www.aapor.org/bestpractices

Anderson, C., Berkowitz, L., Donnerstein, E., Huesmann, L. R., Johnson, J., Linz, D., Malamuth, N., & Wartella, E. (2003) The influence of media violence on youth. *Psychological Science in the Public Interest, 4*(3), 81–110.

BBC News. (2006, November 17). Junk food ad crackdown announced. Retrieved December 7, 2007, from http://news.bbc.co.uk/1/hi/health/6154600.stm

Berry, G., & Asamen, J. (Eds.). (1993). *Children and television: Images in a changing sociocultural world.* Thousand Oaks, CA; Sage Publications.

Bushman, B. J., & Anderson, C. A. (2001). Media violence and the American public: Scientific facts versus media misinformation. *American Psychologist, 56*, 477-489.

Children Now. (2004). *Fall colors: Prime-time diversity report, 2003–04.* Oakland, CA; author. Retrieved December 7, 2007, from: http://publications.childrennow.org/publications/media/fallcolors_2003.cfm

Council of Better Business Bureaus. (2007). *Children's food and beverage advertising initiative.* Retrieved December 7, 2007, from http://us.bbb.org/WWWRoot/SitePage.aspx?site=113&id=dba51fbb-9317-4f88-9bcb-3942d7336e87

Eggerton, J. (2007a, June 28). Obesity task force readies report to Congress. *Broadcasting & Cable.* Retrieved December 7, 2007, fromhttp://www.broadcastingcable.com/article/CA6456259.html?

Eggerton, J. (2007b, September 12). Markey calls on more marketers to trim fat. *Broadcasting & Cable.* Retrieved December 7, 2007 from http://www.broadcastingcable.com/article/CA6477907.html

Eggerton, J. (2007c, September 19). Childhood obesity report delayed again. *Broadcasting & Cable.* Retrieved December 7, 2007, fromhttp://www.broadcastingcable.com/article/CA6479807.html?

Federman, J. (Ed.). (1998). *National television violence study* (Vol. 3): *Executive summary.* Santa Barbara, CA: Center for Communication & Social Policy, University of California, Santa Barbara.

Gawiser, S., & Witt, G. E. (n.d.). 20 questions a journalist should ask about poll results (3rd ed.). Poughkeepsie, NY: National Council on Public Polls. Retrieved 9 October, 2006, from http://www.ncpp.org/qajsa.htm

Gerbner, G., & Gross, L. (1976). Living with television: The violence profile. *Journal of Communication, 26*(2), 173–199.

Gerbner, G., Gross, L., Morgan, M., & Signorielli, N. (1980). The mainstreaming of America: Violence profile No. 11. *Journal of Communication, 30*(3), 10–29.

Greenberg, B., Mastro, D., & Brand, J. (2002). Minorities and the mass media: Television into the 21st century. In J. Bryant & D. Zillmann (Eds.), *Media effects: Advances in theory and research* (2nd ed., pp. 333–352). Mahwah, NJ: Lawrence Erlbaum Associates.

Jordan, A. (2000). *Is the three-hour rule living up to its potential?* Philadelphia, PA: Annenberg Public Policy Center. Retrieved December 7, 2007, from http://www.annenbergpublicpolicycenter.org/NewsDetails.aspx?myId=145

Kunkel, D., & Goette, U. (1997). Broadcasters' response to the Children's Television Act. *Communication Law and Policy, 2,* 289–308.

McGinnis, J., Gootman, J., & Kraak, V. (Eds.). (2006). *Food marketing to children and youth: Threat or opportunity?* Washington, DC: Institute of Medicine, National Academies Press.

National Television Violence Study (NTVS). (1997). *National television violence study* (Vol. 1). Thousand Oaks, CA: Sage.

National Television Violence Study (NTVS) (1998). *National television violence study* (Vol. 3). Thousand Oaks, CA: Sage.

Parents Television Council. (2003a). *The blue tube: Foul language on prime-time network TV.* Retrieved December 7, 2007, from http://www.parentstv.org/PTC/publications/reports/stateindustrylanguage/main.asp

Parents Television Council. (2003b). *Sex loses its appeal: A state of the industry report on sex on TV.* Retrieved December 7, 2007, from http://www.parentstv.org/PTC/publications/reports/stateindustrysex/main.asp

Pinsky, I., & Silva, M. (1999). A frequency and content analysis of alcohol advertising on Brazilian television. *Journal of Studies on Alcohol, 60,* 394–399.

Riffe, D., Lacy, S., & Fico, F. (1998). *Analyzing media messages.* Mahwah, NJ: Lawrence Erlbaum Associates.

Sparks, G. G. (2006). *Media effects research: A basic overview* (2nd ed.). Belmont, CA: Thompson/Wadsworth.

Wartella, E. & Reeves, B. (1985). Historical trends in research on children and the media 1900–1960. *Journal of Communication, 35*(2), 118–133.

Wilson, B., Smith, S., Potter, W. J., Kunkel, D., Linz, D., Colvin, C., & Donnerstein, E. (2002). Violence in children's television programming: Assessing the risks. *Journal of Communication, 52,* 5–35.

Zwarun, L., & Farrar, K. (2005). Doing what they say, saying what they mean: Self-regulatory compliance and depictions of drinking in alcohol commercials in televised sports. *Mass Communication & Society, 8,* 347–371.

15 Advancing the Science of Content Analysis

Amy B. Jordan, Dale Kunkel, Jennifer Manganello, and Martin Fishbein

The mass media are one of the many important factors known to exert influence on people's knowledge, beliefs, attitudes, and behaviors regarding health-related issues. Media depictions, whether fictive or factually grounded, hold great potential to inform and influence the public about a variety of health issues, including the risks of certain behaviors for one's physical and mental well-being, as well as the benefits of different actions for achieving optimal health (Brodie et al., 2001; Brown & Witherspoon, 2002). This potential, coupled with the sheer volume of time the average American spends with media, has created a situation whereby studying patterns of media content is vital to understanding health attitudes, beliefs, and behaviors. Thus, in an increasingly media-rich era, researchers from a range of disciplines have expanded their efforts at studying media messages about health-related topics (Kline, 2003). They pose questions such as: How often do TV portrayals show drinking and driving? How many of the characters who have sexual intercourse in films are shown talking about or using condoms? They answer these questions by quantifying their observations of media messages using the method of content analysis.

As editors, we believe it is important for people studying health messages in the media to carefully weigh the decisions they make when conducting their studies, and to step back to consider how changes in the media landscape may influence their work. For these reasons, we pursue two main goals in this volume. First, we highlight the critical decisions that content analysts working in the area of public health must make in designing research, interpreting data, and disseminating results. It is critical for researchers to not only understand the implications of these decisions, but also to share the reasoning behind their decisions. In doing so, fellow researchers can gain insight into (and perhaps learn lessons from) the approaches used in the studies in this volume. Second, we believe the time has come to consider content analysis methodology in the context of new and continually evolving media technologies. For example, how do portrayals of substance use in music videos airing on YouTube compare to those appearing on a music television channel such as BET? And are the potential effects different due to the medium?

In this concluding chapter, we distill the key themes that emerged from our readings of the authors' contributions, and offer strategies for enhancing the value of future content analysis investigations of health-related topics. These themes emphasize the roles of theory and prior research, the strengths and limitations of content analytic methodology, how changes in technology influence the ways in which audiences receive and process messages, and what unexplored opportunities and responsibilities exist for content analytic researchers examining health messages.

Content Analysis Research Can Benefit Tremendously When Theory and/or Empirical Research Informs Decisions About What to Examine and How to Examine It.

Theories, especially those that explain health behaviors, are widely used in public health research. For studies using content analysis to examine media messages, theories explaining how media can shape attitudes and behavior provide a framework for the reader to understand both the rationale for the research as well as the design (e.g., why certain variables were included rather than others). Content analysis research is often carried out with the assumption that media messages have particular effects on audiences; in such situations, it is clear that empirical findings about effects can and should inform the content categories to be included.

The theories that drive content analysis research may be implicit or assumed. However, as Manganello and Fishbein (Chapter 1) argue, theoretical assumptions and paradigms need to be carefully articulated if they are to be useful as tools to explain and predict patterns of data related to health messages' effects. The application of theory to content analysis studies can provide a strong foundation for research that places observed content patterns into a larger context of media information processing.

Theories other than those used to explain media effects can be useful as well. One question that is important for content analysis research is: What content do people perceive in the same way, and what might they comprehend differently from one another? This question has no simple answer, but is one that each investigator who leads a content analysis study must consider in both designing the study and interpreting its findings.

One of the earliest theorists of content analysis research, Ole Holsti (1969), described content analysis using an encoding/decoding paradigm that emphasized the role of rudimentary contextual factors such as the channel of communication. Today, the consideration of context is viewed as a critical factor in content studies. Indeed, its importance has grown so much that message attributes are now frequently defined and/or measured in a manner that is highly sensitive to contextual features likely to shape the meaning of the message for audiences. As Kunkel notes in Chapter 2, early research examining violence on television (Gerbner, Gross, Morgan, & Signorielli, 1980, 1986) counted all violent acts the same in aggregating data for its central findings, which focused on the widespread prevalence of violence across programs. A slapstick comedy scene in which a character takes a pratfall on an intentionally placed banana peel yields the same "tick on the tally" of violent acts as a fistfight that settles a dispute with both participants left bloody and inca-pacitated. In contrast, investigators who have studied televised violence in recent years have taken a different approach. With a goal of identifying the frequency of violent portrayals that pose a risk of harmful effects such as an increased tendency to aggress, contemporary research (Potter & Smith, 2000; Wilson et al., 1997) has sharpened the message measurement process in a manner that reflects sensitivity to contextual features known from previous effects research to enhance the likelihood of an audience interpretation that is associated with an increased probability of aggression. For example, theory and effects research in the realm of TV violence documents that violence that is shown to be rewarded, or that is depicted without causing pain or suffering for its victims, poses a much greater risk of aggression following exposure than violence that is punished or shown to cause serious harm to victims (Kunkel et al., 1995). Consequently, researchers have differentiated acts of violence with and without these contextual features in an effort to facilitate stronger inferences about likely effects on the audience once the content patterns have been adequately identified.

In Chapter 9, Sorsoli and colleagues discuss the importance of considering context for examining messages about gender and sexual behavior. They point out that this is especially important, as sexual content often consists of subtle innuendos that must be placed into context to be understood as sexual messages. They emphasize that message context is what provides the meaning that results in how messages are interpreted. In their research, they apply feminist theory to highlight the role of gender, and state that "gender—including messages about the ways men/boys and women/girls should feel and act in romantic relationships—is an essential contextual factor to consider" (p. 139).

In addition to greater use of theory and more careful attention to context, the method of content analysis might benefit from empirical data garnered from pilot studies and exploratory research. Such data would help to guide the decisions a content analyst must make, including the operationalization of content variables and the determination of appropriate sample sizes. Most pilot research carried out by content analysts is done in order to test inter-coder reliability. Neuendorf (Chapter 5) describes the very precise and self-reflec-tive steps that must occur during the coder training process, which involves performing trial runs of the coding instrument and testing the reliability of a sub-sample of units. Far fewer studies have the resources necessary to test other elements of the research design. For example, the decision of an analyst to examine two or three episodes of each television series studied is more often based on the hope that such a sample is representative of the overall series than it is based upon empirical evidence to buttress that assumption. Though labor-intensive and expensive, it is useful for researchers to build in the capacity to pursue such studies. They will not only inform the project at hand but could also contribute to a larger base of empirical evidence for optimal content analysis design to better analyze health messages.

Content Analysis Data Have Utility That is Best Appreciated When One Carefully Considers the Strengths and Limitations of the Investigative Tool.

Content analyses of media messages serve many functions. First, they offer important insight into the landscape of health-related information available to audiences. Such analyses are quite useful for providing a first look at whether there are message patterns deserving of further investigation within a larger sample of media or within the population (e.g., Sankofa & Johnson-Taylor, 2007). As a formative research tool, content analysis can shed light on whether media may be misrepresenting, over-representing or under-representing a health-related matter (e.g., Parascoli, 2005).

Second, observed message patterns may reflect or contribute to patterns of change in society at large, and content analysis can help to assess this (e.g., Yanovitzky & Stryker, 2001). For example, Romer, Jamieson, & Jamieson (2006) found that local television and newspaper reports of suicide in six cities were associated with aggregate increases in suicide deaths. Content analyses may also shed light on the impact of regulatory activity designed to address public and policymakers' concerns (e.g., Jordan, 2007). Finally, and perhaps most often, as Kunkel argues in Chapter 2, content analysis is conducted with the assumption that certain kinds of messages may have certain kinds of effects (e.g., Escamilla, Cradock, & Kawachi, 2000; Livingstone, Lunt, & Slover, 1992).

While there are many reasons why content analysis is a useful tool in public health, there are also limitations of content analysis that must be considered. Just as a skilled survey researcher learns early on that social desirability biases may constrain the validity of people's self-report of particular behaviors, a skilled content analyst must recognize that evidence of certain media message patterns is not tantamount to evidence of the *influence* of those messages on health attitudes and behaviors. To understand the potential for message influence, one must first consider the likely interpretation of the substance conveyed. The axiom that the meaning of a message is grounded more in the receiver than in the message itself poses a challenge to content analysis research. One of the leading content analysis theorists, Klaus Krippendorff (2004), embraces a constructivist perspective that underscores the importance of individual differences in the interpretation of media messages. He describes the challenge this way:

> Content is not inherent in communications. People typically differ in how they read texts. The intentions of the senders of broadcast messages may have little to do with how audience members hear those messages. Temporal orderings, individuals' need and expectations, individuals' preferred discourses, and the social situations into which messages enter are all important in explaining what communications come to mean. (Krippendorff, 2004, pp. 9–10)

The axiom that meanings are grounded more in people than in messages has far-reaching implications. Now commonplace are videotapes of police activity, and they occasionally show officers beating suspects that they are in the process of apprehending. In the Rodney King incident in Los Angeles, millions of viewers watched a videotape of officers striking King repeatedly with their batons. Many viewers were convinced that the actions of the officers represented criminal assault rather than anything necessary to subdue the suspect (Baldassare, 1994; Cannon, 1999). But a jury in the California state courts interpreted the behavior differently, ruling that the officers who struck King were justified in their actions and had committed no crime (Mydans, 1992). This outcome triggered extensive rioting in Los Angeles, as many in the community were outraged that the court's interpretation of the video was so dramatically different than their own (Cannon, 1999; Useem, 1997). Strangely enough, in a separate case brought subsequently against the police officers in the federal courts, the same videotape was judged to show abusive criminal behavior, and several of the officers were convicted and jailed (Mydans, 1993). Same video content, different interpretations.

What does all this mean for content analysis research? Is it impossible to do meaningful content analysis research, given that different receivers of each message might make different sense of any given message? The answer is no, and the reason is that there is indeed shared meaning across much of the substance of media messages concerning health topics.

As noted above, audiences bring a great deal of their own selves to the reception and interpretation of mediated messages about health. Content analysts therefore go to great pains to develop clear guidelines by which coders can evaluate media content in a uniform way. Neuendorf (Chapter 5), for example, offers a clear guide to crafting a carefully planned and well-documented coding scheme so that "the data generated by the analysis do not vary regardless of which coder is assigned to analyze any given piece of content" (p. 69). Yet Potter's (Chapter 3) thoughts on defining and measuring content variables are provocative. He argues that when designing a content analysis, "one needs to think carefully about what experiences and perspectives coders bring to the task, and how content characteristics shape the challenges faced by coders" (p. 51). Rather than write more detailed and more complicated coding rules, Potter hopes that content analysis designers can find ways to cue socially shared meanings and schemas as a strategy for increasing reliability and generating data that are more ecologically valid. This may be particularly important as the context of media consumption and the multiplicity of media messages broadens.

Like coders, audiences receive media messages in potentially individualistic ways. Austin (Chapter 12) argues that content analysis might be complemented by a "receiver-oriented message analysis (ROMA)." The ROMA approach explores whether there are systematic differences in how messages are received by the audience(s) of interest, as compared to a content analyst. Her studies of college students' interpretation of alcohol advertisements from magazines reveal a good deal of common meaning between young-adult "receivers" and trained content analysts on measures of manifest content. However, she found interesting differences in receivers' interpretation of messages. Ultimately, Austin argues that "receiver-oriented message analysis data as a complement to traditional content analysis data can help to bridge the gap between content and effects by accounting for the relationships between observed content and received meaning" (p. 206).

Content analysis research is limited in terms of what content patterns can tell us about effects of health messages on the audience. Researchers who look at health-related messages sometimes make the mistake of over-reaching with their results. Discovering that there are fewer movie characters smoking than a decade earlier is an important finding, but it does not say anything about why there are fewer characters smoking or whether this is related to the decrease in new smokers in society. While it is tempting to draw such parallels, one cannot infer effects from a content analysis. However, as Kunkel writes in Chapter 2, a carefully crafted study that employs content categories that are linked to relevant theory and effects research may afford the investigator the opportunity to posit likely effects on those with heavy exposure to the messages being assessed. This of course depends upon the strength of the linkage between the content attributes measured and the existing effects research; the clarity of the patterns identified in the content analysis research; and the generalizability of the content sampled to specific audiences, among other factors.

Nevertheless, the strongest evidence for a relationship between media exposure and beliefs, attitudes, intentions, and health behaviors will come from studies that combine content analytic and effects research. Several chapters in this book integrate these two approaches. While the magnitude of some effects identified may be relatively modest, it is important to consider that small effects can hold significant implications for public health policy when media exposure is involved. Because most people spend huge amounts of time with media, the prospect of cumulative effects across thousands of exposures can render relatively small change in content patterns meaningful from a long-term effects perspective.

Content Analysis Studies Need to Accommodate the Changing Nature of How Media Messages Are Delivered and Received as a Consequence of Rapidly Evolving Technology.

There are many more types of messages in today's multi-media, multi-channel environment than in previous decades. More outlets have led to greater diversity, allowing media-makers to cater to audiences' unique interests. Niche audiences are shaped by demographics, tastes, habits, and preferences and ultimately take on unique contours. In addition, much of the media content that is distributed today is consumed when, where, and how the audiences themselves determine. In fact, a significant proportion of web-based media content is actually created by consumers. It is time for the research community to grapple with the new ways in which audiences receive health content and the implications this holds for how content analysis studies are designed.

Content analysts must be ready to develop new tools and methods to assess the idiosyncratic, interactive (user-controlled), and fleeting health messages in the media landscape. The new media environment offers novel challenges to those who seek to capture what is available in the media and what is consumed by an increasingly individualistic and idiosyncratic audience. Ramasubramanian and Martin (Chapter 7) describe the media experience of one audience—teenagers—as one that has a unique and complex "media ecology." Their media-ecological approach to content analysis takes into consideration the complex relationships between media *content* and media *environments.* For example, they argue that youth audiences often customize their media diet: watching television when, where, and how they want to watch it; listening to music they choose, order, and download to their own personal listening devices; and surfing the web in their own idiosyncratic fashion. Studying teens' exposure to mediated health messages, they argue, requires an extensive effort to determine whether the researchers' conceptualization of a cohesive "audience" is one that even exists in reality. The studies they present in their chapter suggest the need to carry out more genre-based, audience-oriented media sampling techniques.

Video games are known for including much violence, a main area of study for public health researchers. Content analysis of video games, as discussed by Pieper et al. in Chapter 13, is an example of the current challenges facing researchers with respect to studying health messages of interactive media. Game players are the masters of content in many ways. They often have the opportunity to choose their characters, settings, actions, and narrative trajectory, albeit within bounds established by the game producer. Two players of the same video game who start at the same point and who spend the same amount of time with the game may experience dramatically different message environments based upon their individual navigation of the countless options in most interactive games. Similarly, two individuals who spend equivalent time browsing a single, elaborate website may encounter substantially different message content. This variability in the media exposure of individuals who ostensibly have shared the same experience—that is, the same amount of time with the same media target or activity—poses a major challenge for content analysis researchers. In the absence of any consistent protocol for investigating the divergent types of content available within interactive media environments, there is the worry that differences in findings across content studies may be more of a methodological artifact than a function of true differences in health messages. It is therefore critical that content analysis researchers devote time and resources to understanding how the new media environment affects exposure to health-related messages.

Challenges aside, new technologies have opened up new possibilities for the scope and reach of content analysis. Murphy, Wilkin, Cody, and Huang (Chapter 11) describe how digital video recording has exponentially increased the amount of content that can affordably be captured by analysts. Films no longer need to be purchased but can be rented and delivered via mail at a reasonable cost. Television programs no longer need to be videotaped but can be captured on a digital recorder and saved indefinitely with little loss of quality. They might even be watched on internet websites, such as the network website or a TV fan site. Magazines no longer need to sit on shelves and be thumbed through but can be digitized and coded on a computer screen. Such possibilities are limitless, and offer a relief for those who have had to make do with unreliable machines and media titles that come and go all too quickly.

With increased access, however, come some hard decisions. Jordan and Manganello (Chapter 4) describe how, in creating a sampling frame, one is often faced with a choice between sampling "what's available" and sampling "what's consumed." The seemingly limitless universe of "what's available" means that one needs to draw boundaries, however. Boundaries may be defined by tapping into what's available for certain audiences (for example, newspapers in a particular market; programs on a particular cable TV provider). More and more, however, samples are defined by what is most popular (for example, programs with high Nielsen ratings, or songs on *Billboard*'s top 100). And as more content analyses are tied to health-related outcomes for specific audiences, more sampling decisions will need to be carried out based on what the respondents say they are watching, reading, listening to and playing. Ramasubramanian and Martin (Chapter 7) point out how little overlap there was in the media diets of their sample of urban youth; and Collins and colleagues (Chapter 10) write that it was necessary to examine the television favorites of sub-groups of their sample (defined by gender and ethnicity) in order to determine the most appropriate shows to content analyze for possible influence on sexual behavior.

Today's media researchers must recognize that contemporary media audiences "multi-task" and consider how this may attenuate the reception and alter the effects of health messages (Ramasubramanian and Martin, Chapter 7). With the changing media environment have come dramatic changes in how people use available media. Indeed, it is relatively rare for a person to focus exclusively on a single medium. Not only are people using multiple media (e.g., listening to the radio or watching TV while using the internet) but often audiences are also doing something else (e.g., doing homework, grooming, driving, or eating). More important, media may be consumed simply as background while the other activity is in the foreground. Challenges such as these again emphasize the importance of conducting studies that directly link exposure to effects. Clearly, given the amount of multiple media use and multi-tasking that takes place, it cannot be assumed that just because a particular type of content is available in the media, it will be attended to and/or have an influence on a person's attitudes or health behavior.

Content Analysis Offers Unique Insight into the Mediated
Culture That no Other Social Science Research Method Can
Offer—But There Are Opportunities That Have Yet to be
Explored and Responsibilities That Must be Recognized.

As the technology to record, store, and more easily code media content develops, more research can be devoted to analyses of over-time changes in content. Content analyses can offer an important picture of the messages that are available to audiences at any given moment in a society's history. Tracking change—across months, years, decades and centuries—can also be illuminating as it provides a picture of the stability or change in health messages. Such trends can tell the public, policymakers, and health communicators about what publics have ready access to or, alternatively, what may be missing in the information environment.

One of the difficulties of tracking change over time is that relatively few content-based investigations employ the identical measurement framework. For example, differences in defining and measuring sex or violence on television have long proved an impediment to drawing conclusions across disparate studies conducted at different points in time. Simply put, the worry is that higher frequencies of sex or violence at Time 2 compared to Time 1 may be a function of measurement differences as much as of an actual increase in depictions of the target behavior. This issue becomes even more salient as the importance of measuring contextual features takes on added prominence in content-based research. The use of these unique contextual features as an important component in the analysis introduces more opportunity for variance in definitions and measures from one study to the next conducted by different investigators. For example, one study of sex on television might measure the depiction of "safe sex" precautions associated with sexual intercourse, while another might not, because of differing purposes of the research. One example of a content-based research program that has been replicated over time with identical measures is the Kaiser Family Foundation's series of studies of "Sex on TV" (Kunkel et al., 1999, 2001, 2003, 2005). Ongoing programs of research such as this afford the opportunity to track changes in media content over time with greater precision.

The Television Monitoring Project carried out by Murphy and colleagues at the University of Southern California (Chapter 11) offers similar potential. This project examines the health-related content of popular prime-time television shows on an annual basis, tracking messages to which a large segment of Americans are exposed over a period of many years. Another effort, the Hollywood, Health & Society project, which tracks health messages on television has found that breast cancer is often the subject of dramatic television storylines while prostate cancer rarely is (Miller, 2007). Trend data in content analysis may offer insight into how media's agenda-setting function may play a role in establishing audience beliefs and, in this case, cancer-screening behaviors.

For many content analysis efforts, it would be helpful to create a complementary research stream that allows one to draw a connection between the messages to which audiences are exposed and their impact on attitudes, beliefs and behaviors related to health. Collins, Elliott, and Miu (Chapter 10) provide an impressive example of research that effectively combines a content analysis of what a sample of teens watch on television with long-term outcomes for their sexual behavior. Specifically, they evaluated the sexual media content of popular television programs, assessed an adolescent sample's exposure to these messages, and correlated this exposure with earlier initiation of sexual intercourse. Their research design allows them to assess the predictive power of different kinds of sexual messages included in their content analysis.

Like Collins and colleagues, Salazar et al. (Chapter 8) plan to examine connections between media message exposure and sexual behaviors. Their medium of interest—the internet—offers an almost infinite universe of potential messages. Since it was not feasible to analyze every possible web page in the universe of the internet, Salazar and her colleagues designed a content analytic frame that could measure every web page visited by their sample of 530 14- to 17-year-old teens who regularly access the internet. Such a study requires not only a sophisticated use of web browsing tracking technology, but also a clear and expedient way of identifying and analyzing the sites their teens visited. The goal, ultimately, will be to link exposure to particular internet messages to sexual beliefs and behaviors.

As the opportunities for applying the methodology of content analysis for studying health messages advance, researchers simultaneously grapple with the concurrent responsibilities. Signorielli (Chapter 6) writes that researchers must strive to be as careful and ethical with content analysis studies as with traditional human subjects research. Those who code media messages are, in some sense, "human subjects" and may be vulnerable to the pernicious effects of media. Very often one examines media content because one believes that harmful health messages may negatively affect the health beliefs and behaviors of an audience. Content analysis "coders", though taught to carefully deconstruct a message, may need to be monitored or at least debriefed in much the same way one would debrief subjects of a lab experiment. Although many researchers have taken steps to protect coders, they typically are not required to submit content analysis projects to an independent review panel that would evaluate efforts to protect coders (such as a university Institutional Review Board). It may be necessary to take steps to self-monitor, and clearly inform coders and fellow researchers of the strategies used to ensure coder well-being. Salazar and her colleagues studying pornographic content on internet websites take care to inform readers of how they protected their researchers as a critical "decision step" they made in their content analysis (Chapter 8).

Finally, as content analysis researchers produce data that are influential in many domains of public health, they must also recognize that audiences for content analysis research go beyond ivory tower academics—indeed, interested parties include healthcare professionals, policymakers, government workers, educators, parents, and media professionals. Whitney, Wartella, and Kunkel

(Chapter 14) write about the importance of applying content analysis evidence to address real-world problems. Each "non-academic" audience may find the data useful for improving individual, community, and societal health outcomes. With this in mind, they argue that it is critical to develop standards by which a lay public can interpret the validity, accuracy, and scientific merit of content-based research. In addition, it is critical for content analysis researchers to think carefully about how findings are presented, anticipating what might be most interesting to (and even misconstrued by) the press. Scholars are generally not trained to disseminate their findings outside of the academy, yet the press and public are often eager to know the answers to the questions posed by content analysis.

Content analysis of health messages is an important area of research. As more people use this methodology to understand the messages people are exposed to, it is important to ensure that the methodology is used appropriately, that the methods are clearly explained, and that researchers strive to continuously take a "decisions approach" to content analysis.

References

Baldassare, M. (1994). *The Los Angeles riots: Lessons for the urban future*. Boulder, CO: Westview Press.

Brodie, M., Foehr, U., Rideout, V., Baer, N., Miller, C., Flournoy, R., et al. (2001). Communicating health information through the entertainment media. *Health Affairs, 20*, 192–199.

Brown, J. D., & Witherspoon, E. M. (2002). The mass media and American adolescents' health. *Journal of Adolescent Health, 31*(6, Supplement), 153–170.

Cannon, L. (1999). *Official negligence: How Rodney King and the riots changed Los Angeles and the LAPD*. Boulder, CO: Westview Press.

Escamilla, G., Cradock, A., Kawachi, I. (2000). Women and smoking in Hollywood movies: A content analysis. *American Journal of Public Health, 90*, 412–414.

Gerbner, G., Gross, L., Morgan, M., & Signorielli, N. (1980). The "main-streaming" of America: Violence profile No. 11. *Journal of Communication, 30*(3), 10–29.

Gerbner, G., Gross, L., Morgan, M., & Signorielli, N. (1986). Living with television: The dynamics of the cultivation process. In J. Bryant & D. Zillmann (Eds.), *Perspectives on media effects* (pp. 17–40). Hillsdale, NJ: Lawrence Erlbaum Associates.

Holsti, O. R. (1969). *Content analysis for the social sciences and humanities*. Reading, MA: Addison-Wesley.

Jordan, A. (2007, April). Food marketing on children's television: A multi-year comparison. Paper presented at the biennial meeting of the Society for Research on Child Development, Boston, MA.

Kline, K. N. (2003). Popular media and health: Images, effects, and institutions. In T. Thompson, A. Dorsey, K. Miller, & R. Parrott (Eds.), *Handbook of health communication* (pp. 557–581). Mahwah, NJ: Lawrence Erlbaum Associates.

Krippendorff, K. (2004). *Content analysis: An introduction to its methodology* (2nd ed.). Thousand Oaks, CA: Sage Publications.

Kunkel, D., Biely, E., Eyal, K., Farrar, K., Donnerstein, E., & Fandrich, R. (2003). *Sex on TV 3*. Menlo Park, CA: Henry J. Kaiser Family Foundation.

Kunkel, D., Cope, K., Biely, E., Farinola, W., & Donnerstein, E. (2001). *Sex on TV 2: A biennial report to the Kaiser Family Foundation*. Menlo Park, CA: Henry J. Kaiser Family Foundation.

Kunkel, D., Cope, K., Farinola, W., Biely, E., Rollin, E., & Donnerstein, E. (1999). *Sex on TV: Content and context*. Menlo Park, CA: Henry J. Kaiser Family Foundation.

Kunkel, D., Eyal, K., Finnerty, K., Biely, E., & Donnerstein, E. (2005). *Sex on TV 4*. Menlo Park, CA: Henry J. Kaiser Family Foundation.

Kunkel, D., Wilson, B., Donnerstein, E., Linz, D., Smith, S., Gray, T., Blumenthal, E., & Potter, W. (1995). Measuring television violence: The importance of context. *Journal of Broadcasting & Electronic Media, 39*, 284–291.

Livingstone, S., Lunt, P., & Slotover, M. (1992). Debating drunk driving: The construction of causal explanations in television discussion programmes. *Journal of Community and Applied Social Psychology, 2*, 131–145.

Miller, M. (2007, November). Consulting with television writers to encourage cancer and disparities topics in television programs. Paper presented at the annual meeting of the American Public Health Association, Washington, DC.

Mydans, S. (1992, April 30). The police verdict; Los Angeles policemen acquitted in taped beating. *The New York Times*.

Mydans, S. (1993, April 18). Verdict in Los Angeles; 2 of 4 officers found guilty in Los Angeles beating. *The New York Times*.

Nandy, B. R., & Sarvela, P. D. (1997). Content analysis reexamined: A relevant research method for health education. *American Journal of Health Behavior, 21*, 222–234.

Parascoli, F. (2005). Feeding hard bodies: Food and masculinities in men's fitness magazines. *Food & Foodways, 13*, 17–37.

Potter, W. J., & Smith, S. (2000). The context of graphic portrayals of television violence. *Journal of Broadcasting & Electronic Media, 44*, 301–323.

Romer, D., Jamieson, K., & Jamieson, P. (2006). Are news reports of suicide contagious? A stringent test in six cities. *Journal of Communication, 56*(2), 253–270.

Sankofa, J., & Johnson-Taylor, W. (2007). News coverage of diet-related health disparities experienced by Black Americans: A steady diet of misinformation. *Journal of Nutrition Education and Behavior, 39*, S41–S44.

Useem, B. (1997). The state and collective disorders: The Los Angeles riot protest of April 1992. *Social Forces, 76*, 357–377.

Wilson, B., Kunkel, D., Linz, D., Potter, W. J., Donnerstein, E., Smith, S., Blumenthal, E., & Gray, T. (1997). Violence in television programming overall: University of California Santa Barbara study. *National television violence study* (Vol. 1). Thousand Oaks, CA: Sage Publications.

Yanovitsky, I., & Stryker, J. (2001). Mass media, social norms and health promotion efforts: A longitudinal study of media effects on youth binge drinking. *Communication Research, 28*(2), 208–239.

Subject index

Author index

DATE DUE	RETURNED